An Introduction to Histotechnology

An Introduction to Histotechnology

A Manual for the Student, Practicing Technologist, and Resident-in-Pathology

Geoffrey G. Brown, AIMLS, HT(ASCP)

Technical Director of Histopathology Laboratories
Department of Pathology
Indiana University School of Medicine
Indianapolis, Indiana

Foreword by

John M. Budinger, M.D.

Department of Pathology
Lawrence Hospital
Bronxville, New York

ACC

APPLETON-CENTURY-CROFTS/NEW YORK

78 79 80 81 82 / 10 9 8 7 6 5 4 3 2 1

Prentice-Hall International, Inc., London
Prentice-Hall of Australia, Pty. Ltd., Sydney
Prentice-Hall of India Private Limited, New Delhi
Prentice-Hall of Japan, Inc., Tokyo
Prentice-Hall of Southeast Asia (Pte.) Ltd., Singapore
Whitehall Books Ltd., Wellington, New Zealand

Library of Congress
Catalog Card Number: 78-51037

Text design: Jerry Wilke
Cover design: Rodelinde Albrecht

PRINTED IN THE UNITED STATES OF AMERICA
0-8385-4340-5

This book is dedicated to the memory of
PROFESSOR J. W. S. BLACKLOCK, M.D.
Pathologist, Teacher, and Friend

Contents

Foreword

This book is written by an experienced histotechnologist who is also an able and enthusiastic teacher. Workers in this field are no longer content with recipe-books; they want sensible explanations of the many procedures which they must perform. They also expect information adequate for the rational selection of procedures in their laboratory. The current training of pathologists rarely includes much experience of histotechnology, and so the technologist is often left to his own devices.

In the past few years histotechnology has enjoyed rapidly growing educational opportunities. National and state societies have sponsored many workshops and meetings, and the critical certification of schools is underway. Those of us who have participated in these programs are richly rewarded by the enthusiastic, bright inquisitiveness of histotechnologists. The "Ovine-Wheel-Turner" is rightly fading into history. More professional advancement is still to come, and it must rest on a solid understanding of the many standard procedures now available in a good histology laboratory.

The educational levels of histotechnologists are still extremely varied. This is the main challenge to any continuing education program and of course, to any book. Mr. Brown has supervised and trained histotechnologists in several parts of the world, often with very limited facilities and budget. His affectionate, yet critical approach to subject and student are clearly apparent throughout this book. With one or two exceptions, the books of this field are either manuals of technique or treatises on histochemistry. He has carefully walked the middle road, with charity and sympathy for the often limited background of his students. He has successfully written a book for starting off a novice and for advancing the experienced worker.

John M. Budinger, M.D.
Department of Pathology
Lawrence Hospital
Bronxville, New York

Preface

When starting to write this book the first two questions that arose were, "Where do I start?" and "How far do I go?" while staying within the confines of the title. The first question was easily answered, and as a result this text is a natural progression from my *Primer of Histopathologic Technique* published in 1969. Much of that original material is included here and forms the foundation upon which this book was built, because I still believe that we must start with the basic principles and not assume that the student of histotechnology has some prior knowledge of the subject.

As before, I have made use of line drawings or diagrams of equipment to clarify its construction and working parts. It may appear that I have included too many illustrations of too many types of equipment and instruments available to the histotechnologist. This has been done deliberately to familiarize the student with the many pieces of equipment that are available as most laboratories are limited by their budget in what they possess and use.

A new chapter has been included on basic microscopy. It is essential that the histotechnologist and resident in pathology have at least a rudimentary knowledge of how the microscope works and how to care for it. More damage is caused by ignorance than anything else.

Now to try and answer the question of "How far do I go?" This is not so easy. I have tried to compile a book that is not limited by the requirements for the certification of histotechnologists, but that also provides the practicing histotechnologist with a fairly broad selection of techniques with which to meet the day to day requests for stains for diagnostic purposes. This should also be of use to the resident in pathology. Have I answered my second question? Only the reader will know if I have succeeded in filling his needs. To completely cover histotechnique one would require an encyclopedia of methods.

The practice of histotechnology is an art; a discipline requiring manual dexterity and an eye for color. It has not been overtaken by automation, nor will it be for many years. The practitioners of this art, the histotechnologists, exhibit much pride in their chosen profession. As a result they are taking giant strides in upgrading their training, knowledge, and qualifications. This was made apparent when they formed the National Society for Histotechnology, dedicated to the continuing education and professional recognition of the histotechnologist.

I sincerely hope that this book will be a useful tool in helping histotechnologists reach these goals.

It is impossible to write a book such as this without an enormous amount of help, encouragement, and support. Therefore I wish to acknowledge the people and companies who supplied these so necessary ingredients.

First I wish to thank my wife, Veronica, who typed much of the manuscript, often deciphering what must be the worst handwriting in the world, as well as spending many hours proofreading and assisting in indexing this work. Also special thanks go to Dr. John M. Budinger for his encouragement, suggestions, and the foreword; to John P. Koski for his contribution to the appendix; and to Messrs. James Rapp and Ronald Murray who assisted by providing their photographic skills. I must also thank the technologists in the histology laboratory at the University of Texas Medical Branch for acting as a sounding board and for their helpful comments as to what should be included.

The commercial and manufacturing companies supported me by generously supplying illustrations for the text. They are:

American Optical Corporation
Cambridge Medical Instruments Ltd., England.
Curtin Matheson Scientific Inc.
Fisher Scientific Company.
Hacker Instruments Inc.
Lab-Tek Products.

Ernst Leitz Inc., Germany.
Lipshaw Manufacturing Corporation.
LKB Instruments Inc.
Shandon Southern Instruments Inc.
Technicon Instruments Corporation.
Carl Zeiss Inc., Germany.

Finally, thank you to my publishers, who had faith in me.

Geoffrey G. Brown

In keeping with contemporary scientific usage, degree signs are not used in notation for temperatures. Instead, there is simply a number followed by either C (Celsius) or F (Fahrenheit). (**G.G.B.**)

An Introduction to Histotechnology

ONE

The Cell

The study of cell structure and function is termed cytology. When many different types of cells congregate and are held together by various fibers they form tissues, the study of which is called histology.

The cell is the smallest particle of living matter that is able to reproduce. With the advent of tissue culture and the electron microscope, our knowledge of the cell has greatly increased. It is not proposed to go deeply into cytology, but to give a simple description of the cell and some of its structures, thus enabling the student to obtain a better understanding of certain aspects of fixation, or preservation, of the cell in relation to histopathologic technique.

Structure of the Cell

The cell is comprised of protoplasm and consists of a nucleus and cytoplasm. Both the nucleus and the cytoplasm are enclosed in membranes. Table 1 gives some of the more important constituents of the cell that are illustrated in Figures 1 and 2.

THE NUCLEUS

The Nucleus

The nucleus, which could be likened to the heart or brain of the cell, is enclosed by the nuclear membrane. This membrane is not thought

TABLE 1

Constituents of the Cell

Cytoplasm	Nucleus
Cell membrane	Nuclear membrane
Ground cytoplasm	Nucleolus
Centriole	Karyosome
Mitochondria	Chromatin meshwork
Golgi element and/or neutral red vacuole	Ground cytoplasm
Cytoplasmic inclusions	
Vacuoles	

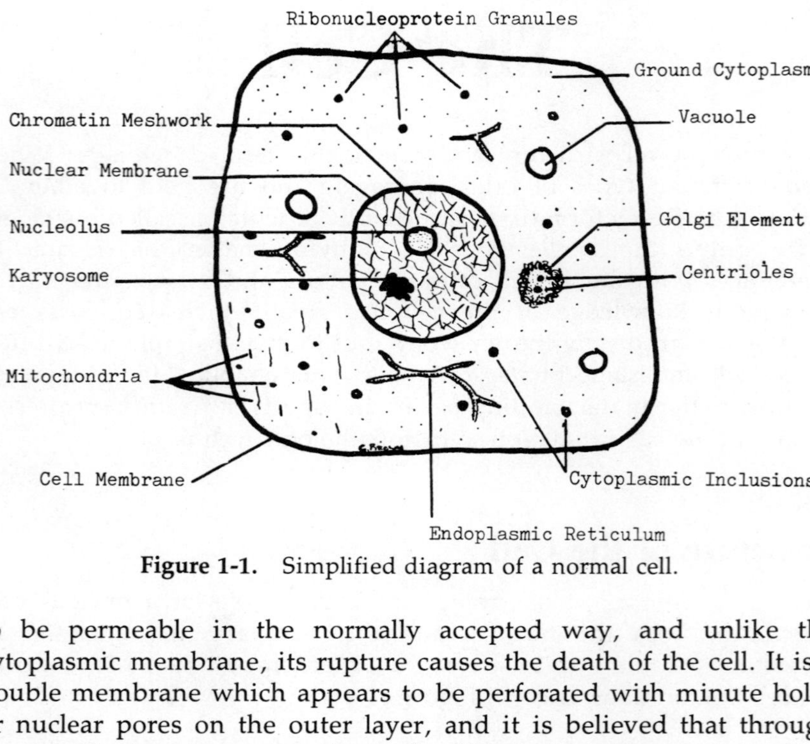

Figure 1-1. Simplified diagram of a normal cell.

to be permeable in the normally accepted way, and unlike the cytoplasmic membrane, its rupture causes the death of the cell. It is a double membrane which appears to be perforated with minute holes or nuclear pores on the outer layer, and it is believed that through these, cytoplasmic contact is made. Every function of the cell is directed from the nucleus. The ground substance of the nucleus is a colloidal solution of proteins and salts, with the proteins often precipitated into a fine meshwork on fixation.

The Nucleolus

The nucleolus is fairly regular in shape and is seen as a paler-staining body than the karyosome. It stains deeply with basic dyes due to its acid reaction and is said to consist of substances other than nucleoproteins, most probably ribonucleic acid (RNA).

The Karyosome

The karyosome, which is often irregular in shape, consists of chromatin or nucleoprotein. This is made up of protein bound to nucleic acids, ribonucleic acid (RNA), and deoxyribonucleic acid (DNA). There is often more than one karyosome present in the nucleus. It stains intensely with basic dyes.

The Chromosomes

The chromosomes are not normally visible in the resting cell, and only during *mitosis*, or cell division, can they be seen and counted. There are 46 chromosomes in each human cell, and during mitosis

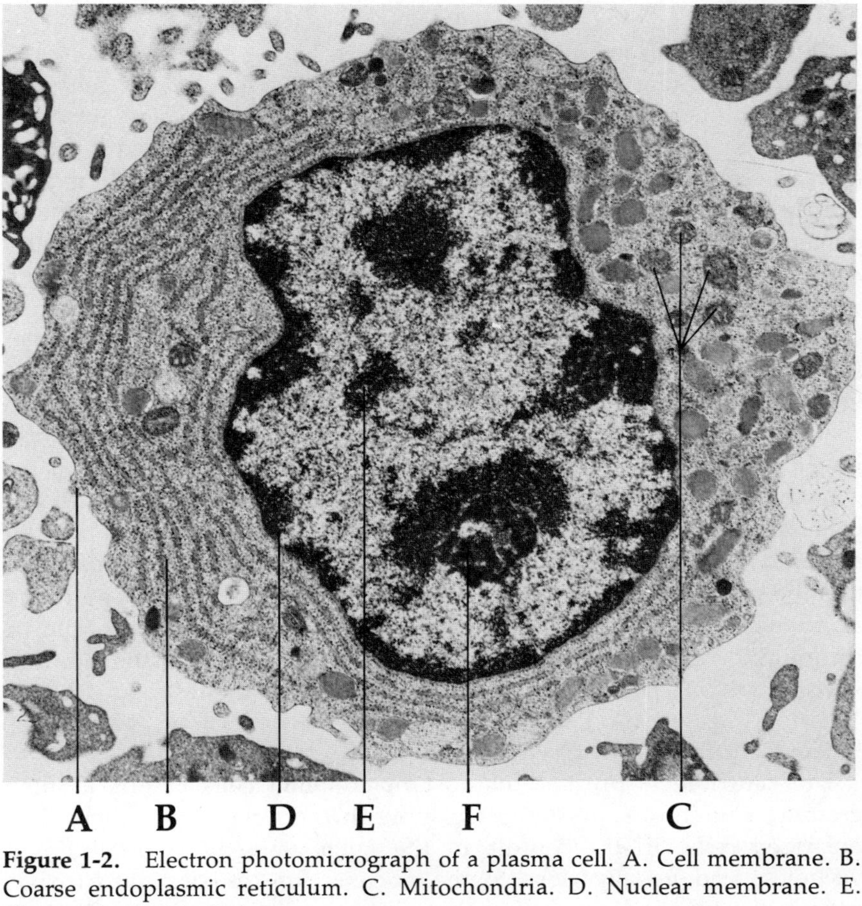

Figure 1-2. Electron photomicrograph of a plasma cell. A. Cell membrane. B. Coarse endoplasmic reticulum. C. Mitochondria. D. Nuclear membrane. E. Chromatin. F. Nucleolus.

these chromosomes are divided equally and carry the ancestral characteristics of the parent to the daughter cell. Chromosomes are extremely rich in deoxyribonucleic acid (DNA).

THE CYTOPLASM

The Cell Membrane

This membrane is an extremely fine skin that completely covers the cytoplasm, retaining it and preventing damage to the cell. It is a semipermeable membrane, which is probably composed of protein and lipid molecules, and allows the passage of food and excretory products by osmosis. It may be pierced with a very fine pipette, allowing substances to be injected into the cytoplasm without causing the death of the cell.

Ground Cytoplasm

Ground cytoplasm is the name given to the whole of the cell with the exception of the nucleus. The cytoplasm may appear granular, reticular, or fibrillar after fixation, but this does not represent the true appearance of the substance during life. In the living cell it is a homogeneous, translucent substance containing water with salts and sugars in true solution and proteins in colloidal solution. The water comprises about 80 percent of the substance by weight, and the dissolved substances produce an osmotic pressure approximately equivalent to an 0.9 percent aqueous solution of sodium chloride. Inorganic salts are also present and can be demonstrated by microincineration, a method that is used for the location of the salt rather than its identification, although some salts may be identified subsequently by the use of a polarizing microscope.

Cytoplasmic structures, such as the golgi element and mitochondria, and cytoplasmic inclusions, such as fat and glycogen, can be seen suspended in the cytoplasm. In some cells ribonucleoprotein particles may be present and their presence or absence is a determining factor as to whether the staining of the cytoplasm will be basophilic or acidophilic. When ribonucleoprotein particles are present the staining is basic.

The Centriole

The centriole is present in most mammalian cells and is a small granule, sometimes double, often lying in the long axis of the cell in polarized cells, in the middle of the golgi element, or neutral red vacuoles, and usually close to the nucleus. Its division into two is usually the first indication that the cell is about to divide. During cell division (mitosis) the spindle on which the chromosomes arrange themselves lies between the two centrioles, and the fibers radiate from it. It has no apparent structure, is resistant to reagents, and stains intensely with many dyes.

Mitochondria

Mitochondria are minute rodlike, filamentous, or granular bodies which have a smooth outline. They occur in the majority of mammalian cells, but not in mature red blood cells, and are among the first structures to disappear on the death of the cell. It is probable that they are semifluid in consistency, and there is evidence that they are composed of a mixture of lipids and proteins in varying proportions. Their function is not yet clearly determined, but it is thought that they are concerned with cellular metabolism.

Golgi Element

The golgi element is present in most cells. It is seen as *neutral red vacuoles* in the living cell, but after death these may be demonstrated as the *golgi element* by silver and osmium tetroxide techniques. Its size and shape may vary, and it may sometimes appear as rodlets, or as a network. During mitosis the Golgi element breaks up into rodlets and separates into roughly equal amounts, although the rodlets themselves do not divide.

Endoplasmic Reticulum

The endoplasmic reticulum is a labyrinth of tiny tubes running in all directions and connecting all parts of the cell. It is the digestive tract and delivery system of the cell, delivering supplies to the vacuoles for storage and nutrition.

Lysosomes

The lysosome, a small body which is similar in shape to the mitochondria, has a finely granular structure and is enclosed in a membrane. The membrane surrounding the particles is probably lipoprotein in nature. It has been demonstrated that the contents of the lysosomes are digestive enzymes. The rupture of the membrane and the subsequent release of these enzymes may be a cause of autolysis.

Cytoplasmic Inclusions

Cytoplasmic inclusions are primarily nutritive substances which are elaborated and stored within the cell. Some of the more important of the cytoplasmic inclusions are:

Fat. Occurs as globules and can be easily recognized *intra vitam* by its extreme refringency.

Glycogen. Exists in a state of solution within minute cytoplasmic droplets of a watery nature.
Yolk. Found in the form of granules or small discs.
Mucin. May be demonstrated in the mucin producing cells in a granular form known as "mucigen."

Mitosis

Mitosis, or cell division, is the normal method of cell reproduction except in a few highly specialized cells such as nerve cells. It usually takes about one hour for the process of mitosis to be completed, but this time is dependent upon several conditions, the most important being heat. Mitosis can be induced and stopped by a variety of agents; for example, x-rays in large doses stop cells from reproducing.

The process of mitosis can be divided into four distinct phases (Fig. 3): (1) prophase, (2) metaphase, (3) anaphase, and (4) telophase.

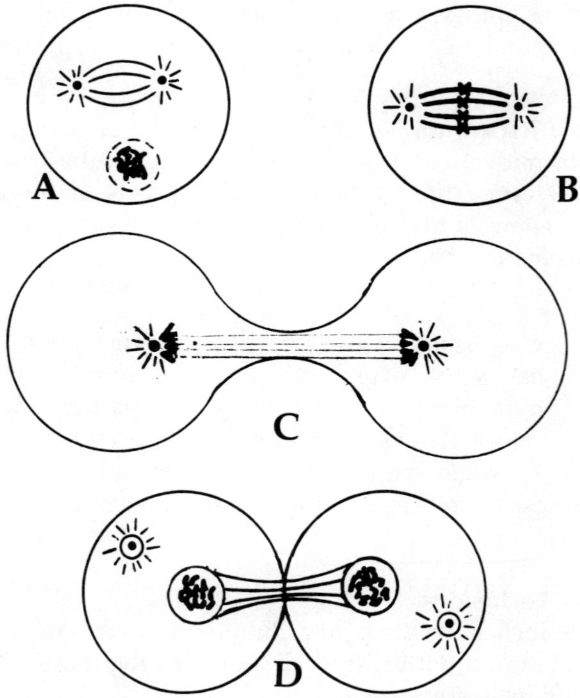

Figure 1-3. Mitosis. **A**. Prophase. **B**. Metaphase. **C**. Anaphase. **D**. Telophase.

Prophase

The centrioles start to move to opposite poles of the cell, and the nuclear membrane starts to disappear. The chromosomes appear to thicken and shorten by entangling themselves into closely wound spirals. Fibers appear between the centrioles forming the achromatic spindle on which the chromosomes will arrange themselves.

Metaphase

The nuclear membrane has completely disappeared, and the centrioles are at opposite poles of the cell. The chromosomes now arrange themselves in the center of the spindle and the two chromatids of each chromosome start to repel each other, forcing the chromosomes to separate and move towards the centriole at either end of the spindle.

Anaphase

The chromosomes continue to move in opposite directions towards the two centrioles, and the spindle elongates into a cylindrical body. By now the chromosomes will have traveled most of the way along the spindle towards opposite poles.

Telophase

The chromosomes are now at opposite poles, and the spindle stem starts to disappear. Nuclear membranes are being formed, and the chromosomes now unravel and dissolve into the new nucleus. The cytoplasmic membrane, which has become elongated and constricted, now divides. The two cells are connected by a fine thread which separates as the new cells move apart.

TWO

Preparing Specimens for Examination

Specimens may be prepared for histologic examination in a variety of ways to suit both the nature of the specimen and the type of technique that may be requested.

The following methods are those in most common usage:

1. Sectioning
2. Smears
3. Dissociation
4. Microincineration
5. Vital staining
6. Autoradiography

Sectioning

Sectioning is the most common method of preparing tissues for histologic examination, whether for routine purposes or research. As the name implies, an extremely thin slice or section is taken from the tissue and mounted on a slide for examination under the microscope. The advantage of this method is that cells can be studied in their relationship to one another in the tissue and not divorced from their natural background. I refer to this as the microanatomic picture.

Tissue which is to be sectioned is usually embedded in a material that will give it support during sectioning, and the embedding medium employed will depend on both the type of tissue and the techniques to be used for staining. Paraffin wax is the most common of the embedding media, and this, or one of the commercial waxes containing additives, is the usual medium employed in routine histologic procedures. Other common embedding media are celloidin, low-viscosity nitrocellulose (LVN), ester wax, gelatin, methacrylate, and resins.

PARAFFIN SECTIONS

The tissue is fixed to preserve its natural structure in as lifelike a manner as possible, and because most fixatives are aqueous solutions and therefore not miscible with paraffin wax, the water must be removed. This process is called dehydration, and is accomplished by passing the tissue through ascending grades of alcohol. The alcohol is now replaced with another reagent that is miscible with paraffin wax, a procedure known as clearing, after which the tissue is soaked in molten paraffin wax until all of the clearing agent has been removed and the specimen is saturated with wax. A mold is then filled with molten wax in which the specimen is arranged in a precise position. This is cooled rapidly to solidify the block, and the tissue is now ready for sectioning.

CELLOIDIN SECTIONS

Celloidin, like paraffin wax, is not miscible with water, and tissue to be embedded in this medium needs dehydrating as for wax, but is not cleared in the same way. It is a form of purified nitrocellulose (gun cotton) and is soluble in equal parts of absolute ethyl alcohol and ether. When solidified it has a somewhat rubbery consistency. Celloidin tends to give greater support to the tissue than does paraffin wax, and is therefore often used for delicate specimens such as eyes, and when it is advisable to avoid heat, which tends to make tissue hard and brittle.

There are two techniques for celloidin embedding, namely "wet" and "dry." The major disadvantage of the "wet" method is that the cut sections and the blocks must be stored in dilute (80 percent) alcohol, while both the block and the knife must be kept moistened with alcohol during cutting. The disadvantage of the celloidin techniques is the time necessary to impregnate the tissue. This is measured in weeks rather than hours.

Celloidin sections are normally cut at 10μ–15μ as opposed to the 4μ–6μ routinely cut from paraffin blocks.

Low-viscosity nitrocellulose (LVN) is comparable to celloidin.

DOUBLE EMBEDDING

Double embedding is a combination of paraffin and celloidin embedding, thus taking advantage of the best qualities of each method. The tissue is first impregnated with celloidin and then with paraffin wax, the block being cast as for the paraffin technique. Double embedding is mainly used for very delicate tissues such as eyes.

WATER-SOLUBLE WAXES

The obvious advantages of these waxes are the time and expense saved by eliminating the necessity of dehydrating and clearing the tissue processed by these methods. However, the waxes are rarely used for routine histologic procedures as they do not allow the production of sections comparable to those produced by the paraffin wax method.

The main disadvantage of these waxes is the difficulty encountered in removing creases and in flattening sections prior to mounting. It is obvious that water cannot be used to float out the sections, and dilute alcohols have not been used with any great success in an effort to overcome this major problem.

Some workers have found sectioning easier when the tissue has been freeze-dried before impregnation.

FROZEN SECTIONS

Fresh or fixed tissue can be sectioned while frozen. The technique is used when sections are required urgently for a rapid diagnosis, in many of the neurologic methods, for demonstrating substances which are soluble in alcohol and other fat solvents, and histochemical techniques.

Sections are cut on the freezing microtome, where the tissue is frozen on the block holder with carbon dioxide gas or in the cryostat, a cold chamber containing a microtome and kept at approximately −20 C. The cryostat often contains a mechanism for the rapid freezing of tissue.

If tissue is friable, that is fragile, it may be impregnated with gelatin or a commercial preparation prior to freezing.

THICK SECTIONS

For urgent sections, when freezing equipment is not available, a very thin slice of fresh or fixed tissue is cut freehand with a razor or scalpel. Staining is restricted to the surface layers of cells.

A greal deal of experience is required for this technique, and it is only used in extreme emergencies. Impression smears may give better results.

GROUND SECTIONS

Ground sections are sometimes prepared from bone, which is ground until it is paper thin and almost transparent, and mounted as either stained or unstained preparations.

PLASTIC EMBEDDED SECTIONS

Plastic embedding is employed as the method of choice for preparing sections of undecalcified bone. The embedding medium is much harder than paraffin wax, thereby giving greater support to the tissue, and the procedure takes much less time than the celloidin method.

Special knives and a heavy duty microtome should be used.

Plastic may also be used for soft tissue specimens, either as the primary embedding medium or as a secondary medium where very thin (1μ–2μ) sections are required. These may be sectioned on a standard rotary microtome.

SECTIONS FOR ELECTRON MICROSCOPY

Tissue to be sectioned for electron microscopy is embedded in a resinous medium. This is very hard and gives excellent support to the specimen. Sections are cut on a special microtome, an ultramicrotome, as thick sections (1μ) for screening purposes and as ultrathin sections (500–1000 Å) for study under the electron microscope. The knives are specially made, and may be glass or diamond.

The thick sections may be mounted onto glass slides and stained by biological stains, while the ultrathin sections are mounted onto copper grids and stained by metallic impregnation techniques.

Smears

Smears can be made by either pressing the cut surface of tissue onto a slide, an impression smear; spreading material with a wire loop; crushing it between two slides; or by smearing with another slide as in making blood films. The preparations are then fixed, stained, and mounted.

This technique allows greater detail to be studied than by using wet or teased preparations, but has similar disadvantages.

Dissociation

The tissue is teased with needles in a watchglass containing an indifferent medium such as normal saline. The preparation can be left in the watchglass or transferred to a microscope slide for examination under the microscope, where the cells are studied either stained or unstained. The main advantage of the method is that the cells are examined while still alive, and the disadvantage is that they are divorced from their normal surroundings, the anatomic relationship of the cells being destroyed during teasing.

Microincineration

Microincineration is used to locate the presence and position of mineral elements in the tissue. Alcohol-fixed tissue is sectioned and duplicate sections taken. One section is incinerated in a special oven, a muffle furnace, at an extremely high temperature, and the other section is stained in the normal way. The ash residue of the incinerated section is examined alongside the stained preparation, and the incidence and location of any mineral deposits is noted. A polarizing microscope is often used to examine the ash residue of the incinerated section, and sometimes it is possible to identify some of the mineral deposits found in the tissue.

A great deal of experience is required to be able to interpret the results of this technique, and in view of the limited field of application, this technique is not normally used in the routine histology laboratory.

Vital Staining

Certain cytoplasmic granules may be stained in living cells, and some cells (phagocytes) actually ingest minute particles of dye.

The cells may be stained by dissociating tissue in a simple staining solution (*supra vitam staining*), a method often used to stain reticulocytes in hematology, or in the living organism by injecting a dye into the tissue (*intra vitam staining*). Mitochondria and neutral red vacuoles may be demonstrated by vital staining, and one of the useful ways of employing this technique is the demonstration of nerve endings in tissue.

Autoradiography

Radioactive isotopes are injected into organs that are then fixed and sectioned. The sections are mounted in contact with a photographic emulsion, which is blackened by the isotopes when it is developed. The sections may be stained by routine methods, permitting the relationship and location of the isotopes and cells to be studied.

THREE

Fixation

Fixation is the rapid killing, hardening, and preservation of tissue, thus maintaining its existing form and structure and all of its constituent elements. Correct and adequate fixation is the fundamental criterion for all histologic preparations, and without this any work will be of mediocre quality.

Tissue for histologic studies should be fixed as quickly as possible after death or its removal from the body by surgical procedures. Some laboratories prefer to receive fresh tissue from the operating room in order that they may place the specimen in a fixative themselves, while others request that the tissue be placed in a fixative immediately when removed. In the first instance, the tissue should be placed in a plastic bag, which can then be sealed and taken to the laboratory as soon as possible. If there is likely to be any delay the specimen must be refrigerated until it can be delivered. In the second case, all jars for routine specimens should contain sufficient fixative to allow the volume of the fluid to be at least 20–30 times the bulk of the tissue. When an extended period of time for storage is expected, as is the case with specimens intended for museum preparations, the volume of the fixative should never be less than 50 times, and preferably 100 times, the bulk of the specimen. Whole organs should be injected with fixative as well as immersed in it, and hollow organs must be packed with absorbent cotton wool soaked in fixative before immersion.

It is the responsibility of the histology laboratory to ensure that there is an adequate supply and choice of fixatives available at all times.

Correct fixatives for subsequent techniques are essential, and although 10 percent neutral formalin is an adequate fixative for most routine procedures, other fixatives may well permit better results. Therefore, a decision must be made as to what methods may be required before fixation is started. It is important to remember that in some instances it is difficult, if not impossible, to change the ongoing procedure, and although secondary fixation is possible for many techniques, it does not allow the excellent results which could have been achieved with correct primary fixation. Remember that in histologic technique it is difficult, if not impossible, to "kill two birds with one stone," and unlike some of the clinical laboratories we cannot go back for another specimen.

The Aim of Fixation

When fixed, the appearance of the cell is an imitation of its appearance in a living state.

H. M. Carleton[1] defined the aim of fixation as follows: "To preserve the cell and tissue constituents in as lifelike a manner as possible after death." As well as preserving the appearance of the cell and tissue constituents, fixation should prevent putrifaction and autolysis.

Once these changes have commenced, and this happens rapidly, particularly in postmortem tissue, the cell no longer appears as it would in a living state. For this reason fixation should commence and be completed as soon and as rapidly as possible.

Effects of Fixation

Following fixation the cell and tissue constituents undergo fairly rigorous treatment before being examined by the pathologist. The major effect of fixation is to make the cell and tissue constituents resistant to damage and distortion during this processing by rendering them insoluble. Fixation has several other effects, the most important of which are:

Hardening of Tissue. This effect is reinforced by the dehydrating action of high grade alcohol. This allows easier handling of soft and friable tissue.

Rendering Cells Insensitive to Hypo- and Hypertonic Solutions.

Altering the Optical Density of Some Cells. This occurs when the refractive index is raised in varying degrees, enabling cell and tissue constituents to be optically differentiated from one another more easily, sometimes in unstained preparations.

Aiding or Inhibiting Staining. Some fixatives act as mordants or accentuators to certain dyes, eg, formaldehyde intensifies hematoxylin, while others inhibit certain dyes, eg, osmium tetroxide inhibits hematoxylin.

Osmosis in Fixation

It would appear that osmosis plays an important part in fixation and that fixatives should be in isotonic solution. This is not strictly true, for many of the reagents used in fixation have their own effect on the tissues and cells. Formaldehyde is commonly used in an isotonic solution as formol saline, but most of the other agents are not in isotonic solution. For example, glacial acetic acid, which is of higher osmotic pressure than cells and should therefore cause shrinkage, actually causes swelling in certain tissue, while picric acid, which has a lower osmotic pressure and should cause swelling, causes cells to shrink during fixation.

These effects are usually balanced to some degree, and an agent that causes shrinkage will be used in conjunction with one which causes swelling; for example, Bouin's fluid contains picric acid, which causes shrinkage, and glacial acetic acid, which causes swelling.

When formol saline is used as an isotonic solution, the isotonicity need only be approximate. There is nothing to be gained by having an exact physiologic solution of saline.

Common Reagents Used in Fixation

FORMALDEHYDE

Formaldehyde is a gas produced by the oxidation of methyl alcohol. It is soluble in water to the extent of 40 percent (approximately) by weight and is sold commercially as a solution of formol or formaldehyde, usually containing 10–15 percent methanol, which is added to prevent polymerization. Commercial formaldehyde (37–40 percent) is treated as a concentrated (100 percent) solution for all calculations in dilution.

Formaldehyde frequently turns acid during storage due to the formation of formic acid. This is easily neutralized by the addition of magnesium or calcium carbonate to a 10 or 15 percent solution of formalin or by buffering a 10 percent solution by adding sodium phosphate monobasic (4 g) and sodium phosphate dibasic, anhydrous (6.5 g), per liter with a resultant pH of 7.0. Formalin is best used as a neutral solution as it has a tendency to leave a golden brown precipitate in blood containing organs and neutralizing the solution helps to reduce the frequency of such deposits which form more easily in an acid solution. The concentrated solution of formaldehyde should never be neutralized as there is a grave danger of an explosion.

Commercial formalin frequently becomes cloudy on standing, especially if it is stored in a cold place, due to the formation of a white precipitate of paraformaldehyde. This has no adverse effect on the properties of the solution and may be removed by filtering before use.

Pure formalin (40 percent formaldehyde) is unsatisfactory as a fixative and is usually employed as a solution diluted 1:10 or 1:20 with water or saline, or as a constituent of a compound fixative.

Ten percent formalin is an excellent agent for fixing gross specimens prior to cutting up, which is made easier by primary fixation. The natural color of the specimen may be restored by immersing the tissue in 70 percent alcohol for 1 hour, which is extremely useful if color photographs are required. If the specimen is to be kept for any length of time, it may be wise to add some cadmium or cobalt salts to the fixative to prevent the fat in the tissue from dispersing out into the fluid. Lengthy storage requires that the fluid be changed every three months, and also tends to bleach the specimen.

Formalin preserves proteins by forming additive compounds with them by the production of linkages with the tissue constituents, some of which may be removed by subsequent washing in water, while others are quite insoluble. Because proteins are thus preserved and not precipitated, formalin is a valuable fixative for demonstrating enzyme activity.

Glycogen is preserved, and some compound lipids are fixed. Neutral fats are preserved in the sense that formalin does not dissolve them, but it does not render them resistant to subsequent treatment in fat solvents. After fixation in formalin, fat may be demonstrated in frozen sections.

All rooms in which concentrations of formalin are used must have extremely good ventilation, and an exhaust fan is an excellent accessory to such a room. The vapor of formaldehyde is injurious to the eyes and nasal mucosa and should be avoided as far as possible. Gloves should be worn when handling tissue fixed in formalin as it has an unpleasant effect on the hands, and prolonged exposure is likely to cause dermatitis.

GLUTARALDEHYDE

Glutaraldehyde is normally used as a buffered solution for electron microscopy techniques and is almost always followed by secondary fixation in osmium tetroxide. It acts on tissue in a manner similar to that of formaldehyde, giving excellent morphologic detail and good preservation of enzyme activity.

It may be used as a fixative for small pieces of tissue such as renal biopsies for paraffin sections but tends to make the tissue more brittle than does formalin.

PARAFORMALDEHYDE

Paraformaldehyde is a white powdery polymer of formaldehyde available from commercial sources in a chemical grade.[2] Used in solutions with buffers it fixes tissue up to 0.5 mm in thickness with excellent morphologic detail. Fixation time does not appear to be critical and may vary from several hours to several weeks without any apparent deterioration of detail. It is especially useful for fixing tissue that may possibly require study by electron microscopy (EM) in addition to regular histologic studies. In such instances the reserve tissue may be postosmicated and processed for EM.

The vapor from paraformaldehyde is occasionally used as a fixative for some techniques.

MERCURIC CHLORIDE

Mercuric chloride is a salt soluble in water to approximately 7 percent at room temperature, 53 percent in boiling water, and 33 percent in cold alcohol.

Mercuric chloride ions are believed to act in the same way as many other metallic ions in combining with the acid groups of proteins, especially the carboxyl and hydroxyl, and the phosphoric acid of nuclear proteins. It is a general protein precipitant, but differs from chromium in not forming complexes capable of binding together adjacent protein chains. The protein precipitates are soluble in sodium chloride and potassium iodide.

Fats and lipids are neither attacked nor dissolved, but the presence of mercuric chloride prevents the adequate freezing of tissue for frozen sections. Because it is radiopaque, the use of x-rays to ascertain the degree of decalcification is prevented.

Mercuric chloride permits brilliant staining of the cytoplasm, and the results with metachromatic methods are excellent. It may be used following fixation in formalin to brighten cytoplasmic staining. The slides are immersed in a saturated solution of mercuric chloride for 20 minutes prior to staining.

Because of the excessive shrinkage of tissue caused by mercuric chloride, it is rarely used alone, its main use being as a constituent of a compound fixative. It penetrates and hardens tissue rapidly, but, unfortunately, it hardens the outside of the specimen so quickly that unless very thin (4–5 mm) pieces of tissue are used the center may be improperly fixed.

Mercuric chloride leaves a black deposit in the tissue which must be removed before staining. This may be done during dehydration by adding iodine to the first two alcohols, or immediately before staining. The procedure for removing the pigment from sections is as follows:

1. Sections to water.
2. Lugol's iodine for 5 minutes.
3. Rinse in water.
4. Five percent sodium thiosulfate until the sections appear colorless. Allow up to 5 minutes.
5. Wash in running water for 5 minutes.
6. Commence staining.

Mercuric chloride is extremely corrosive to metals and the use of metal caps on containers is to be avoided. If this is not possible the inside of the cap should be coated with paraffin wax. Technicians should be warned of the corrosive effect of this salt, especially to personal jewelry, because it will attack gold or silver.

Note. Because of the environmental problems encountered in the disposal of mercury salts, it is being suggested that zinc chloride be substituted for mercuric chloride in Zenker-type fixatives. Zinc chloride is less toxic than mercuric chloride and does not leave artifact pigments in the tissue.[3]

OSMIUM TETROXIDE

Osmium tetroxide is a very costly reagent and is usually kept as a stock 2 percent aqueous solution in the dark. The solution will be reduced by light, but the addition of one drop of saturated aqueous mercuric chloride to every 10 ml of stock solution will help to prevent reduction. It is used as an aqueous solution from 0.5 to 2 percent, or in conjunction with other reagents, usually chrome salts.

Osmium tetroxide forms additive compounds with proteins, while the Golgi element, mitochondria, conjugated lipids, and fat are fixed by it. Fat is not only fixed but is also demonstrated by it, the fat being stained black by the formation of hydrated osmium dioxide.

Some tissue, for example adrenal, may be fixed in the vapor; the vapor gives better fixation than the fluid and does not require washing out. The vapor is very irritating and can cause conjunctivitis and blindness. Because of this the crystals should be dissolved in cold water.

Osmium tetroxide penetrates poorly and slowly, and only very small pieces of tissue should be fixed. Hematoxylin is inhibited, but brilliant nuclear staining is given with safranin.

CHROMIC ACID

Chromic acid is mostly employed as a 1–2 percent aqueous solution, often in compound fixatives containing osmium tetroxide or potassium dichromate. It precipitates all proteins and is probably the only fixative that preserves carbohydrates, rendering them insoluble in water.[4]

Tissues fixed in chromic acid (chromium trioxide) must be washed before dehydration, because unless the excess chromic acid is removed, an insoluble precipitate of a suboxide may be formed. The washing must be thorough, in running tap water for 24 hours, or at least overnight.

Because chromic acid is a powerful oxidizing agent, such reagents as formaldehyde, a reducing agent, should only be added to fixatives containing this as a constituent immediately before use.

POTASSIUM DICHROMATE

Potassium dichromate is frequently used as a constituent of compound fixatives or as a 3 percent aqueous solution, and is saturated at approximately 12 percent at room temperature. Tissue fixed in potassium dichromate requires thorough washing in running tap water before dehydration.

It gives homogenous fixation of the cytoplasm without precipitation, its action being similar to that of formaldehyde, but nuclear proteins are dissolved. Lipids are preserved, and it is the usual fixative employed for mitochondria.

When acidified beyond the crucial point, pH 4.2–5.2, both the cytoplasm and chromatin are precipitated as meshworks and chromosomes are well fixed, but the mitochondria are destroyed.

PICRIC ACID

Picric acid is highly explosive in a dry state and must be kept moist, preferably stored under distilled water. It is normally kept in the laboratory as saturated aqueous or saturated alcoholic solutions, approximately 0.5–1.0 percent at room temperature. The supernatent fluid of the stored picric acid is a ready source of saturated solution.

It precipitates and combines with proteins to form picrates, the majority of which are water soluble. To prevent the loss of these picrates, the tissue must be passed directly to alcohol. Picric acid is mainly used in Bouin's fluid, a compound fixative containing glacial acetic acid and formaldehyde, or with alcohol for the fixation of glycogen. The trichrome methods stain brilliantly after fixation in picric acid. Because of the yellow coloration it imparts to tissue, picric acid is extremely useful in locating fragments of tissue that might otherwise be overlooked.

GLACIAL ACETIC ACID

Glacial acetic acid is so called because it solidifies at 17 C. It produces marked swelling in unfixed collagen fibers, and because of this property it is used in many compound fixatives to counteract the shrinking qualities of other reagents such as formaldehyde and mercuric chloride.

Proteins are not fixed, but nuclear proteins are precipitated. It is therefore used in fixatives for chromosomes. Mitochondria and the Golgi element are either distorted or destroyed, and because of this acetic acid is rarely incorporated in cytoplasmic fixatives.

TRICHLORACETIC ACID

Trichloracetic acid is a deliquescent solid best left as such and weighed out when required. Like glacial acetic acid it causes swelling in tissue and is therefore used in compound fixatives to counteract the shrinking properties of other reagents. It may sometimes be used as a weak decalcifying agent, but only for very small pieces of tissue or delicate bone. Trichloracetic acid is a general protein precipitant.

ETHYL ALCOHOL

Used mainly for dehydration, ethyl alcohol is occasionally employed as a fixative, usually in Carnoy's fluid. Its chief uses are for histochemical methods with particular reference to enzymes, and for fixing smears. Penetration is slow, except when it is used in Carnoy's fluid when fixation is extremely rapid, and it shrinks and hardens tissues considerably.

Fats and lipids are dissolved, especially by the higher grades of alcohol, protein is denatured and made insoluble by the rearrangement of the protein molecule, and glycogen is precipitated. When used at ordinary temperatures (room temperature) alcohol has a tendency to cause polarization or streaming to one pole of the cell.

TABLE 1

Effect on Cellular Substances of Reagents Used in Fixatives

	Proteins	Nucleoprotein	Neutral Fat	Glycogen	Golgi & Mitochondria	Enzymes
Formaldehyde	Additive Compounds	Additive Compounds	Preserved	Preserved	Fixed	Preserved
Mercuric Chloride	Precipitated	Precipitated	Preserved	Preserved	Preserved	—
Osmium Tetroxide	Additive Compounds	Additive Compounds	Fixed	—	Fixed	—
Chromic Acid	Precipitated	Precipitated	Preserved	Preserved	Preserved	—
Potassium Dichromate	Preserved	Dissolved	Preserved	Preserved	Preserved	—
Picric Acid	Precipitated	Precipitated	—	Precipated	—	—
Glacial Acetic Acid	Not Fixed	Precipitated	—	Preserved	Destroyed	—
Trichloracetic Acid	Precipitated	Precipitated	—	—	—	—
Ethyl Alcohol	Denatured	Denatured	Dissolved	Precipitated	Dissolved	Preserved
Acetone	Preserved	Preserved	Dissolved	Very Poor	Dissolved	Preserved

ACETONE

Acetone is very similar in action to ethyl alcohol, and is also a dehydrating agent, but does not preserve glycogen well. Its use as a fixative is in histochemical techniques for the demonstration of enzymes such as lipases and phosphatases.

METHYL ALCOHOL

Methyl alcohol is mainly used for fixing smears of blood and bone marrow, often during staining, for example, with Leishman's stain and Wright's stain.

Essentials of Fixation

1. Commence fixation as soon as possible.
2. The bulk of the fixative must exceed that of the tissue by at least 20–50 times. Exceptions to this are fixatives containing osmium tetroxide which require only 5–10 times the bulk of the tissue.
3. Do not exceed the time required for complete fixation. Specimens to be kept for any length of time should be placed in 10 percent formalin or Kaiserling's fluid:

40 percent formaldehyde	40 ml
Potassium acetate	6 g
Potassium nitrate	3 g
Tap water	200 ml

4. Use the correct fixative for subsequent techniques.
5. Many fixatives require thorough washing to remove excess salts, and some need treatment to remove pigments prior to staining.

The effect on cellular substances of reagents used in fixatives is shown in Table 1.

REFERENCES

1. Carleton HM, Drury RAB: Histological Technique, 3rd ed. Oxford University Press, London, 1957, p. 11.
2. Lynn JA, Martin JH, Race GJ: Recent improvements of histologic technics for the combined light and electron microscopic examination of surgical specimens. Am J Clin Pathol 45:704–713, 1966.
3. Barszcz CA: Use of zinc chloride in Zenker type fixatives. Histo-Logic 6:87, 1976.
4. Bauer H: Mikroskopisch-Chemischer Nachweiss von Glykogen und Einigen Anderen Polysacchariden. Z Mikrosk Anat Forsch 33:143–159, 1933.

FOUR

Compound Fixatives

Choice of Fixative

When tissue is to be processed it is necessary to determine what cell or tissue constituents are to be demonstrated, and by which techniques. Once this is decided the choice of fixative is made easy.

Fixatives fall into three main groups:

1. Microanatomic.
2. Cytologic. This group may be further divided into *nuclear* and *cytoplasmic*.
3. Histochemical.

It is possible for some fixatives to serve in some degree for all three groups, eg, Bouin's fluid, but in the majority of cases something will have to be sacrificed in order to demonstrate specific substances. This may be excessive shrinkage of the tissue, or ease of handling of the sections. Despite these disadvantages, it is best to pick the correct fixative for the substance to be demonstrated.

A selection of the more common and reliable fixatives is given on the following pages with their advantages and disadvantages.

Microanatomic Fixatives

Microanatomic fixatives aim at preserving the relationship of cells and tissue to each other in as lifelike a manner as possible. This group of fixatives is the most widely used in routine histologic technique.

A microanatomic fixative may contain glacial acetic acid, but will never contain osmium tetroxide because the latter inhibits hematoxylin.

· TEN PERCENT FORMOL SALINE

40 percent formaldehyde	10.0 ml
Sodium chloride	0.9 g
Tap water	90.0 ml

Fixation time for tissue measuring 3.0 × 1.5 × 1.5 cm is 24 hours.

Advantages

1. Tissue may be left for an indefinite period of time, provided that the fluid is changed every three months. This is because formol saline not only fixes tissues but preserves tissue elements, thereby allowing secondary fixation if and when required. The addition of cadmium or cobalt salts will help to prevent the lipids from oozing out into the fixative.
2. Fat is preserved, and although not fixed it may be demonstrated in frozen sections.
3. It gives even fixation with little shrinkage.
4. It allows good results on the nervous system, and as a neutral solution is used for many histochemical techniques.
5. It gives good results with most staining methods, including the silver techniques.
6. It is the best fluid for dissection specimens as it allows the color of the tissue to be regained after immersion in 70 percent alcohol.

Disadvantages

1. It is slow, and does not harden tissue sufficiently to resist shrinkage during dehydration.
2. When used on postmortem tissue, and when acid, a deposit may be formed in the tissue, particularly in blood-containing organs. This may be removed with saturated alcoholic sodium hydroxide or picric acid.
3. The metachromatic reaction of amyloid is reduced, and acid dyes stain less brightly than after fixation in a fluid containing mercuric chloride.

TEN PERCENT FORMALIN

Ten percent formalin is formol saline minus the sodium chloride. The fixation time, advantages, and disadvantages are the same.

TEN PERCENT NEUTRAL BUFFERED FORMALIN

40 percent formaldehyde	100.0 ml
Distilled or deionized water	900.0 ml
Sodium phosphate, monobasic	4.0 g
Sodium phosphate, dibasic (anhyd.)	6.5 g

This solution has all of the advantages of formol saline, but is less likely to leave formalin deposits in tissue. It is strongly recommended for routine use.

FORMOL CALCIUM

40 percent formaldehyde	10 ml
Calcium chloride	1 g
Distilled or deionized water	90 ml

This solution is strongly recommended for studies on lipids.

FORMALIN-AMMONIUM BROMIDE (FAB)

40 percent formaldehyde	15 ml
Ammonium bromide	2 g
Distilled or deionized water	85 ml

Recommended as the fixative for neurologic tissue, especially when silver or gold impregnation techniques are to be employed.

FORMOL CORROSIVE

Sat. aq. mercuric chloride	90 ml
40 percent formaldehyde	10 ml

Fixation time for tissue measuring $3.0 \times 1.5 \times 1.0$ cm is 3–24 hours.

Advantages

1. There is rapid fixation with little or no shrinkage or hardening of tissue.
2. Cytologic detail and RBCs are well preserved.
3. It allows most staining methods, including the silver reticulum methods. Cytoplasmic staining is brighter than after formalin fixation, and metachromatic staining is sharper.

Disadvantages

1. Slices of tissue should not exceed 1.0 cm in thickness and preferably be no thicker than 0.5 cm.
2. It leaves a deposit of mercuric chloride in the tissue that must be removed before staining.
3. It will not allow the cutting of frozen sections.
4. It inhibits the use of x-rays in determining the end point of decalcification.

ZENKER'S FLUID

Mercuric chloride*	5.0 g
Sodium sulfate (optional)	1.0 g
Potassium dichromate	2.5 g
Distilled water	100.0 ml

Add 5 ml glacial acetic acid *immediately* before use. Fixation time for tissue measuring 3.0 × 1.5 × 0.5 cm is 12–24 hours.

Advantages

1. It is excellent for liver, spleen, connective tissue fibers, and nuclei.
2. It gives fairly rapid and even fixation.
3. It gives excellent results with the trichrome methods.
4. Stock solution keeps well.

Disadvantages

1. Tissue should not exceed 0.5 cm in thickness.
2. Tissue tends to become brittle if left in fixative for more than 24 hours.
3. It does not allow the cutting of frozen sections.
4. It requires washing in running water for 8–12 hours to remove the excess dichromate.
5. It leaves a deposit of mercuric chloride which must be removed before staining.
6. It is not stable after the addition of the acetic acid.

* Note: See page 19, Chapter 3, for possible substitution of zinc chloride for mercuric chloride in Zenker-type fixatives.

HELLY'S FLUID (ZENKER FORMOL)

Although this fluid contains both an oxidizing agent (potassium dichromate) and a reducing agent (formaldehyde), it gives excellent microanatomic fixation.

Mercuric chloride	5.0 g
Sodium sulfate (optional)	1.0 g
Potassium dichromate	2.5 g
Distilled water	100.0 ml

Add 5 ml of 40 percent formaldehyde *immediately* before use.

Fixation time for tissue measuring 3.0 × 1.5 × 0.5 cm is 12–24 hours.

Advantages

1. It is recommended for pituitary, bone marrow, spleen, and nuclei.
2. Cytoplasmic granules are well preserved.
3. It gives better results with nuclear staining than Zenker's fluid.

Disadvantages

Identical to those of Zenker's fluid.

BOUIN'S FLUID

Sat. aq. soln. picric acid	75 ml
40 percent formaldehyde	25 ml
Glacial acetic acid	5 ml

Fixation time for tissue measuring 3.0 × 1.0 × 1.0 cm is 6–24 hours.

Advantages

1. It is recommended for embryos.
2. It produces very little microanatomic distortion.
3. It preserves glycogen.
4. It permits brilliant staining results.
5. It is useful for minute fragments of tisse as the yellow color given to the tissue makes it easier to locate the specimen.
6. Tissue may be transferred directly to 70 percent alcohol.

Disadvantages

1. There is poor penetration and therefore it should only be used with small pieces of tissue.

2. The picrates formed during fixation are water soluble.
3. Kidney tissue is badly distorted and should never be fixed in Bouin's fluid.
4. Cytoplasmic structures such as mitochondria are distorted or dissolved.

GENDRE'S FLUID

Sat. alc. (95 percent) soln. picric acid	80 ml
40 percent formaldehyde	15 ml
Glacial acetic acid	5 ml

Gives better fixation of glycogen than does Bouin's fluid, possibly due to the higher concentration of picric acid.

HEIDENHAIN'S "SUSA"

Mercuric chloride	45 g
Sodium chloride	5 g
Trichloracetic acid	20 g
Glacial acetic acid	40 ml
40 percent formaldehyde	200 ml
Distilled water	800 ml

Fixation time for tissue measuring 3.0 × 1.5 × 1.0 cm is 6–12 hours.

Advantages

1. It is recommended for biopsies, tumors, and particularly skin.
2. There is rapid and even penetration with a minimum of shrinkage and hardening.
3. It allows brilliant staining with good cytologic detail.
4. Tissue may be transferred directly to 90 percent alcohol.

Disadvantages

1. Tissue should not exceed 1.0 cm in thickness as *prolonged* fixation causes shrinkage, hardening, and bleaching of the tissue.
2. There is poor penetration of RBCs and some cytoplasmic granules are dissolved.
3. It leaves a deposit of mercuric chloride that must be removed before staining.
4. It is impossible to stain elastic by Weigert's method after fixation in "Susa."

Cytologic Fixatives

A cytologic fixative is one which is primarily concerned with the fixation of the cell and cellular constituents. This group of fixatives is usually divided in two, one group for nuclear fixation and the other for cytoplasmic fixation. This is because the chemical reactions of the reagents used in the solutions make it virtually impossible to get first-class fixation of the nucleus and the cytoplasm simultaneously.

Cytoplasmic Fixatives

A cytoplasmic fixative will never contain glacial acetic acid, because mitochondria and golgi elements are destroyed by it. Osmium tetroxide is frequently employed for the demonstration of these.

FLEMMING'S FLUID (MINUS ACETIC ACID)

1 percent chromic acid	15 ml
2 percent osmium tetroxide	4 ml

Fixation time for specimens measuring 1.0 × 0.5 × 0.2 cm is 26–48 hours.

Advantages

1. It demonstrates and fixes fat permanently.
2. Only a small amount of fixative is required, 5–10 times the bulk of the tissue.
3. The omission of acetic acid improves the cytoplasmic detail, especially mitochondria.

Disadvantages

1. There is poor penetration, often with excessive blackening of the outside of the tissue while the center is barely fixed. Because of this only small pieces of tissue may be used.
2. Tissue requires washing for 24 hours in running water to remove excess salts. Failure to do this may result in an insoluble pigment.
3. The solution deteriorates rapidly, but not so rapidly as with the addition of acetic acid.
4. It is very expensive.

CHAMPY'S FLUID

3 percent potassium dichromate	7 ml
1 percent chromic acid	7 ml
2 percent osmium tetroxide	4 ml

Fixation time for tissue measuring 1.0 × 0.5 × 0.2 cm is 24–48 hours.

Advantages

1. It preserves mitochondria, the golgi element, and fat, which is also demonstrated.
2. Only a small amount of fixative is required, 5–10 times the bulk of the tissue.
3. Often gives better results with tissue of invertebrates and lower vertebrates than with those of mammals.

Disadvantage

The same as for Flemming's fluid minus acetic acid.

REGAUD'S FLUID

3 percent potassium dichromate	80 ml
40 percent formaldehyde	20 ml

Fixation time for tissue measuring 3.0 × 1.5 × 1.0 cm is 12 hours.

Advantages

1. It is more penetrating than the chrome-osmium fixatives.
2. Mitochondria and yolk are preserved.

Disadvantages

1. Fat is not preserved.
2. It needs postchroming.
3. It requires washing in running water for 24 hours prior to dehydration.
4. It deteriorates rapidly and should be mixed immediately before use.

MULLER'S FLUID

2.5 percent potassium dichromate.

Fixation time for tissue measuring 3.0 × 1.0 × 1.0 cm is 24 hours.

Advantages

The same as for Regaud's fluid.

Disadvantages

1. Fat is not preserved.
2. It requires washing in running water for 24 hours prior to dehydration.

ALTERNATIVES

A few of the microanatomic and nuclear fixatives may be used as cytoplasmic fixatives. Those most usually employed as such are:

1. Helly's fluid.
2. 10 percent formalin or formol saline plus postchroming.
3. Carnoy's fluid for demonstrating glycogen.
4. Bouin's fluid, also for glycogen.

Nuclear Fixatives

A nuclear fixative will invariably contain glacial acetic acid because nuclear chromatin has an affinity for this.

FLEMMING'S FLUID

1 percent chromic acid	15 ml
2 percent osmium tetroxide	4 ml
Glacial acetic acid	1 ml

Fixation time for tissue measuring 1.0 × 0.5 × 0.2 cm is 24–48 hours.

Advantages

1. It gives excellent nuclear fixation including chromosomes.
2. It demonstrates fat, and fixes it permanently.

3. Only a small amount of fixative is required, 5–10 times the bulk of the tissue.

Disadvantage

See Flemming's fluid minus acetic acid.

CARNOY'S FLUID

Absolute ethyl alcohol	60 ml
Chloroform	30 ml
Glacial acetic acid	10 ml

Fixation time for tissue measuring 3.0 × 1.0 × 1.0 cm is ½ = 3 hours.

Advantages

1. It is recommended for lymph glands, biopsies, and chromosomes.
2. It preserves glycogen.
3. It fixes and dehydrates simultaneously.
4. It is extremely rapid, probably the most rapid of all fixatives.

Disadvantages

1. It causes excessive shrinkage and hemolysis of RBCs.
2. Only small pieces of tissue may be used.

BOUIN'S FLUID

Sat. aq. picric acid	75 ml
40 percent formaldehyde	25 ml
Glacial acetic acid	5 ml

Fixation time for tissue measuring 3.0 × 1.0 × 1.0 cm is 6–24 hours.

Advantages

1. It gives better nuclear fixation than Flemming's fluid.
2. As previously stated for microanatomic fixatives.

Disadvantages

As previously stated for microanatomic fixatives (p 28).

NEWCOMER'S FLUID

Isopropyl alcohol	60 ml
Propionic acid	30 ml
Petroleum ether	10 ml
Acetone	10 ml
Dioxane	10 ml

Fixation time for tissue measuring 3.0 × 1.0 × 1.0 cm is 12–18 hours at 3C. Tissue measuring 3 mm in thickness is fixed in 2–3 hours.

This fluid is recommended for the fixation of mucopolysaccharides and nuclear proteins. It allows a better Feulgen reaction than does Carnoy's fluid.

Advantages

1. It is very rapid.
2. It fixes chromosomes.
3. It preserves nuclear proteins, giving better results for Feulgen's reaction than does Carnoy's fluid.
4. It is recommended for mucopolysaccharides.
5. Tissue requires only one change of absolute alcohol before clearing.

Disadvantages

1. It causes excessive shrinkage.
2. Only small pieces of tissue should be used.

Fixatives for Smears

SCHAUDINN'S FLUID

Sat. aq. mercuric chloride	66 ml
Absolute ethyl alcohol	33 ml
Glacial acetic acid	1 ml

This fluid gives excellent cytologic fixation. Wet smears should be placed into this fluid immediately after they are made and left for 5–30 minutes, depending on the thickness of the smear. It is important that the smear should not be allowed to dry before being placed in the fixative. A deposit of mercuric chloride is left on the smear, and this must be removed before staining.

CLARKE'S FLUID

Absolute ethyl alcohol	75 ml
Glacial acetic acid	25 ml

Gives excellent nuclear fixation. Recommended for fixing smears, tissue culture coverslip preparations, and chromosome studies. Fixation time is 10–20 minutes. Smears should be washed for 5 minutes in 70 percent alcohol to remove the excess acetic acid.

ETHER/ALCOHOL

Petroleum ether and absolute ethyl alcohol are mixed in equal parts and poured into a coplin jar. Fresh wet smears should be made and placed in the mixture for 30–60 minutes depending on the thickness of the smear. Wash in distilled water before staining.

METHYL ALCOHOL

Methyl alcohol is usually used to fix dried blood films and is often incorporated in the stain. It is employed for both thick and thin preparations. Fresh frozen tissue cut on the cryostat is usually fixed in methyl alcohol immediately when cut; the coagulation of the proteins making the section adhere to the slide.

Histochemical Fixatives

Histochemical fixatives aim at preserving the chemical constituents of the cells and tissues. In the majority of cases it is normal to have to sacrifice all other aspects of fixation to this end.

TEN PERCENT FORMOL SALINE

Used as a neutral solution, to help prevent the formation of pigment, formol saline is a better fixative than alcohol in that it preserves microanatomic and cytologic detail without excessive distortion due to shrinkage. Besides preserving enzymes and nucleoproteins, it allows the demonstration of fats and lipids, which are dissolved by high grade alcohol.

ABSOLUTE ETHYL ALCOHOL

Ethyl alcohol is commonly used at 4C for the demonstration of enzymes. Nucleoproteins and nucleic acids are preserved, but methyl alcohol gives better fixation for these. Glycogen is precipitated but tends to stream to one pole of the cell (polarization), and fats are dissolved.

ACETONE

Acetone is used in a range of from −5 C to +4 C for the fixation of enzymes, particularly phosphatases. It tends to leave reactive groups of enzymes closer to their original state than does alcohol. Fat is dissolved and glycogen poorly preserved.

NEWCOMER'S FLUID

Newcomer's fluid is recommended for the fixation of mucopolysaccharides and nuclear proteins. It permits a better Feulgen reaction than does Carnoy's fluid.

Secondary Fixation

This is the term used when tissues are placed into a second fixative to facilitate the demonstration of a specific substance. It is mainly used with tissues or organs that have been placed in a primary fixative for storage purposes, and for specimens that require further techniques, having already been fixed for routine procedures. The usual primary fixative is either 10 percent formalin or 10 percent formol saline.

This method of fixation is not to be recommended when primary fixation for specific observations is possible in the first instance.

Postchromatization

Postchromatization is the treatment of tissue in a 3 percent aqueous solution of potassium dichromate for 24 hours following fixation, and it is normally used as a method of mordanting. It is most often done immediately following fixation, usually with 10 percent formol saline, and prior to dehydration, but can also be done on deparaffinized cut sections prior to staining. When the method is utilized at this time, the period of immersion in dichromate is much reduced.

Techniques Used for the Fixation of Gross Specimens

In some cases extra care must be taken during fixation to ensure proper penetration of the fixative and the prevention or reduction of shrinkage, and to avoid contamination of the specimen with precipitates caused by the reduction of the fixative. The latter is of great importance when using osmium tetroxide.

The following techniques should be used when fixing gross specimens:

Hollow Organs

Hollow organs, i.e., the stomach, should be packed with absorbent cotton that has been saturated with fixative. The entire organ is then immersed in a sufficient quantity of fixative. Care must be taken not to overstuff the organ thereby causing stretching and distortion (flattening) of the interior surfaces.

Skin and Intestine

Intestine should be opened along its entire length and flattened out, mucosal surface uppermost. Both skin and intestine should be pinned out flat on cork or wax sheets and floated face down in the fixative. When using fixatives containing mercuric chloride it must be remembered that this salt will corrode metal pins. Wooden slivers, hedgehog spines, or porcupine quills should be used instead of pins.

Whole Organs

The fixative for whole organs, i.e., kidney and liver, must be injected into the main arteries, and these vessels and the veins tied off when full. The specimen, either lying on a thick pad of absorbent cotton wool or suspended by a thread tied to the vessels, is then immersed in a sufficient quantity of fixative.

Lungs

Since the lungs contain air they will normally float on the surface of the fixative and must be held under the surface by some means or other to ensure proper coverage. The easiest way of surmounting this problem is to cover the specimen with several layers of cotton gauze.

Lungs may also be filled with fixative by injecting the fluid into the bronchi and tying off when they are fully distended. Do not overfill or the specimen will be distorted.

Eyes

Under *no* circumstances should the globe be injected with fixative, nor should "windows" be cut in the schlera. The entire globe should be placed into 20–30 times its own volume of fixative for 48 hours.

Bone Marrow

A small quantity of marrow should be placed in a conical centrifuge tube containing Zenker formol. After standing for two hours the tube is centrifuged, the specimen forming a compact "button" at the tip of the tube. The button is processed in the normal way.

Brain

Whole brains should be suspended by a cord passed under the basilar artery. This prevents flattening of the organ where it would rest on the bottom of the jar. Brain, being dense tissue, takes a long time to fix properly.

Spinal Cord

The dura should be opened along the entire length of the specimen, and the cord should then be suspended in a tall jar (gas jar), with the bottom end weighted to keep the cord stretched out straight. This helps prevent shrinkage. If it is not possible to suspend the cord, the specimen may be pinned to a large board in the manner previously described for skin and intestine.

When Using Osmium Tetroxide

Osmium tetroxide, or osmic acid as it is sometimes called, has a tendency to reduce and form a black precipitate that settles on the bottom of the jar. Because of this, tissue should be suspended in the fluid. The easiest method of doing this is to wrap the tissue in cotton gauze and suspend it by means of a length of thread. The gauze and the thread should be thoroughly rinsed with distilled water before use.

FIVE

Decalcification

Decalcification, a form of ionization, is the complete removal of calcium salts from the tissue following fixation, with particular reference to bones and teeth. Without the removal of these salts, normal sectioning is impossible, and although ground sections can be made, these sections have a limited use. The microanatomic detail of such sections is often obscured by bone dust and debris.

The calcium is removed by the use of acids, alone or in combination with other substances such as alcohol or formaldehyde. Ion exchange resins, chelating agents, or electrophoresis are also commonly employed methods of decalcification. The use of mineral acids is the method most usually employed in routine histology laboratories.

Tissue should be suspended in the decalcifying agent by a waxed thread to ensure that the reagent has the fullest access to it. Waxing of the thread is essential to prevent its being attacked by the acid. This procedure also keeps the specimen above any precipitates that may form in the bottom of the container. Metal-capped containers should not be used for decalcifying solutions.

The criteria for good decalcifying solutions are:

1. Complete removal of the calcium salts.
2. The absence of harmful effects on cells and connective tissue fibers.
3. The absence of harmful effects on subsequent staining, especially on the staining of the nuclei.

Selection of Agents

The reagents that are most commonly employed in routine laboratories contain either nitric acid, hydrochloric acid, or formic acid. These may be used alone or as constituents of compound decalcifying fluids. Some establishments prefer to use a chelating agent such as ethylene-diamine-tetra-acetic acid disodium salt, commonly abbreviated to EDTA, the way most technicians identify it. It is manufactured commercially as Versene. The majority of technicians prefer to employ one of the acids mentioned above, these having the advantage of being readily available, stable, and relatively inexpensive, or one of the commercially prepared decalcifying fluids for routine histologic procedures.

The properties of the more important of these reagents, in connection with decalcification, are discussed below.

NITRIC ACID

Nitric acid is a decalcifying agent that is very rapid but destructive to tissue, especially when used in high concentrations. This effect is suppressed somewhat when it is used in conjunction with alcohol, much better nuclear staining being obtained. Nitric acid is normally used as a 5 or 10 percent aqueous solution, or in conjunction with other reagents.

Note. The nitric acid used should be pure and stabilized with urea. 1–2 g/2000 ml is adequate. Nitric acid that has started to discolor (yellow) tends to accelerate decalcification.

HYDROCHLORIC ACID

Hydrochloric acid is not quite as rapid as nitric acid but is still rather destructive. It allows fairly good nuclear staining and does not require washing out of the tissue prior to dehydration. As a 1 percent solution in 70 percent alcohol it is extremely good for surface decalcification of blocks.

FORMIC ACID

Formic acid is fairly rapid in action and not nearly as destructive as either nitric or hydrochloric acid. It is not recommended for urgent work and requires neutralizing and thorough washing to remove the acid from the tissue prior to dehydration. Nuclear staining is better than after decalcification in nitric or hydrochloric acid.

TRICHLORACETIC ACID

Trichloracetic acid is a weak decalcifying agent similar in action to formic acid, but—due to its high molecular weight as compared to formic acid—much larger quantities are necessary. It is extremely slow in action and therefore unsuited for urgent work.

SULFUROUS ACID

Sulfurous acid is a very weak acid, used only with minute spicules of bone.

PHENOL (CARBOLIC ACID)

Phenol is not actually a decalcifying agent, but is included here for convenience. It is extremely useful for softening hard tissues such as uterine fibroids. Following fixation the fixative is washed out and the specimen is placed in a 4 percent aqueous solution of phenol for 1–3 days. There is definite softening of the tissue thus making sectioning much easier, and there are no marked harmful effects on subsequent staining.

Decalcifying Fluids

PHLOROGLUCIN-NITRIC ACID

Conc. nitric acid	10 ml
Phloroglucin	1 g

Mix under a fume hood. When the dense brown fumes abate add:

10 percent nitric acid	100 ml

Decalcification time for a block of bone 5 mm in thickness is 12–24 hours.

Advantage

It is a very rapid decalcifying agent, probably the most rapid of all.

Disadvantages

1. Nuclear staining is very poor.
2. It is extremely destructive to tissue if they are left for too long.
3. It needs neutralizing with 5 percent sodium sulfate followed by thorough washing in running tap water for at least 24 hours.
4. The chemical test cannot be used to ascertain the degree of decalcification.

AQUEOUS NITRIC ACID

Conc. nitric acid	5–10 ml
Distilled water	to 100 ml

Decalcifying time for a block of bone 5 mm in thickness is 12–24 hours.

Advantages

1. It is a rapid decalcifying agent.
2. It causes less damage to the tissue, and gives better nuclear staining than does formol nitric acid.
3. Tissue is passed directly to 70 percent alcohol to remove the acid.

Disadvantages

Decalcification time must be carefully controlled to prevent any damage to the tissue.

FORMOL NITRIC ACID

40 percent formaldehyde	5 ml
Conc. nitric acid	10 ml
Distilled water	85 ml

Decalcification time for a block of bone measuring 5 mm in thickness is 1–3 days.

Advantages

1. It is a rapid decalcifying agent.
2. It allows better nuclear staining than does phloroglucin-nitric acid.
3. It is recommended for urgent biopsies.
4. It is not nearly as destructive as 5 or 10 percent aqueous nitric acid.

Disadvantages

1. It does not permit as good nuclear staining as a slower acting agent.
2. It requires neutralizing with 5 percent sodium sulfate followed by thorough washing in running tap water for at least 12 hours.

PERENYI'S FLUID

10 percent nitric acid	4 parts
0.5 percent chromic acid	3 parts
Absolute ethyl alcohol	3 parts

Decalcification time for a block of bone 5 mm in thickness: 2–7 days.

Advantages

1. It is a gentle decalcifying agent, probably due to the presence of the chromic acid and alcohol-suppressing maceration.
2. It allows good nuclear staining and cytoplasmic detail.
3. It is recommended for routine decalcification.
4. It does not require neutralizing and washing out of the tissue. The specimen may be transferred directly to 90 percent alcohol.

Disadvantages

1. It is slow, and therefore of no use for urgent work.
2. The routine chemical test cannot be used to ascertain the degree of decalcification. A modified test may be used.

VON EBNER'S FLUID

Saturated aq. soln. sodium chloride	50 ml
Distilled water	50 ml
Conc. hydrochloric acid	8 ml

Decalcification time for a block of bone 5 mm in thickness is 3–7 days.

Advantages

1. It is fairly rapid.
2. It permits reasonably good nuclear staining.
3. It may be dehydrated without washing out the acid first.
4. It is recommended for teeth.

Disadvantages

The chemical test cannot be used to ascertain the degree of decalcification.

FORMIC ACID

Formic acid (S.G.1.20)	10 ml
10 percent formol saline	90 ml

Decalcification time for a block of bone 5 mm in thickness: 3–7 days.

Advantages

1. It fixes and decalcifies simultaneously.
2. It permits fairly good nuclear staining.
3. It is recommended for small pieces of bone and teeth.

Disadvantages

1. It is slow, and therefore not suitable for urgent work.
2. It requires neutralizing with 5 percent sodium sulfate and removal with thorough washing in running tap water.

FORMIC ACID-SODIUM CITRATE

20 percent aq. sodium citrate	50 ml
45 percent formic acid	50 ml

Decalcification time for a block of bone 5 mm in thickness: 3–14 days.

Advantages

1. It is recommended for autopsy material, cartilage, bone marrow, and research tissue.
2. It permits good nuclear staining.

Disadvantages

1. It is slow, and not recommended for routine specimens.
2. It is not recommended for dense bone.
3. It requires neutralizing with 5 percent sodium sulfate followed by washing in running tap water for at least 18 hours.

TRICHLORACETIC ACID

Trichloracetic acid	5 g
10 percent formol saline	95 ml

Decalcification time for a block of bone 5 mm in thickness: 5–8 days.

Advantages

1. It permits good nuclear staining.
2. It is removed by alcohol, and therefore does not require washing out.

Disadvantages

1. It is slow, and only recommended for minute spicules of bone.
2. It is not recommended for dense bone.

FLEMMING'S FLUID

1 percent chromic acid	15 ml
2 percent osmium tetroxide	4 ml
Glacial acetic acid	1 ml

Although a fixative, Flemming's fluid may be used as a decalcifying fluid for minute spicules of bone. The solution must be renewed frequently as it tends to reduce, and will also form a precipitate in the bottom of the container. Because of the insoluble pigments that may be formed if passed directly to alcohol, the specimen must be thoroughly washed in running tap water to remove any excess chrome salts.

The chemical test cannot be used to ascertain the degree of decalcification, and nuclear staining with hematoxylin is inhibited.

Commercial Decalcifying Solutions

There are several commercial decalcifying solutions available on the market today. Whether one should use one of the solutions prepared in the laboratory or a commercial product (and which one) is a matter of personal choice.

A selection of these reagents is given below (this list is for information only and is not an endorsement of any particular product):

Cal-Ex II	Fisher Scientific Co.
D-calcifier	Lerner Laboratories
Decal	Omega Chemical Corp.
Decalcifying Fluid	Harleco
Decalcifying Solution, S/P	Scientific Products
Formic Acid Reagent	Wood Scientific, Inc.
RDO	Du Page Laboratories

Chelating Agents

Chelating agents are substances that have the property of combining with calcium ions. The usual agent employed in decalcification is Versene, which is manufactured commercially as a water-softener. In addition to calcium ions, other salts are removed, for example, iron and magnesium deposits. Most technicians refer to this substance by its abbreviation EDTA, the full name being ethylene-diamine-tetra-acetic acid disodium salt:

EDTA	5.5 g
10 percent neutral formalin	100.0 ml

Decalcification time for a block of bone 5 mm in thickness: 7–21 days.

Advantages

1. It allows good staining results.
2. There is very little structural damage to the tissue.
3. The end point of decalcification can be ascertained by the chemical test.

Disadvantages

1. It is extremely slow, and therefore unsuitable for routine specimens.
2. It tends to harden tissue slightly.

Ion Exchange Resins

These resins are used to remove calcium ions from the decalcifying fluid thereby speeding up the process of decalcification. They are not used with fluids containing mineral acids, but give good results with those containing formic acid. The physical test, or preferably x-rays should be used to ascertain the degree of decalcification because it is impossible to use the chemical test.

Decalcification by Electrophoresis

Theoretically, this technique is based on the calcium ion being attracted to a negative electrode. This removes calcium ions from the electrolyte in much the same way as ion exchange resins remove calcium from the decalcifying fluid.

Decalcification time is reduced considerably by electrophoresis, but this is probably due more to the heat produced by the passage of the current than to the electrolytic reaction, although the latter does help by keeping the electrolyte relatively free of calcium. If the electrolyte is kept cool, the reaction is a little slower but the subsequent staining is improved.

The technique is not widely used as a routine method of decalcification.

Tests to Ascertain the Degree of Decalcification

If tissues are exposed to decalcifying fluids for too long a period, the net result is maceration and destruction of the tissue, while too short an exposure will result in unremoved calcium. Because of these possibilities a specimen should be left in decalcifying fluid for as long as is necessary to remove the calcium and no longer.

There are three types of test available to determine this end point. They come under the headings: physical tests, chemical tests, and x-ray.

PHYSICAL TESTS

Experienced technicians often rely on their sense of touch in determining when tissue is decalcified. They do this by bending the tissue in their fingers or needling it, that is, probing into the specimen with a needle. The first method is unsatisfactory in that small foci of calcium may not be detected, especially in the center of the tissue. Although the second method will often detect these pockets of calcium, needle-tract artifacts are left in the tissue, possibly destroying some very important detail necessary for diagnosis. For these reasons physical testing is not recommended, although in some instances it may be unavoidable.

CHEMICAL TESTS

The chemical test relies on the detection of calcium in the decalcifying solution. When no further calcium is detected decalcification is complete. During decalcification the fluid should be changed every 24–48 hours, 24 hours being recommended in the early stages. The test is performed on the fluid about to be discarded.

Method

1. To 5 ml of decalcifying fluid (to which has been added a piece of litmus paper) add concentrated ammonia drop by drop, until the fluid is neutralized.
2. If at this stage the solution goes cloudy due to the formation of calcium hydroxide, decalcification is not complete and it is not necessary to proceed further.
3. Add 0.5 ml of saturated aqueous ammonium oxalate.
4. If cloudiness occurs due to the presence of calcium oxalate then decalcification is not complete.
5. If the solution remains clear, leave for 30 minutes. Should the fluid remain clear at the end of this time then it is safe to assume that decalcification is complete.

A modification of this method by Crawford[1] allowed the use of the chemical test following decalcification in Perenyi's fluid. He dissolved the precipitate formed by the addition of ammonia with glacial acetic acid and then proceeded with the ammonium oxalate.

Some technicians neutralize the decalcifying solution with 2N sodium hydroxide and add 1 ml of 5 percent sodium or ammonium oxalate. An absence of cloudiness indicates that decalcification is complete.

X-RAYS

X-rays are the most reliable method of checking on the end point of decalcification as even the smallest pocket of calcium can be detected. The obvious disadvantage of this method for routine checking is the cost involved, and unless large numbers of specimens may be tested simultaneously it is uneconomical. Figure 1 shows varying degrees of the removal of calcium from a large specimen of bone as seen by x-ray.

Effects of Heat on Decalcification

Heat will speed up the process of decalcification considerably. However, this is hazardous to the specimen; the loss of calcium salts occurs

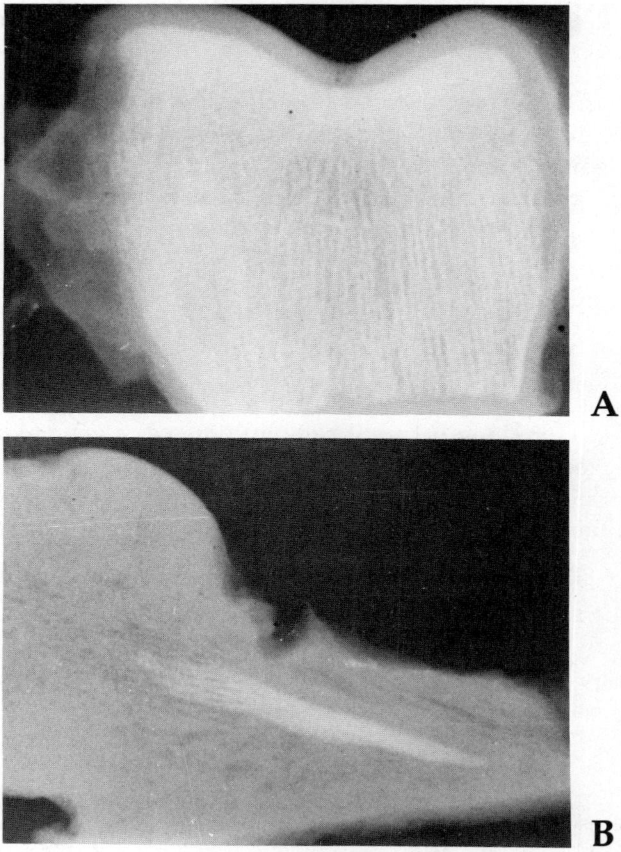

Figure 5-1. Photograph of an x-ray showing varying degrees of decalcification. A. Undecalcified bone. B. Partially decalcified bone.

very rapidly and is followed by marked swelling and hydrolysis of the bone matrix, soon resulting in complete digestion of the specimen.

At 37 C nuclear staining and the staining of collagen fibers with Van Gieson's stain are impaired.

At 55 C complete digestion occurs in:

8 percent hydrochloric acid in 24 hours.

10 percent formic acid/hydrochloric acid mixture in 24 hours.

5 percent formic acid in 48–72 hours.

Decalcification is best done at room temperature.

Surface Decalcification and Softening of Hard Tissues

Difficulties are often encountered in sectioning due to the hardness of the tissue, or to an unexpected pocket of calcium. These can often be a major problem in autopsy specimens, causing considerable damage to the edge of a microtome knife. Once discovered, however, these problems are often easily overcome by the use of one of the following reagents.

PERENYI'S FLUID

This fluid was originally used to soften hard tssues and remove small deposits of calcium long before it came into use as a general decalcifying fluid. Fixed tissue should be left in the fluid for 12–24 hours and then dehydrated in the routine manner, or the cut surface of a block may be submerged in the fluid for an hour or two prior to sectioning Figure 2.

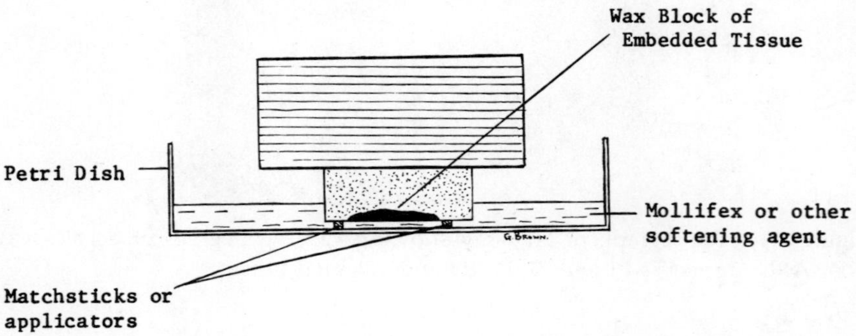

Figure 5-2. Diagram showing how blocks may be placed in tissue softeners or "surface decalcified."

LENDRUM'S METHOD

Following fixation and after washing out the fixative, tissue should be placed in 4 percent aqueous phenol for 1–3 days. The method may also be used for tissue that has already been embedded, the cut surface of the block being immersed in phenol for a few hours prior to cutting. Lendrum (1951) also advocates that the exposure of the cut surface of a block to 2 percent hydrochloric acid for a few hours is sufficient for decalcification when unexpected deposits of calcium are encountered during sectioning. I find that 1 percent hydrochloric acid in 70 percent alcohol works equally well in the same circumstances.

MOLLIFEX

Mollifex* is used to soften hard tissue in the block. It will also work on minute deposits of calcium. The cut surface of the block is immersed in the reagent for a few hours before cutting. The tissue may swell slightly and have a soapy look to it, but this does not have any effect on subsequent staining of the section.

REFERENCE

1. Crawford RA: A chemical test for the detection of calcium when using Perenyi's fluid. J Med Lab Technol 14: 111, 1957

* Product of the British Drug House, Chadwell Heath, Essex, England.

SIX

Processing of Tissue

With the exception of tissue for frozen or ground sections, which does not normally require embedding, all specimens must be dehydrated, cleared, impregnated, and embedded in a suitable medium to facilitate ease of sectioning. As a general rule, material that has been embedded can be cut in much thinner sections than is possible without this procedure. For example, paraffin sections can be cut routinely at 4 microns. The common exception to this is that frozen sections can be cut in the cryostat at 4–5 microns with relative ease.

Dehydration

Before tissue can be impregnated with certain embedding media, it requires dehydrating and clearing. This is because many of the embedding media are not miscible with water. Dehydration is the term used to define the *complete removal* of water from the tissue, either with reagents or by freeze-drying.

The three most common reagents that are used as dehydrating agents are alcohol (the agent in most common use), acetone, and dioxane (diethylene dioxide). In addition to being a dehydrating agent, dioxane is an excellent clearing agent as it is miscible with both water and paraffin wax. It causes little shrinkage of the tissue, but its fumes are *extremely toxic* in confined spaces. Unfortunately, it does not allow good ribboning of sections.

It is possible to utilize accessory agents such as calcium oxide and anhydrous copper sulfate, but the use of these is really to dehydrate the dehydrating reagent, thus accelerating the process while at the same time effecting an economy. Anhydrous copper sulfate can also be used as an indicator to show when the dehydrating fluid is saturated with water. When this point is reached the copper sulfate crystals turn a bright blue.

Routine dehydration is facilitated by bringing the tissue through a succession of alcohols of increasing strength, usually ranging from 70 percent to absolute, until all of the water has been removed from the specimen. The tissue should be allowed to remain in each strength of alcohol for just as long as is necessary for complete saturation, as prolonged immersion in the higher grades of alcohol will result in excessive shrinkage and hardening of the tissue.

The following reagents are commonly used as dehydrating agents:

1. Acetone—a very rapid dehydrant.
2. Butyl alcohol—a slow dehydrant that is miscible with paraffin and therefore excludes the use of a clearing agent.
3. Dioxane—not routinely used. It is miscible with paraffin and therefore excludes the use of a clearing agent. It is *very toxic* in confined spaces.
4. Ethyl alcohol—considered the best routine dehydrant.
5. Ethylene glycol monoethyl ether (Cellosolve)—a rapid dehydrant that does not require graded dilutions.
6. Isopropyl alcohol—frequently used as a substitute for ethyl alcohol, but cannot be used for celloidin techniques.
7. Tetrahydrofuran—a rapid dehydrant without causing excessive shrinkage.

Clearing

Clearing is not the making of the tissue transparent as the title implies, although this may occur in some instances, but is the replacement of the dehydrating fluid with a substance that is miscible with the embedding medium to be employed.

Although most routine laboratories rely on only a few basic reagents for clearing, there are many readily available. The properties of some of the more common clearing agents are discussed in the following section.

Clearing Agents

XYLENE (XYLOL)

Clears objects up to 5 mm in thickness in ½–1 hour.

Advantages

1. It is a rapid dealcoholization agent, probably the most rapid of all.
2. It does not dissolve celloidin.
3. It does not extract aniline dyes.
4. It is easily eliminated from wax.

Disadvantages

1. It will only clear from absolute alcohol.
2. It will make tissue brittle and hard if it is left for too long.
3. It has a tendency to go acid in partially filled vessels.

TOLUENE

Clears objects up to 5 mm in thickness in 1–2 hours.

Advantages

1. It will not make tissue as brittle or as hard as xylene. Tissue may be left in toluene for as long as 12 hours without undue ill effects.
2. It is rapid and can be used for routine and urgent specimens.

Disadvantages

1. It will only clear from absolute alcohol.
2. It has a tendency to go acid in partially filled vessels.
3. Prolonged exposure to high concentrations of the fumes will have toxic effects.

BENZENE

Clears objects up to 5 mm in thickness in 1–3 hours.

Advantages

1. It is fairly rapid.
2. It does not make tissue as brittle as does xylene or toluene.
3. It causes a minimum of shrinkage.
4. It is easily eliminated from wax.

Disadvantage

Highly inflammable.

CEDARWOOD OIL

Clears objects up to 5 mm in thickness in 2–3 days.

Advantages

1. It clears readily from 95 percent alcohol.
2. It is very tolerant, producing little or no shrinkage and brittleness, even if the tissue is left immersed indefinitely.
3. It does not extract aniline dyes.
4. It clears celloidin sections in 5–6 days.

Disadvantages

1. It is difficult to remove from paraffin wax.
2. It is too slow for routine purposes.
3. It is too expensive for use as a routine clearing agent.

Note

1. If cedarwood oil becomes milky with age it may be cleared by filtering.
2. Cedarwood oil that has been used to clear tissue previously fixed in acetic–alcohol fixatives may sometimes crystallize, only a small quantity being necessary to affect the entire batch. The mass resulting from this crystallization has a melting point of approximately 35 C. The oil may be restored to its normal state by heating it to 200 C.
3. Tissue tends to float on cedarwood oil, and as clearing proceeds it sinks into the oil. To prevent the tissue from drying out before it has a chance to clear, a layer of absolute alcohol should be superimposed on the surface of the oil. When the specimen is saturated it must be transferred to fresh cedarwood oil.

CHLOROFORM

Clears objects up to 5 mm in thickness in 12 to 24 hours.

Advantages

1. It is very tolerant and does not harden tissue as does toluene or xylene. It is recommended for tough tissue such as skin, fibroids, and decalcified specimens.
2. It is extremely useful for large specimens.

Disadvantages

1. It is difficult to ascertain when the tissue is cleared.
2. Tissue has a tendency to float on chloroform and must be held under the surface by some means, usually absorbent cotton gauze.
3. It is difficult to remove from paraffin wax, which it causes to deteriorate.

CARBON TETRACHLORIDE

Clears objects up to 5 mm in thickness in 8–15 hours.

Advantage

It is similar in action to chloroform, but much cheaper.

Disadvantages

1. It is *very* toxic in confined spaces.
2. Similar to those of chloroform.

LEGROIN

Clears objects up to 5 mm in thickness in 12 hours.

Advantages

1. It does not harden tissue as much as toluene or xylene.
2. It is easily eliminated from paraffin wax.

Disadvantages

1. It is difficult to ascertain when the tissue is cleared.
2. It is slow and therefore not recommended for routine use.

ANILINE OIL

This reagent is not normally used as a clearing agent in routine histologic procedures. It is more often used for clearing embryos and insects.

Aniline oil could be used to advantage with extremely delicate specimens. Its main advantage is that it can clear from 70 percent alcohol and that it does not cause excessive shrinkage or hardening of tissue.

Impregnation

Impregnation is the process of completely saturating the specimen with the medium to be used for embedding. In the method for paraffin sections this means complete removal of the clearing agent, usually toluene or xylene, and its replacement with paraffin wax or one of the commercial waxes containing some additive. The additives are designed to improve the waxes, especially in regard to the sectioning qualities. Some of the additives improve the supporting power of the wax and the elasticity of the blocks, thereby making sectioning much easier.

Most of the embedding media in common use are discussed in the following section.

Embedding Media

PARAFFIN WAX

Paraffin wax is available in a wide range of melting points, ranging from 45 to 60 C. The waxes with the lower melting point are softer than those with a higher melting point. In temperate climates it is normal to use waxes with melting points ranging from 55 to 60 C, depending on personal choice, or even to mix a 55 C wax and a 60 C wax in equal parts. The high melting point waxes are used in tropical climates, especially in those with a high humidity. In West Africa, I used waxes containing ceresin with a melting point of 58–60 C.

It is essential that paraffin wax used for impregnation and embedding be of the highest quality, and that it be free from grit, dust, water droplets, and other foreign matter. All fresh wax should be filtered before use. The molten wax may be filtered through ordinary filter paper in the wax oven, which is kept at a temperature 2 C higher than the melting point of the wax. It is unfortunate that the commercial paraffin wax dispensers (Figure 1) do not, as yet, have an efficient filtering system built in.

Tissue may be impregnated with paraffin wax by any one of these three methods: (1) manual processing; (2) automatic processing using an automatic tissue processing machine (Figures 2–9); and (3) vacuum embedding.

During manual processing at least four changes of wax are required at 15 minute intervals in order to ensure the complete removal of the clearing agent from the tissue. The specimen is allowed to remain in

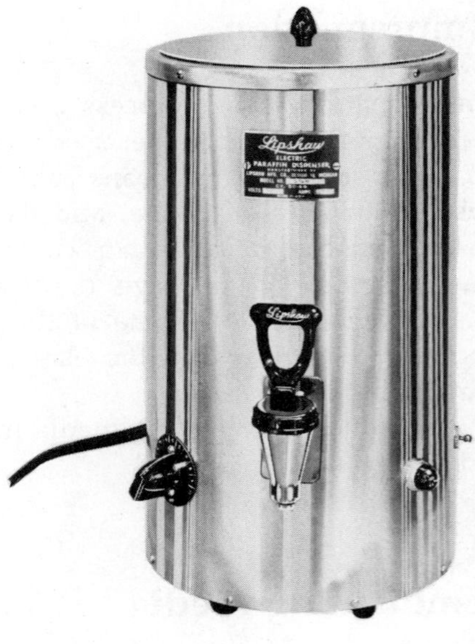

Figure 6-1. *Opposite:* A paraffin dispenser. (*Courtesy of Lipshaw Manufacturing Co. Detroit, Mich.*)

Figure 6-2. *Below:* Lipshaw Vacutherm #1050 automatic tissue processing machine. (*Courtesy of Lipshaw Manufacturing Co. Detroit, Mich.*)

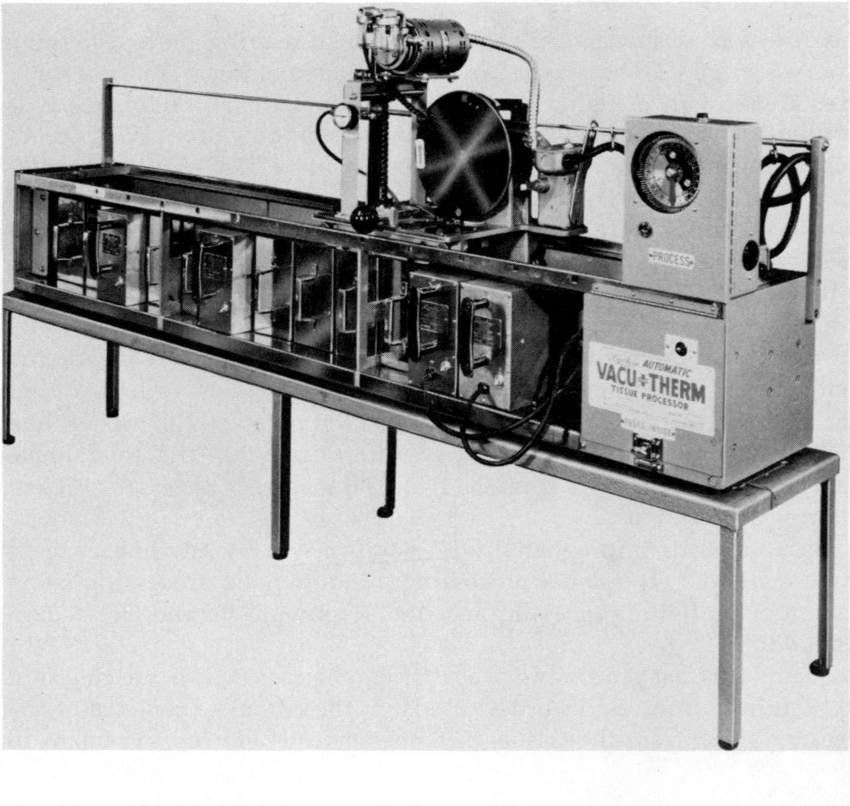

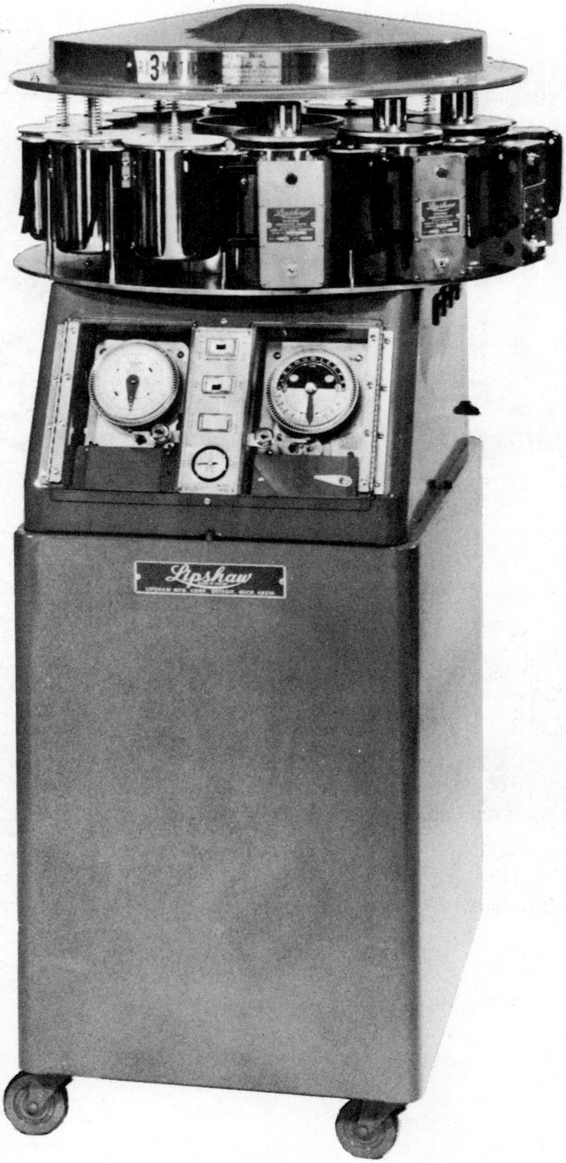

Figure 6-3. The TRI 3 MATIC automatic tissue processing machine (*Courtesy of Lipshaw Manufacturing Co., Detroit, Mich.*)

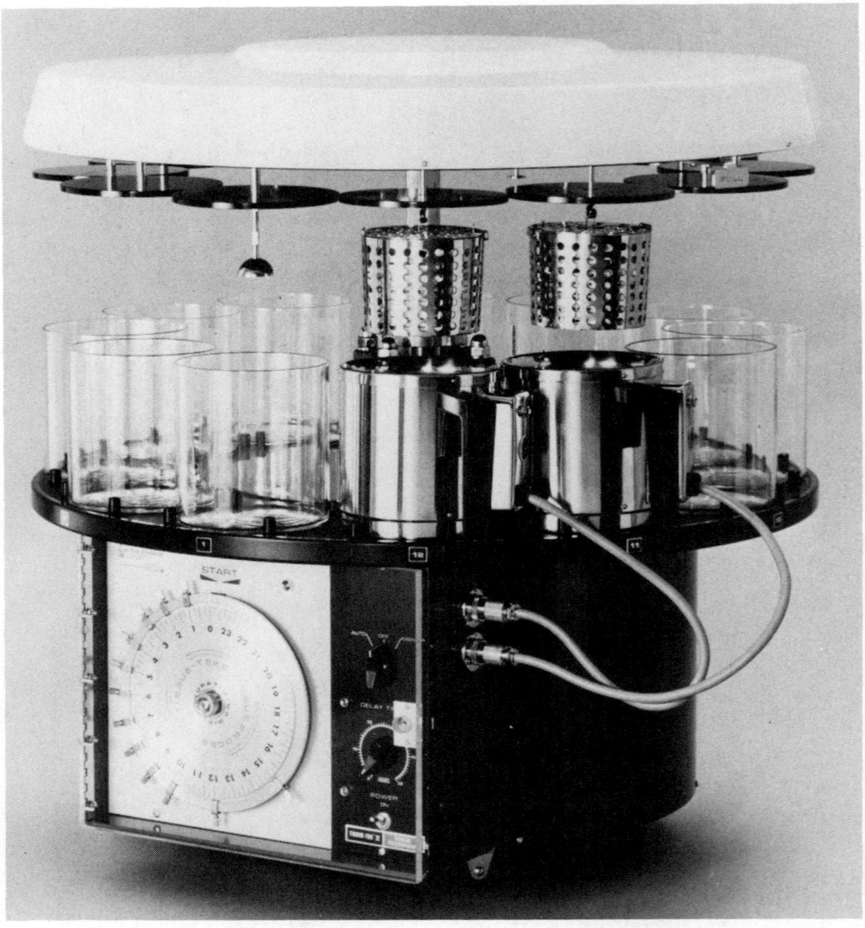

Figure 6-4. The TISSUE-TEK II automatic tissue processing machine. (*Courtesy of Lab-Tek Products, Division Miles Laboratories, Inc., Naperville, Ill.*)

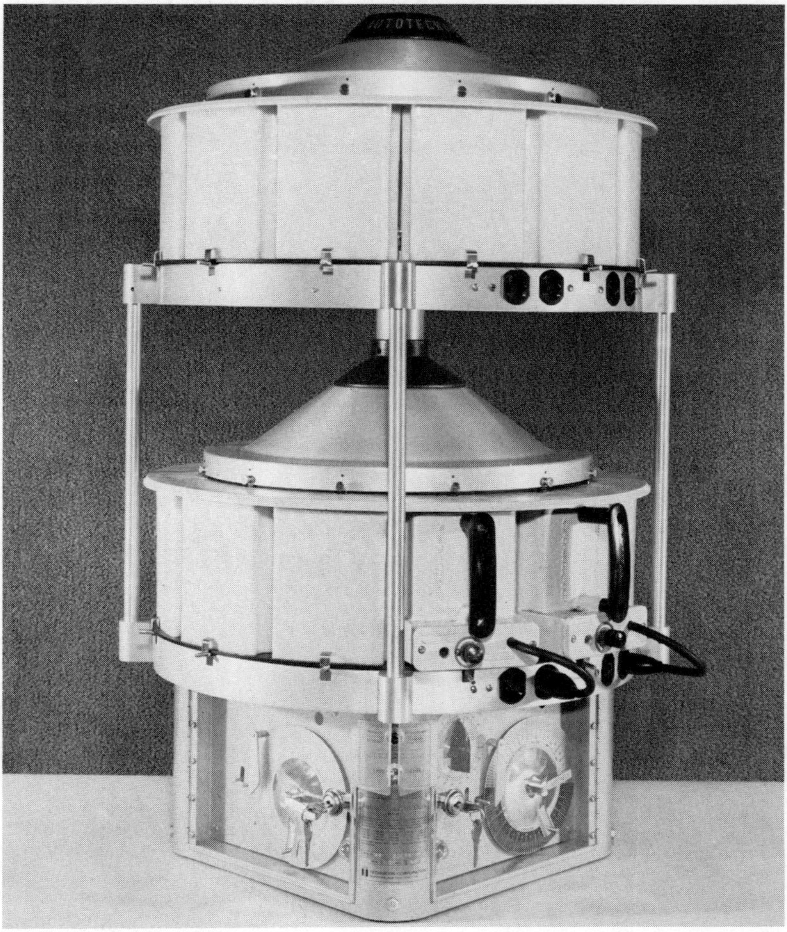

Figure 6-5. The Autotechnicon Duo automatic tissue processing machine. (*Courtesy of Technicon Instruments Corp., Tarrytown, N.Y.*)

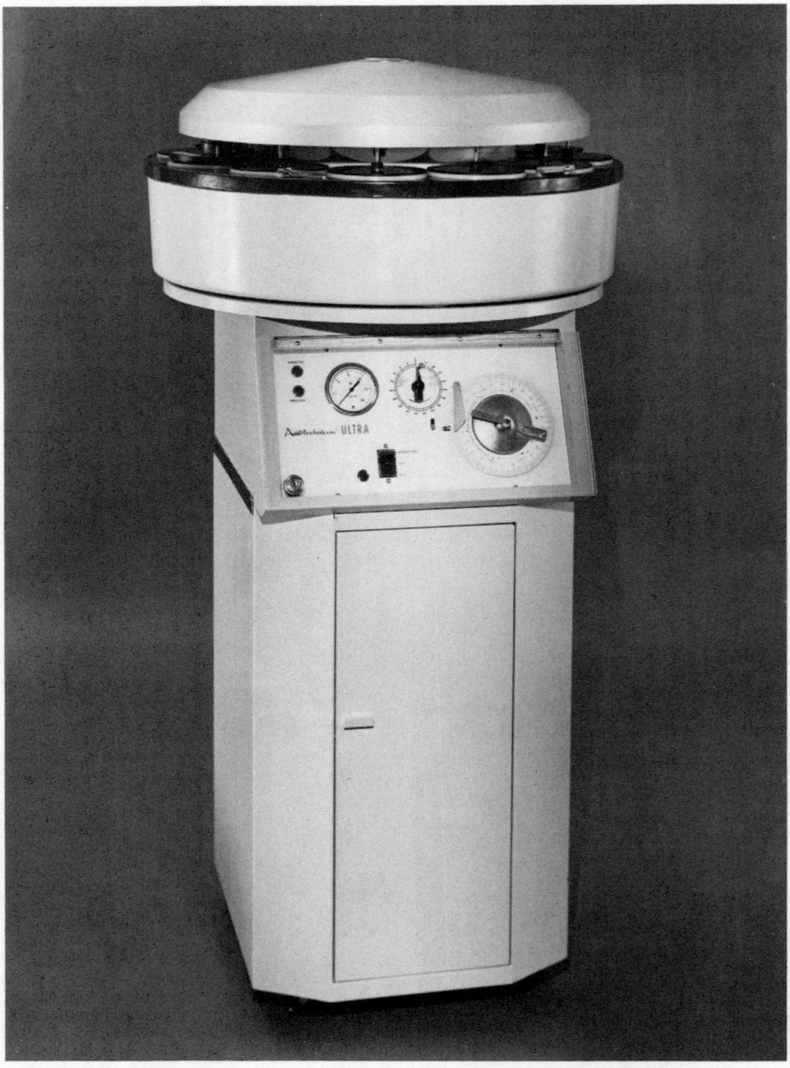

Figure 6-6. The Autotechnicon ULTRA automatic tissue processing machine. (*Courtesy of Technicon Instruments Corp., Tarrytown, N.Y.*)

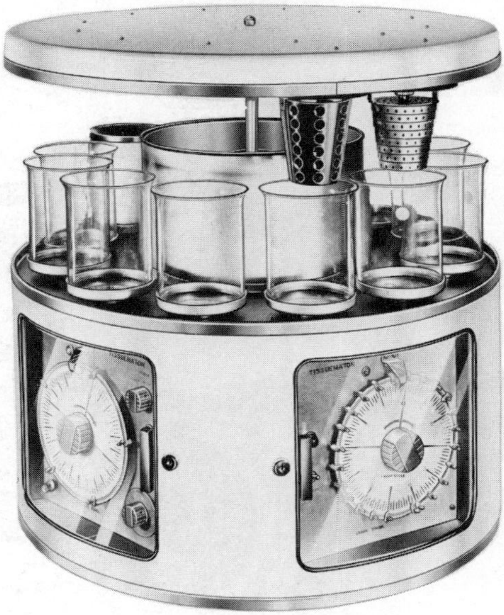

Figure 6-7. The Tissuematon automatic tissue processing machine. (*Courtesy of Fisher Scientific Co., Pittsburgh, Pa.*)

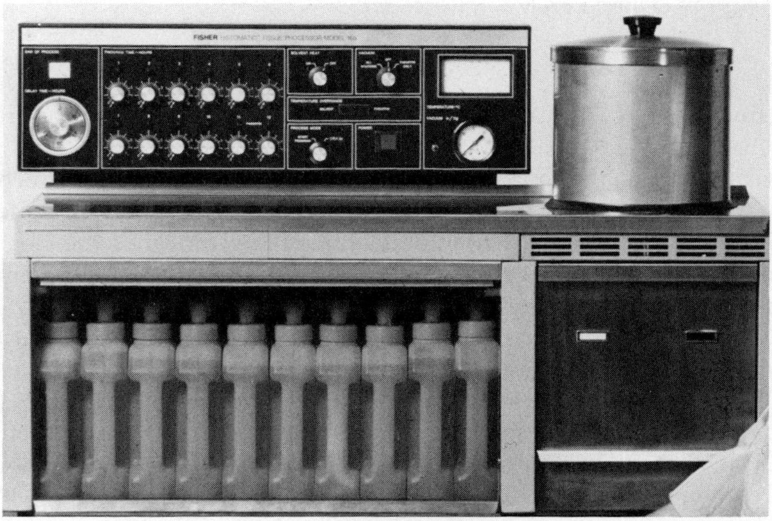

Figure 6-8. The Fisher HISTOMATIC Model 165 automatic tissue processing machine. (*Courtesy of Fisher Scientific Co., Pittsburgh, Pa.*)

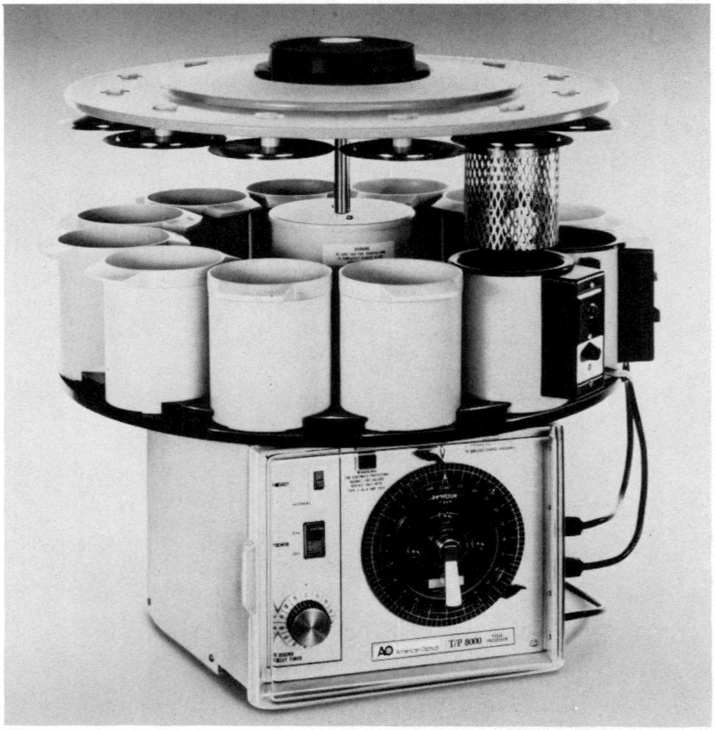

Figure 6-9. The T/P 8000 automatic tissue processing machine. (*Courtesy of the American Optical Corp., Buffalo, N.Y.*)

the final change of wax until it is embedded, a period of approximately 3 hours.

During automatic processing, using a tissue processing machine only two changes of wax are required because the tissues are agitated in the wax, a procedure which accelerates the removal of the clearing agent. The second change of wax is used to impregnate the specimen.

In both of these methods (Table 1) it is vitally important that the tissue has an adequate period of time in the molten wax, but that this is not too prolonged. Tissue that has been immersed in molten wax for too long before being embedded suffers excessive shrinkage and hardening, which can, and does, cause great difficulty when sectioning. When a specimen has not been left in molten wax for long enough the following effects are apparent:

1. The clearing agent is retained in the tissue and the block is soft and crumbly.
2. The wax has failed to penetrate the tissue thoroughly.

TABLE 1-A

Timetable for Tissue Processing for Paraffin Wax

	Manual Processing	Automatic Tissue Processing
10% Formalin	24 hr	2 hr
10% Formalin in 70% alcohol	—	2 hr
70% Alcohol	6 hr	—
90% Alcohol	Overnight	—
95% Alcohol	—	2 hr
95% Alcohol	—	2 hr
Absolute alcohol	2 hr	1 hr
Absolute alcohol	1 hr	1 hr
Absolute alcohol	—	1 hr
Absolute alcohol + copper sulfate[a]	1 hr	—
Xylol or toluene	1 hr	1 hr
Xylol or toluene	1 hr	1 hr
Paraffin wax	15 min	2 hr
Paraffin wax	15 min	—
Paraffin wax	15 min	—
Paraffin wax	15 min	—
Paraffin wax	3 hr	2 hr
	Embed	Embed
Total time	58 hr	17 hr

[a] Anhydrous copper sulfate is optional.

3. The tissue will not section well and the section will break up when being floated out on the waterbath.

Certain tissues, for example, bone, skin, lung, and any dense or tough specimens, will benefit by being impregnated with wax under negative pressure in the vacuum-embedding bath (see Vacuum Embedding). This method has the advantage of very rapid impregnation with a minimum of exposure to heat, which has a tendency to harden tissue. The time required for complete removal of the clearing agent and thorough impregnation of the tissue may be reduced by 50–75 percent, depending on the size of the specimen.

Following impregnation, the tissue is embedded in molten wax at a temperature somewhere between 5 and 10 C above its melting point, and then cooled rapidly. Some blocks may need to be trimmed to a suitable size for sectioning, depending on the type of embedding mold used.

TABLE 1-B

Timetable for Rapid Processing for Paraffin Wax

	Rapid Manual Technique	Ultra-technicon	Ultra-technicon[a]
10% Formalin	30 min at 60 C	40 min	—
10% Formalin in 70% alcohol	30 min at 60 C	20 min	20 min
95% Alcohol	30 min at 60 C	10 min	10 min
Absolute alcohol	30 min at 60 C	20 min	10 min
Absolute alcohol	15 min at 60 C	20 min	10 min
Absolute alcohol	—	20 min	10 min
Absolute alcohol + acetone	15 min at 60 C	—	—
Acetone	15 min at 60 C	—	—
Xylol or toluene	15 min at r.t.[b]	10 min	10 min
Xylol or toluene	15 min at r.t.	15 min	10 min
Xylol or toluene	15 min at r.t.	20 min	10 min
Paraffin wax	15 min	20 min	10 min
Paraffin wax	15 min	—	—
Paraffin wax	15 min	—	—
Paraffin wax	15 min	—	—
Paraffin wax	1 hr	45 min	20 min
	Embed	Embed	Embed
Total time	$5\frac{1}{2}$ hr	4 hr	2 hr

[a] Prefixed biopsies.
[b] Room temperature.

PARAPLAST

Paraplast is a mixture of highly purified paraffin and several plastic polymers, which give it the advantage of being more elastic due to its plastic content. It is similar to paraffin wax, and some technicians like a mixture of Paraplast and paraffin, allowing serial sections to be cut with ease at 4μ. Results with paraplast are as good as those obtained by double embedding. No special techniques have to be employed for its use and it is soluble in the common clearing agents. Impregnation and embedding methods are the same as those employed for paraffin wax.

TISSUEMAT

Tissuemat is a product of paraffin containing rubber and is used in the same way as paraffin wax and Paraplast.

BIOLOID

Recommended as the embedding medium for thin-walled and circular specimens. Its elasticity allows the original shape of the specimen to be regained after processing and sectioning, see page 166.

GELATIN

Gelatin is usually employed as an embedding material for friable specimens and tissue fragments requiring frozen sections. As it is water soluble, the specimens do not require dehydrating and clearing, although the fixative, usually 10 percent formalin, must be completely removed from the tissue by thorough washing in running tap water for 12–24 hours.

Gelatin has a low melting point and specimens embedded by this method do not suffer from the hardening effects of heat on tissue. All impregnation is performed at 37 C in the following manner:

After washing out the fixative:

1. Place into 10 percent gelatin plus 1 percent phenol for 24 hours.
2. Transfer to 20 percent gelatin plus 1 percent phenol for 12 hours.
3. Embed in 20 percent gelatin plus 1 percent phenol and allow to cool, preferably in a cold room or refrigerator.
4. Trim the block to the desired size.
5. Harden the block by immersing it in 10 percent formalin for 12–24 hours.

The 1 percent solution of phenol is added to the gelatin to prevent the growth of molds.

Tissue processed by this method should not exceed 2–3 mm in thickness as gelatin has a tendency to inhibit freezing.

ESTER WAX

Ester wax is an embedding medium that is harder than paraffin wax but with a much lower melting point: 46–48 C. The formula in most common use is Ester Wax 1960.*

Ester wax is not water soluble, but it is soluble in 95 percent ethyl alcohol and the usual clearing agents. Because the wax is soluble in 95 percent alcohol, it is possible to impregnate the specimen without using any of the routine clearing agents. When clearing agents are

* Manufactured by British Drug Houses, Poole, Dorset, England.

used, those usually employed are ethylene glycol monoethyl ether (Cellosolve), or xylene. Tissue is not transferred from the clearing agent to concentrated wax as in the paraffin technique, but to a 50:50 mixture of the clearing agent and ester wax and left for 3–6 hours. The specimen is then placed into pure wax and given three or four changes at suitable intervals of time. Embedding is done in exactly the same way as for paraffin wax, except that the blocks must not be placed in water. It is best to cool the blocks in the refrigerator. Due to contraction of the wax, a central depression often forms in the block and it may be necessary to "top up" to prevent exposure of the tissue.

Sectioning of ester wax blocks should be done on a heavy duty microtome, such as the sliding or sledge type, because of the hardness of the wax. Sections may be cut from 3μ–15μ and mounted in the usual manner, but they should be dried at 37 C and not at room temperature or the sections will crumble.

WATER-SOLUBLE WAXES

Several types of water-soluble waxes are available, the majority of which are polyethylene glycols. They are graded for use by their molecular weight, the ones in most common use being 1000 and 1500 with melting points of 38–42 and 45–56 C, respectively. These temperatures are approximate as the melting points vary slightly with each batch of wax.

The merits of polyethylene glycols over paraffin wax are:

1. They cause relatively little shrinkage. Tissues do not require dehydrating and clearing in the manner necessary for paraffin wax embedding.
2. Tissues do not become brittle, and are not exposed to such high temperatures as those required for paraffin wax embedding.
3. They are very useful for work on enzymes, which are frequently destroyed at the temperatures required for paraffin wax embedding.
4. They are useful for the demonstration of lipids, which are soluble in the reagents employed for processing paraffin sections.
5. Polyethylene glycols tend to give better support to the tissue than does paraffin wax.

In spite of these advantages over paraffin wax, polyethylene glycols are not used routinely because of the difficulty in "floating out" and mounting the sections. Not only are they readily soluble in water, but also in the usual dehydrating and clearing agents. The addition of a trace of soap to the water, or the use of a 10–20 percent solution of polyethylene glycol 900 in water, minimizes the disintegration of the sections and allows them to be flattened and picked up in the normal manner.

After fixation, and washing out the fixative if this is necessary, tissues are impregnated by the following technique:

1. 70 percent polyethylene glycol in water: 45 minutes.
2. 90 percent polyethylene glycol in water: 1 hour.
3. 100 percent polyethylene glycol: 25 minutes.
4. 100 percent polyethylene glycol: 25 minutes.
5. 100 percent polyethylene glycol: 25 minutes.

The tissues are embedded in pure (100 percent) polyethylene glycol and the blocks cooled at 5 C in the refrigerator.

CELLOIDIN

Celloidin is a useful embedding medium for hard or fragile specimens, and although it is not employed very frequently in routine histologic techniques, it is extremely useful in neurologic work. Tissues receive far greater support from celloidin than from paraffin wax, and as a result much larger specimens may be sectioned when this medium is used. Because no heat is required during processing, it causes a minimum of shrinkage and hardening of the tissue, and this can be extremely important when cutting large sections of bone.

In spite of the apparent advantages over paraffin wax, the disadvantages outweigh them and the use of celloidin as a routine embedding medium is very limited. The time taken to impregnate the tissue must be measured in days and weeks rather than in hours, and sections can seldom be cut thinner than 10μ, the usual thickness being 15μ. In addition, the blocks normally require storing in 70 percent alcohol and the sections and knife must be continually moistened with 70 percent alcohol during cutting.

Celloidin, a purified form of nitrocellulose (gun cotton), is normally supplied as a wool or in shreds moistened with alcohol, and is used in three concentrations. It is dissolved in equal parts of ether and alcohol. The three concentrations are:

1. 2 percent solution (thin).
2. 4 percent solution (medium).
3. 8 percent solution (thick).

Preparation of Solutions

The celloidin is dried overnight on filter paper in the incubator at 37 C. The dried wool is now weighed out and soaked in absolute ethyl alcohol for several hours to soften it. An equal volume of ether is added and the solution is mixed thoroughly and allowed to stand. Any lumps will dissolve if the solution is left overnight. Celloidin solutions must be kept in bottles with ground-glass stoppers to prevent evaporation of the solvent. It is important to keep the neck and stopper of the bottle free of celloidin by wiping it clean with absolute alcohol. Solutions of celloidin should be stored well away from any source of flame as they are *extremely flammable*.

Impregnation

1. Following dehydration the tissue is placed into equal parts of ether and alcohol for 12–24 hours. This is the clearing process.
2. Place into thin (2 percent) celloidin solution for 5–7 days.
3. Place into medium (4 percent) celloidin solution for 5–7 days.
4. Place into thick (8 percent) celloidin solution for 3–5 days.

Note. All of the above procedures must be done in wide-mouthed bottles with ground-glass stoppers.

Embedding

1. Position the specimen in a paper boat (page 83) and fill to the brim with thick celloidin.
2. Place under a bell jar with one edge of the jar raised very slightly by means of a matchstick or applicator stick, or in a desiccator. If the boat is placed in a desiccator the top should be removed for a few seconds each day to admit fresh air to assist in hardening the block. It may be necessary to "top up" the block to prevent the exposure of the tissue. This sometimes occurs as the celloidin shrinks on hardening.
3. When the finger, *not the nail*, no longer leaves an impression on the surface of the block, hardening is complete.
4. Store the blocks in 70 percent alcohol until ready for cutting.

Note. Chloroform vapor may be used to accelerate the hardening of the block.

Mounting the Block for Cutting

When required for cutting the celloidin block must be trimmed to the required size and mounted on a vulcanite or wooden block. The vulcanite blocks are available with a diamond pattern cut into the surface, but the wooden blocks must be roughened with a saw to assist in the adhesion of the celloidin block.

The surface of the mounting block is covered with a liberal quantity of 2 percent celloidin and the celloidin block is firmly pressed into position. The two blocks must be held in close contact for at least an hour and this is accomplished with a vise or weights. At the end of this time the seal is hardened by immersing the block in 70 percent alcohol and leaving it for at least 30 minutes before cutting.

The "Dry" Celloidin Technique

The dry celloidin technique was evolved to obviate the necessity of using 70 percent alcohol for the storage of blocks and during cutting. The tissue is dehydrated in exactly the same manner as for the "wet" celloidin method, impregnated and then cast in a mold and left to harden. When the celloidin is nearly set, but not quite as hard as described earlier, it is placed in Gilson's mixture:

Chloroform	1 part
Cedarwood oil	1 part

Fresh cedarwood oil is added, daily for large objects and every two hours for small specimens, until the mixture is 90 percent cedarwood oil. The celloidin block should be quite transparent at the end of this process. It is now exposed to the air until perfectly dry and stored in an airtight container, preferably a glass jar with a screw cap or ground-glass stopper.

This method is not used frequently and the "wet" celloidin technique still remains the method of choice in a great many laboratories.

Low-Viscosity Nitrocellulose (LVN)

Low-viscosity nitrocellulose has a lower molecular weight than celloidin and forms a 20 percent solution with ease. It penetrates tissue fairly rapidly and forms a harder block than does celloidin, permitting sections to be cut dry. Sections often have a tendency to crack when embedded in pure LVN, and to prevent this a small amount of celloidin is added to give elasticity to the block. The following formula will give a stock 20 percent solution of LVN:

Celloidin	4 g
LVN	140 g
Ether	250 ml
Absolute ethyl alcohol	210 ml

Preparation

1. Soften the celloidin in 50 ml of absolute alcohol and add 50 ml of ether. Stand to dissolve.
2. Make a paste of the LVN in the remainder of the alcohol and add the remainder of the ether.
3. Mix the two solutions together and leave overnight.

Impregnation

Following dehydration place the specimen into:

1. Ether/alcohol mixture (50:50) for 12–24 hours.
2. 5 percent solution of LVN for 3–5 days.
3. 10 percent solution of LVN for 2–4 days.
4. 20 percent solution of LVN for 12–24 hours.

When the specimen is thoroughly impregnated with 20 percent LVN, it is cast in a mold and embedded in exactly the same manner as for the celloidin method. The blocks are stored in 70 percent alcohol until required for sectioning, then they are mounted in the same way as celloidin blocks except that 20 percent LVN is used as the adhesive.

Low-viscosity nitrocellulose should always be handled with care and never allowed to dry. It is *highly explosive*.

Special Processing Techniques

VACUUM EMBEDDING

Certain tissues are dense and difficult to impregnate by routine methods. These tissues require extra exposure to wax and will subsequently suffer from the effects of excessive exposure to heat. When possible, such specimens should be impregnated by the vacuum-embedding technique: that is, impregnated with wax under negative atmospheric pressure. The advantages of the method are in the reduction of the time required for complete impregnation, which can range from 25 to 75 percent of the time required for normal processing depending on the size of the specimen. This reduction in time means that the tissue is not overexposed to heat, which has a tendency to cause brittleness and increases the shrinkage and hardening of tissue.

All tissue would benefit from vacuum embedding, but the method is strongly recommended for certain types of tissue, which may be classified as follows:

1. Tough (fibrous tissue)
2. Dense (brain)
3. Hard (bone)
4. Air-containing (lung)
5. Blood-containing (spleen)
6. Poorly penetrating (skin)
7. Delicate (eye)

The vacuum-embedding oven (Fig. 10) consists of a heavy brass chamber with a lid of thick plate glass. The lid rests on a wide rubber

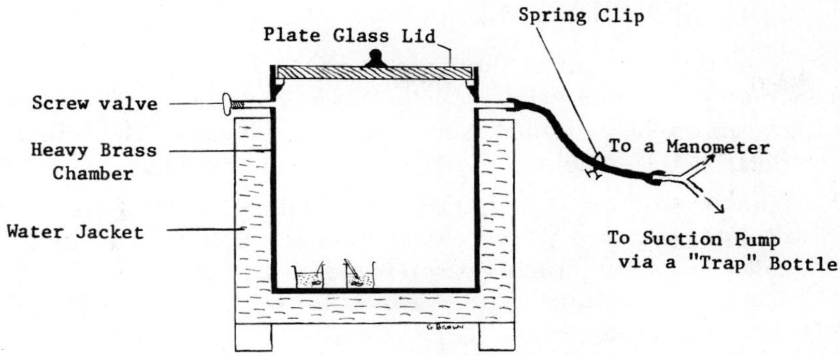

Figure 6-10. Diagram of a vacuum-embedding oven.

washer to effect an airtight seal when the chamber is in use. There are two screw valves in the upper part of the chamber to allow the exhaustion and readmission of air. The greater part of the chamber is enclosed in a water jacket, the temperature of which is thermostatically controlled. When in use, the internal temperature of the chamber should be 2–4 C above the melting point of the wax. Some of the more recent automatic tissue processing machines have a vacuum chamber built into them (see Figs. 2, 3, 6–8).

Method

After fixation and dehydration proceed as follows:

1. Clear in two changes of xylene, 1 hour in each.
2. Place the tissue in molten wax in the vacuum chamber and make airtight.
3. Exhaust the air slowly by means of a vacuum pump or a Venturi suction pump until there is a negative pressure of 400–500 mm Hg.
4. Leave for 15 minutes, then slowly readmit air until normal atmospheric pressure is reached.
5. Place the tissue in fresh wax.
6. Repeat steps 3 and 4.
7. Place the tissue into fresh wax.
8. Repeat step 3 and leave for 30–45 minutes.
9. Bring to normal atmospheric pressure and embed the tissue.

Note. The exhaustion and readmission of air must be gradual or the specimen may be ruined.

PETERFI'S DOUBLE-EMBEDDING METHOD

Peterfi's method combines the support given by celloidin with the ease of manipulation of paraffin sections. The method's chief use is for cutting sections of delicate tissue such as eyes where the retina is easily detached. The method of impregnation is as follows:

1. Following routine dehydration the specimen is transferred from absolute alcohol to a 1 percent solution of celloidin in methylbenzoate. This solution must be prepared well in advance.
2. Change the celloidin solution every day for 2–3 days depending on the size of the tissue. Large pieces require at least 3 days.
3. Clear in benzene for 2–3 days changing the solution every 6 hours. Clearing must take the same time as impregnation with celloidin, ie, if impregnation took 3 days then clearing must take 3 days. At the end of this time the tissue should be quite transparent.
4. Transfer the tissue to equal parts of benzene and paraffin wax for 2 hours.
5. Impregnate with paraffin wax in the usual manner. Allow three changes of wax at 20 minute intervals and embed 1–2 hours after the third change. Embedding is as for paraffin wax blocks.

FREEZE-DRYING

Basically freeze-drying is the rapid freezing of tissue (preservation) followed by desiccation (dehydration) and embedding. The process has four stages:

1. Quenching: initial freezing and preservation
2. Desiccation: dehydration
3. Embedding, sectioning, and mounting
4. Treatment before examination: fixation and staining

Technique

1. Plunge small pieces of absolutely fresh tissue into isopentane that has been cooled to −160 to −180 C with liquid nitrogen. The entire bulk of the tissue must be frozen rapidly to prevent the formation of ice crystals. This rapid freezing preserves the tissue by preventing autolysis and putrifaction.
2. Transfer the frozen tissue to the drying apparatus and establish a high vacuum, 10^{-3} mm Hg, maintaining the temperature at −30 to −40 C. Drying is usually complete in 24–48 hours, depending on the size of the specimen. Dehydration occurs as water vapor

passes from the tissue to the vapor trap where it is condensed. The vapor trap is kept at a lower temperature than the chamber containing the specimen. If the trap is cooled with acetone/carbon dioxide mixture the temperature will be approximately −70 C, or −180 C if cooled with liquid nitrogen.

3. Following dehydration the specimen is embedded. The embedding media may be either paraffin wax, water-soluble waxes, or celloidin. Many workers prefer to use either pure paraffin wax or Peterfi's double-embedding technique. Impregnation may be done in the vacuum-embedding oven or in the drying apparatus.
4. Embed in the normal manner.
5. Sections may be cut on any standard microtome, the usual thickness of the sections being 10μ. Thinner sections may be taken, but it is difficult to flatten them, especially if contact with water is to be avoided.
6. Fix and stain the sections.

Although this technique is time consuming and expensive, and therefore not suited to routine histologic procedures, it has several advantages over routine fixation and paraffin processing. The advantages of the method are:

1. There is very little shrinkage of the tissue.
2. Tissues are processed in a fresh state. This is particularly important when working on enzyme demonstration.
3. There is little chemical alteration of the proteins.
4. There is much less displacement of cell constituents. A good example of this is the fact that there is virtually no loss of glycogen in specimens processed by this technique.

FREEZE SUBSTITUTION

Freeze substitution is a variation on the freeze-drying technique and is much cheaper and more suitable for routine laboratories. The procedure has three steps:

1. Quenching.
2. Fixation.
3. Routine dehydration and processing for paraffin wax.

Technique

1. Plunge small pieces of tissue into isopentane which has been cooled to −160 to −180 C with liquid nitrogen.
2. Transfer the frozen tissue to either of the following fixatives:

A. *Rossman's Fluid*

Sat. picric acid in 95 percent alcohol	80 ml
Formaldehyde	15 ml

or

B. 1 percent osmium tetroxide in acetone[1].

The specimen should be left in the fixative for 1–6 days and kept at −60 to −70 C. Return to room temperature slowly, see step three.

3. Dehydrate as follows:

   Fixative A. In absolute ethyl alcohol at room temperature.
   Fixative B. In acetone at −70 C.

4. Clear and embed as for paraffin sections.

Embedding or Casting

Embedding is the process of placing the impregnated tissue in a precisely arranged position into a mold containing the embedding medium, and causing this medium to solidify.

With paraffin wax, or one of the alternatives such as Paraplast or Tissuemat, this is achieved by cooling the block rapidly on a cold-plate at −5 C (Fig. 11), in the refrigerator, or by immersing the mold in cold

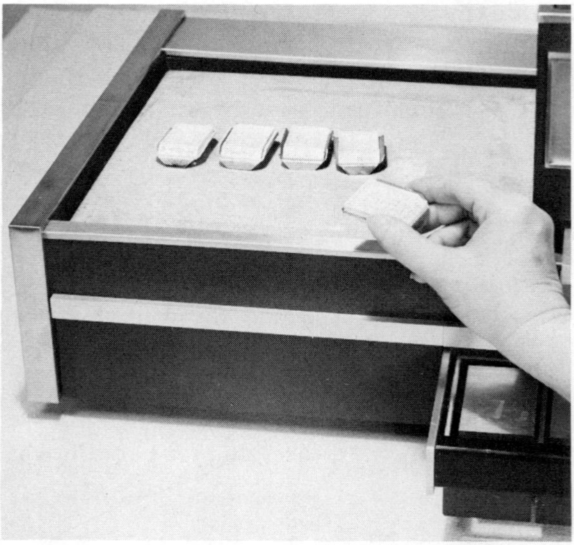

Figure 6-11. Using a cold plate to cool blocks. (*Courtesy of Lab-Tek Products, Division of Miles Laboratories, Naperville, Ill.*)

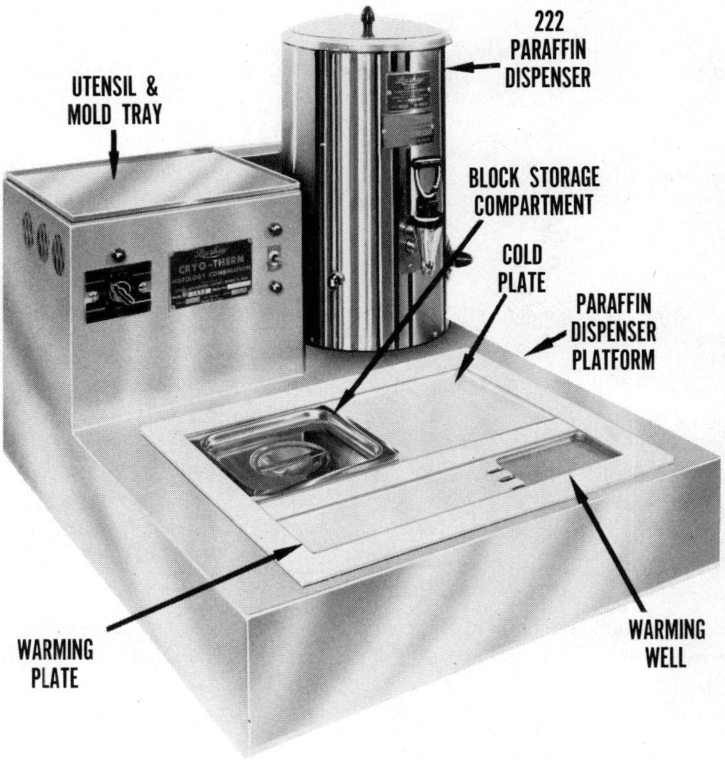

Figure 6-12. The Cryotherm. (*Courtesy of Lipshaw Manufacturing Co., Detroit, Mich.*)

water as soon as a firm skin has formed on the surface of the wax. When the block has solidified it is removed from the mold.

A valuable asset to wax embedding is a piece of equipment having a warm plate to keep the impregnated specimen manageable, and a cold-plate at −5 C to solidify the blocks rapidly. The Lipshaw Cryo-Therm (Fig. 12) and the Tissue-Tek II tissue embedding center (Fig. 13) are such pieces of equipment. While the Cryo-Therm does not have a wax dispenser incorporated in the design, there is a large area provided as a stand for the dispenser of choice, and it does have a cold storage-well designed to keep blocks cool while awaiting sectioning. The Tissue-Tek II has a wax dispenser built into the equipment and a vacuum infiltrator may be added as an accessory. This can be plugged into the embedding center or any ordinary electrical outlet.

Techniques for embedding with other media are discussed under the appropriate headings in the section on embedding media.

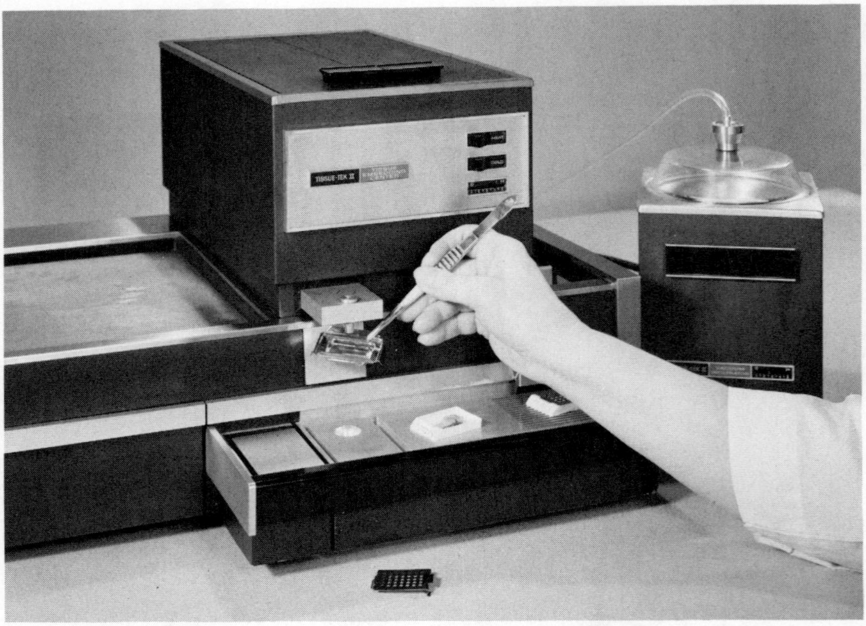

Figure 6-13. The Tissue-Tek II tissue-embedding center complete with a vacuum infiltrator. (*Courtesy of Lab-Tek Products, Division of Miles Laboratories, Naperville, Ill.*)

Orientation

Orientation is the term applied to the placing of the tissue in a precisely arranged position in the mold (Fig. 14). This positioning should be decided upon before the tissue is processed. If there is likely to be any doubt as to which surface is to be cut, the opposite side of the tissue should be marked in order that it can be easily identified. This may be done by spotting the back or opposite surface of the tissue with India ink, or by cutting a shallow groove in it. It is wise to embed tissue so that the softer part of the specimen is cut first and the harder or tougher portion at the end of the cutting pass. This applies especially to skin and bone.

The term orientation is also applicable to the positioning of the block on the microtome prior to cutting, and to the positioning of the sections on the slide.

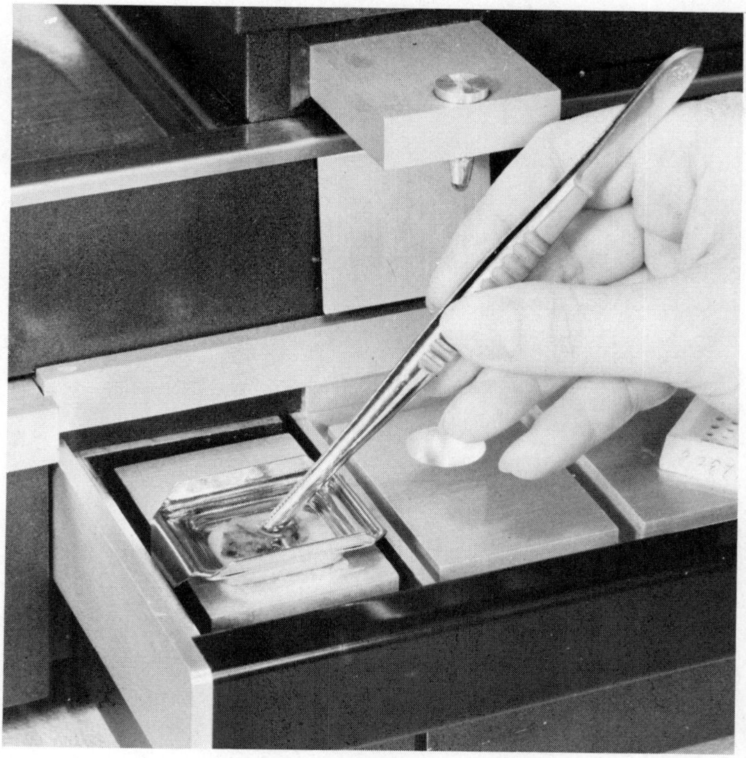

Figure 6-14. Orientating tissue in the mold. (*Courtesy of Lab-Tek Products, Division of Miles Laboratories, Naperville, Ill.*)

Molds

One of the oldest and still most widely used molds is Leuchhart's "L" pieces (Fig. 15. These are two L-shaped pieces of metal resting on a flat metal plate. The "L" pieces can be moved to alter the size of the block so that it will match the size of the specimen being embedded.

The compound embedding unit (Fig. 16) consists of a series of interlocking plates resting on a flat metal base. The interlocking plates are available in two sizes, and form either 25 or 36 compartments. By leaving one of the pieces out a longer block may be cast. For routine histological purposes this type of mold has the advantage over Leuchhart's "L" pieces as many more specimens can be embedded at

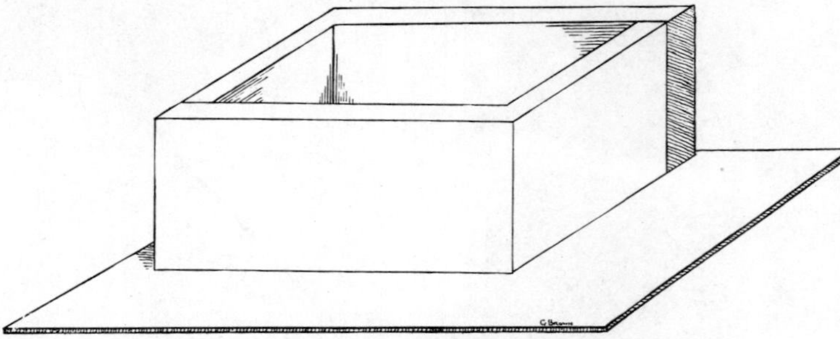

Figure 6-15. Leuchhart's "L" pieces.

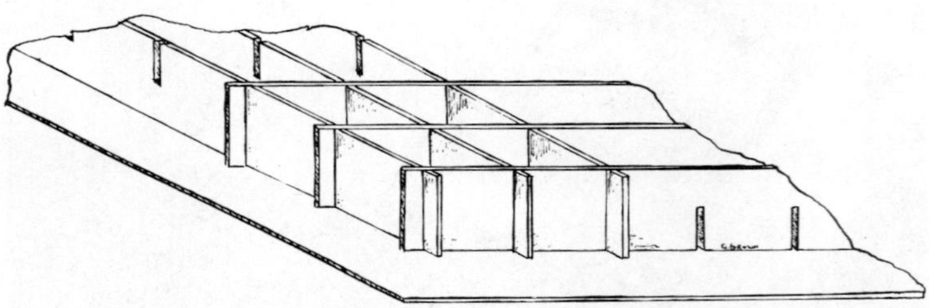

Figure 6-16. Compound embedding unit.

one time, a fact that can be fully appreciated when large numbers of autopsy specimens are embedded.

In the past few years several types of embedding molds have come into general use. Lab-Tek Products, a Division of Miles Laboratories, Inc., have been responsible for two of these systems. The first system is a base mold consisting of a stainless-steel trough onto which fits a plastic top called an embedding ring (Fig. 17). This forms that part of the block that is held in the chuck of the microtome. The specimen is orientated in wax in the base mold and the embedding ring is placed in position and filled up with wax. The block is then allowed to harden and the base mold removed. These molds are available in several sizes and two depths to accommodate most routine requirements. Blocks made in this manner have the advantages of not requiring trimming or mounting onto wooden blocks prior to cutting, and are more easily orientated for resectioning at some later date. I find that these molds are very convenient for routine purposes. The same company has also produced another mold which utilizes a tissue cassette as the embedding ring (Fig. 18A). The molds are available in five sizes (Fig. 18B) and should meet the requirements of most

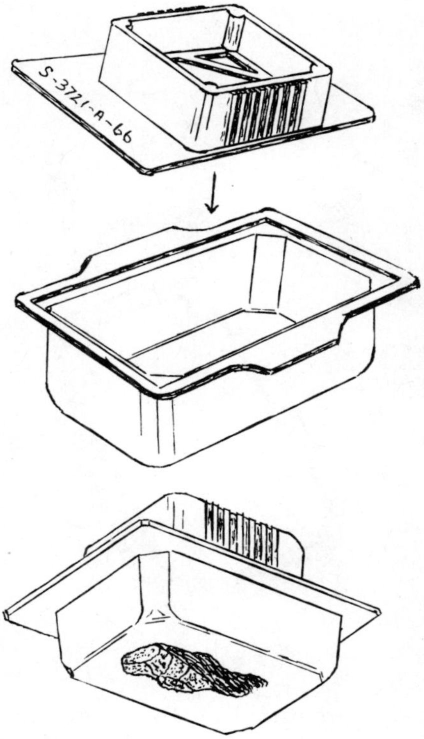

Figure 6-17. *Opposite:* Tissue-Tek embedding ring and base mold. (*Courtesy of Lab-Tek Products, Division of Miles Laboratories, Naperville, Ill.*)

Figure 6-18. *Below:* A. Tissue-Tek II tissue cassette that may be used as an embedding ring. B. Base molds for use with the tissue cassette in A. (*Courtesy of Lab-Tek Products, Division of Miles Laboratories, Naperville, Ill.*)

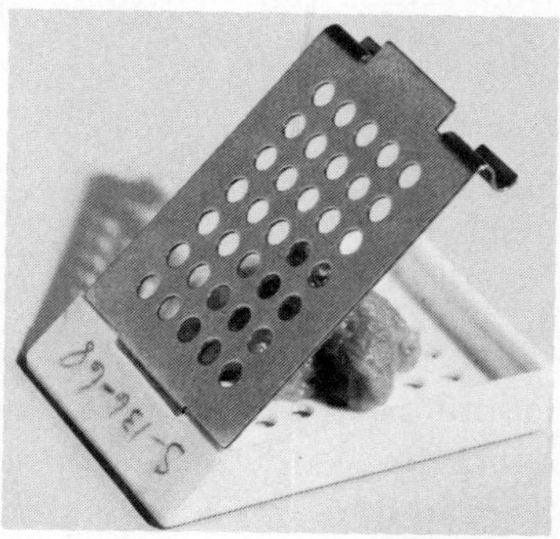

A

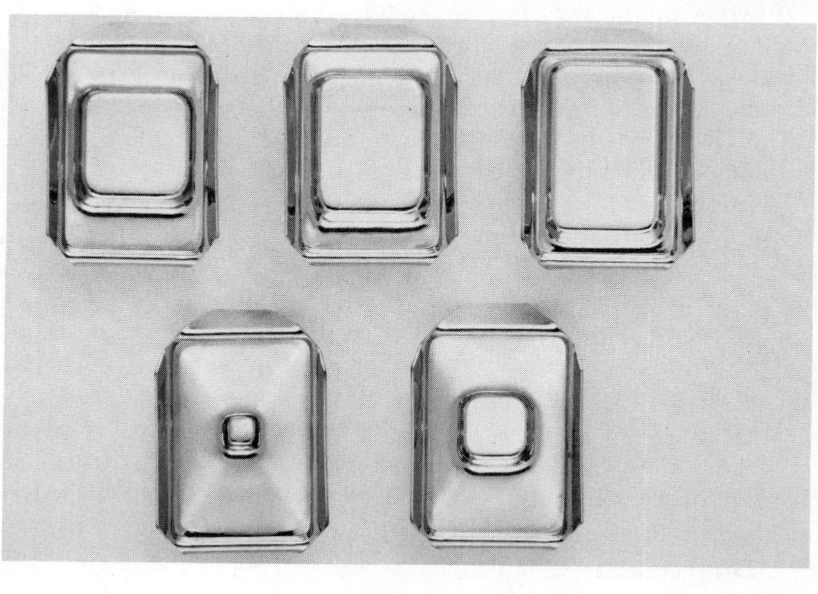

B

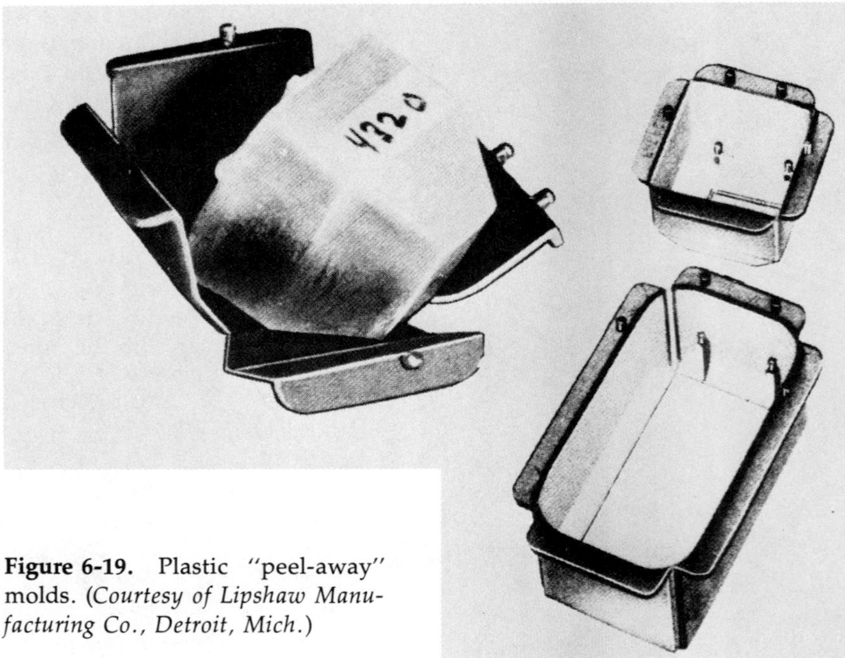

Figure 6-19. Plastic "peel-away" molds. (*Courtesy of Lipshaw Manufacturing Co., Detroit, Mich.*)

laboratories. A special adapter is usually required on the microtome chuck to accommodate these blocks, but in all other respects they are used in the same way as those described in the previous paragraph.

If two of the plastic cassettes are glued together they may be placed into the microtome chuck as a *spacer* positioned behind the block. The thickness of this spacer is such that the finished block fits perfectly into the chuck and negates the necessity of the special adapter.

The TIMS system* utilizes a plastic tissue cassette that is then used as the mold when the specimen is embedded.

Mention should be made of disposable embedding molds. These are made of a plastic and are peeled off of the block after it has been cast and hardened (Fig. 19). These blocks may require mounting onto blockholders prior to sectioning.

Paper boats (Fig. 20) are normally utilized for embedding celloidin blocks, but they are equally useful for paraffin wax blocks. They have the advantage that they can be made to suit any size of tissue.

A great variety of other objects have been found to be extremely useful as embedding molds. They range from Petri dishes, small cardboard boxes, and cover glass boxes to gelatin capsules. I have

* LAB-LINE Biomedical Products, Inc.

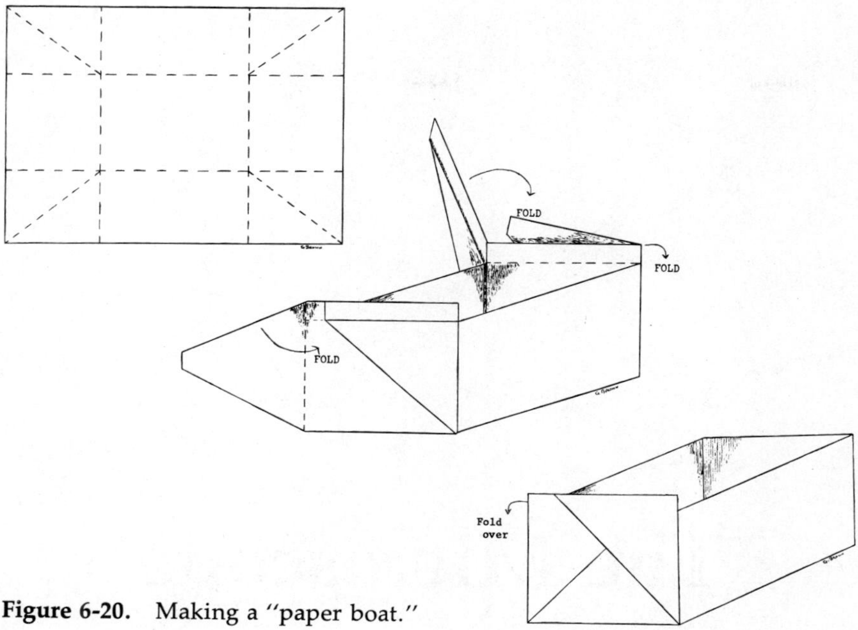

Figure 6-20. Making a "paper boat."

found the latter to be invaluable for embedding extremely small specimens. The capsule is easily removed from the block by soaking it in water.

REFERENCE

1. Feder N, Sidman R: Methods and principles of fixation by freeze-substitution. J. Biophys. Biochem. Cytol. 4:593–603, 1958.

SEVEN

The Microscope

Historical Background

The science of optics, and the knowledge that lenses have the capability of enlarging or magnifying an object, has been known to man for many centuries. Inscriptions so fine that they had to be magnified in order that they could be read and deciphered were discovered in the ruins of Nineveh, the ancient capital of Assyria, along with convex lenses made out of quartz. This city existed from 700 to 612 B.C., thus dating the lenses and making them about 2600 years old.

The practice of microscopy had its beginnings in the early seventeenth century. At this time a Dutch spectacle maker named Hans Lippershey constructed a simple telescope, and another Dutchman named Janssen built a microscope. Galileo heard about these in 1609 and made several simple telescopes using the principles that the Dutchman had pioneered.

The seventeenth century was an extremely fruitful era for the microscopist, who made many observations and discoveries. However, it was equally full of pitfalls and errors, as many of the observations were faulty, mainly due to the poor resolution of the optics and a lack of knowledge in the techniques and art of preparing specimens for examination. What was described often turned out to be artifact.

A Dutch naturalist, Anton van Leeuwenhoek (1632–1723), built the first really practical microscope, and was the first to observe blood cells, sperm, and protozoa. He is also credited with being the first microscopist to employ a biological stain.

In 1733 an Englishman, Chester Moor Hall, invented the achromatic objective, which was capable of bringing the red and blue components of light to a common focus. It was not until 1824 that this discovery was put to practical use with the introduction of a microscope using achromatic optics, a development resulting from the work of two French opticians and instrument makers, Vincent and Charles Chevalier. Achromatic objectives were soon incorporated into the optical systems of most microscopes. Today, even the most inexpensive microscope uses achromatic optics.

Definition

What is a microscope? The microscope is an optical instrument used to magnify very small (microscopic) objects, in particular, those objects that are not normally visible to the human eye.

An ordinary magnifying glass, usually having a magnifying power of less than twenty diameters, is a *simple microscope*. As you can see from Figure 1, Anton van Leeuwenhoek's microscope is a simple microscope with a mechanism for raising and lowering the specimen and another mechanism for focussing. Today the simple microscope may be used for the gross examination of specimens, and it may be mounted in an adjustable stand with a built-in illumination.

We are more interested in the type of microscope that we use in the laboratory for the examination of slides. This is the *compound microscope*. The compound microscope (Fig. 2) usually has three separate and distinct optical systems, each having a specific function. It may also be a monocular or binocular microscope (Figs. 3 and 4), and may even be a double-headed version, which allows two people to examine a specimen simultaneously.

Parts of the Microscope

ESSENTIALS

It is essential that the instrument be rigid, firm, and free from any vibration, not only when upright, but also when inclined at an angle or in the horizontal plane. Joint movements and rack-and-pinion movements must work smoothly and precisely and be free from such

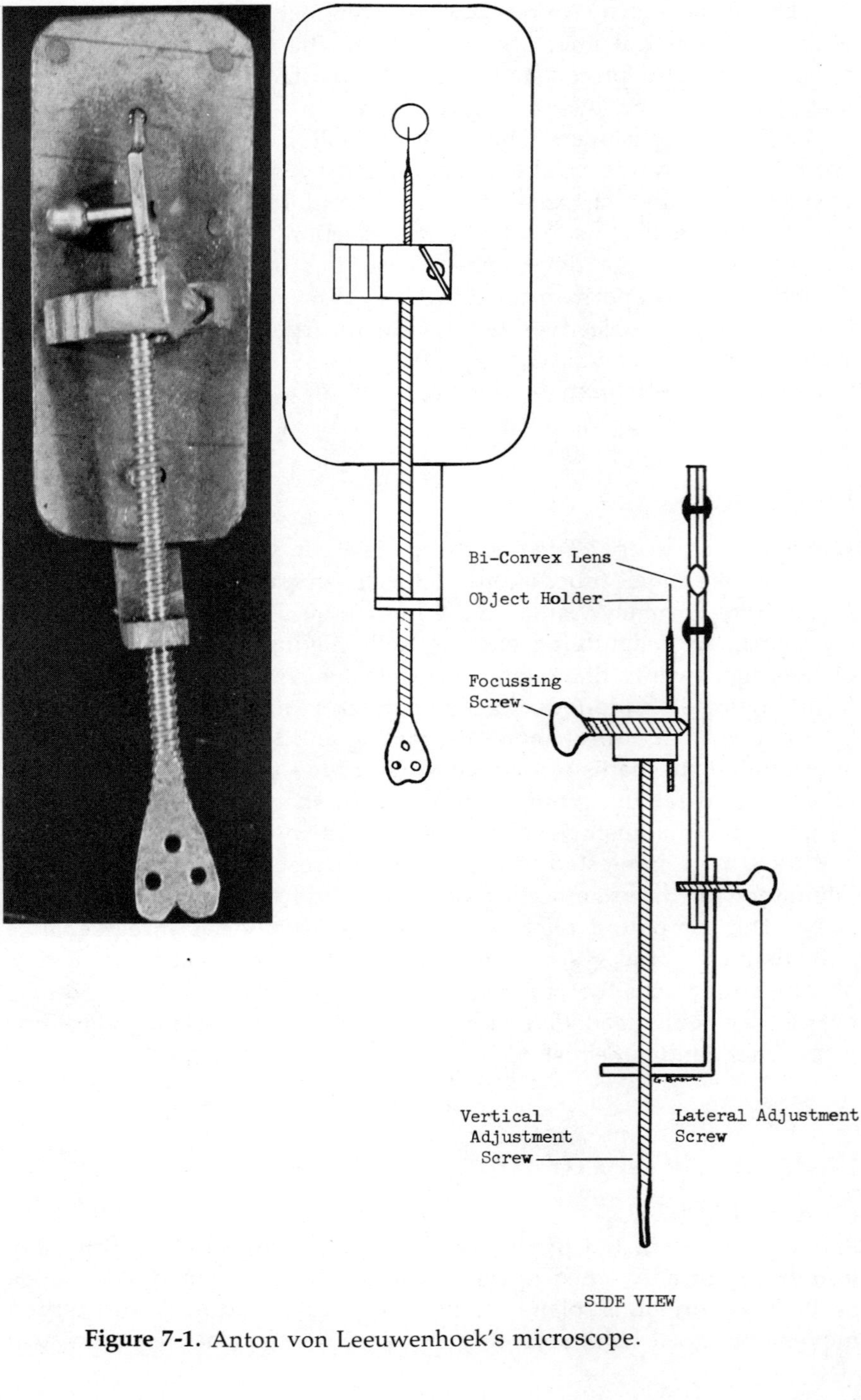

Figure 7-1. Anton von Leeuwenhoek's microscope.

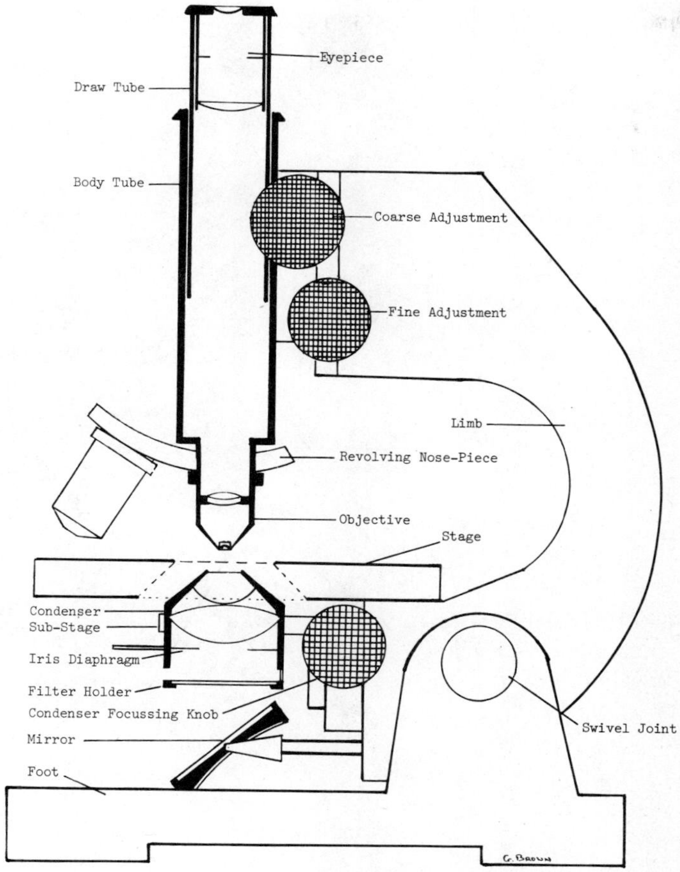

Figure 7-2. Diagram of a compound monocular microscope.

defects as "slipping" and "shake." The optical parts must be of good quality and a large stage is desirable.

The microscope is best used on a heavy, level table or bench, and should not be placed on the slide-out leaf of a desk or table.

THE BASE OR FOOT

There are two types which may be used: (1) the tripod and (2) the modified horseshoe. Both should ensure stability. This is attained in the tripod by the spread of the three feet, which, although not universally used, is mechanically the more correct form and will

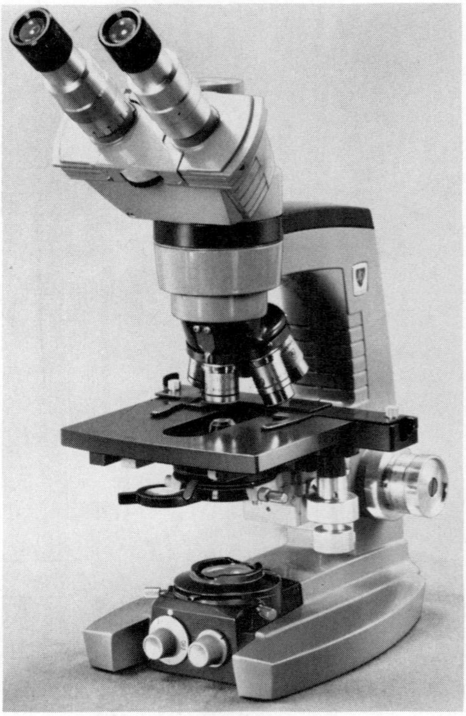

Figure 7-3. The compound binocular microscope. (*Courtesy of American Optical Corp., Buffalo, N.Y.*)

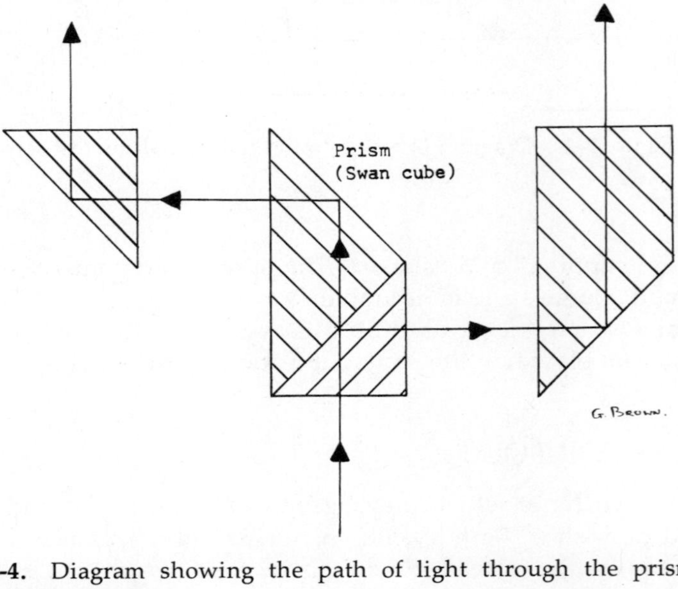

Figure 7-4. Diagram showing the path of light through the prisms of a binocular microscope.

ensure stability even on an uneven surface. The modified horseshoe that is normally used gives stability by dead weight.

THE LIMB

This must be of the optical bench-type and should be of a solid casting to ensure alignment and rigidity.

The limb carries the body tube, the stage, the substage, and the mirror. In some instances it is attached to the base by means of a swivel joint that allows the microscope to be inclined at an angle. On microscopes with an inclined head, the limb and base are either constructed from one solid casting, or the two parts are bolted together through the base. The single casting is best as it is more rigid.

THE BODY TUBE

The body tube is attached to the limb and exists to carry, at opposite ends, the occular (eyepiece) and the objective. The length of the body tube, referred to as the mechanical tube-length, is 160 mm. This is the distance from the top lens (eye lens) of the occular (eyepiece) to the point where the objective is screwed into the revolving nosepiece. The Leitz microscopes have a mechanical tube-length of 170 mm.

The older monocular microscopes were often fitted with a removable draw tube (Fig. 5) which had graduations engraved up the length. By extending the draw tube, the final image could be magnified further,

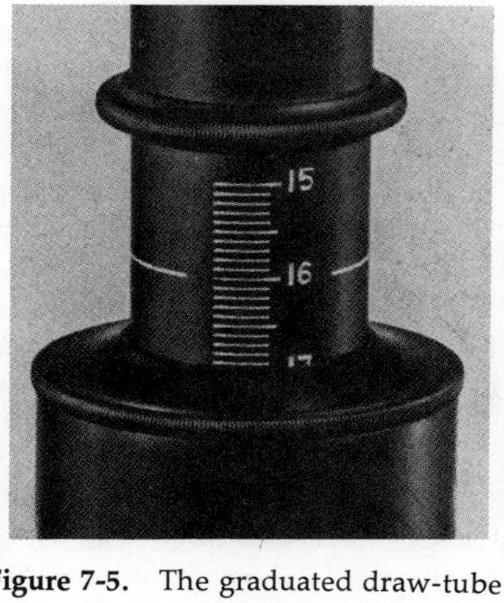

Figure 7-5. The graduated draw-tube.

but its primary purpose was the elimination of the spherical aberration when using cover glasses of incorrect or uneven thickness. Objectives are usually corrected for use with standard number 1 cover glasses, which are 0.13–0.16 mm in thickness. A shorter tube-length is desirable when using low grade cover glasses, which are thicker.

The draw tube should be threaded at its lower end to allow the attachment of accessories for photographic purposes, or the attachment of a very low powered objective to produce a simplified compound microscope.

THE NOSEPIECE

This consists of a circular plate attached to the lower end of the body tube and having a circular aperture corresponding to the lumen of the body tube. To the under surface of this plate is pivoted a similarly curved plate that has from three to five threaded tubulars. The objectives are threaded into these tubulars.

By rotating the lower plate each objective can be brought into the optical axis of the microscope in succession. The objectives should be positioned so that each brings a higher magnifying power into use in series. It is essential that the nosepiece be centered accurately so that the variance in position of the object, when central with the lowest powered objective, is not greater than one half of the radius of the field when viewed with the highest powered objective. This is usually the oil-immersion (2 mm) objective.

THE STAGE

The stage may be either circular or square in shape, and preferably, will have a large flat area. The majority of stages are square. It is absolutely essential that the surface of the stage be flat, smooth, and rigid. All stages should be equipped with either spring clips for holding a slide in position, or a mechanical stage that will allow the operator to move the slide about. A mechanical stage of the built-in type is preferable to the clip-on variety.

To ensure rigidity the stage should be mounted on supports that have been cast solid with the limb, and not attached to the small central projection. However, many microscopes today have stages that may be raised and lowered to focus the object, rather than raising and lowering the body tube, and are therefore attached by slides to give mobility.

Most mechanical stages have two large scales set at right angles to each other, with a small scale facing each of them (Fig. 6). The purpose

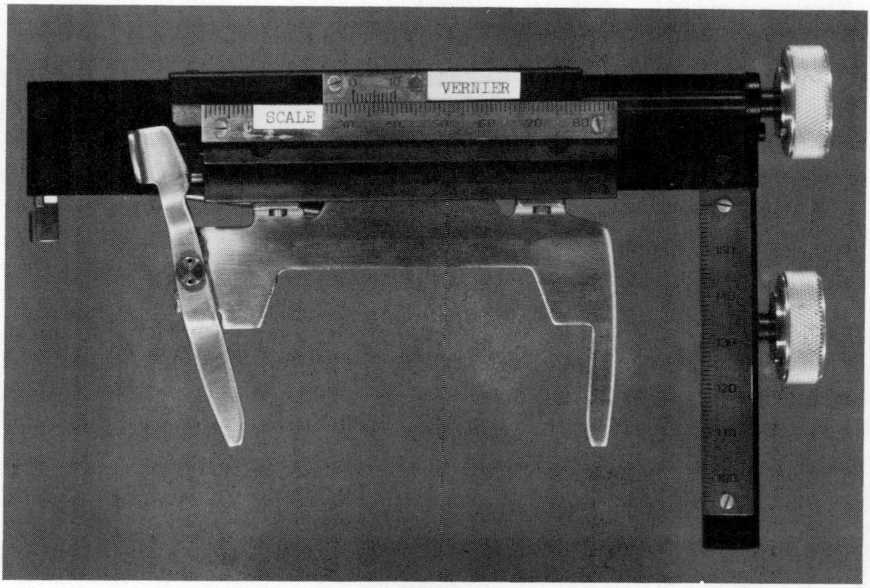

Figure 7-6. The mechanical stage and vernier scale.

of these is to enable the operator to record the position of any desired field on the slide for future reference. The small scale is called a vernier.

The *vernier scale* was introduced by Paul Vernier (1580–1637), who utilized the ability of the human eye to detect a displacement equal to a quarter of the width of a broken line when one part is displaced sideways in respect to the other.

The large scale is graduated in centimeters and subdivided into millimeters, while the vernier scale is nine millimeters in length and divided into ten equal divisions. It can be utilized to read linear measurements smaller than 1 mm.

The centimeter scale and the vernier scale slide opposite to each other, but face to face. The centimeter scale is fixed.

Reading the Vernier

The zero line indicates the whole number on the fixed centimeter scale. When it points between two numbers on the centimeter scale, the lower number is the whole number. Examine the graduations on the vernier scale and determine which division corresponds most exactly to division on the centimeter scale. The number of this graduation line on the vernier scale indicates the decimal figure to be added to the whole number.

To locate a specific field, the readings from both scales are recorded on the slide. It is essential that the readings be identified as horizontal and vertical, and that the slide be placed on the stage in the same position as when the readings were taken, ie, with the label to the left- or right-hand side.

THE SUBSTAGE

The substage is located below the stage, hence its name, and carries the condenser. It may be raised and lowered by means of a rack-and-pinion mechanism.

The substage should be equipped with the means to center the condenser, ie, centering screws, and also some device or mechanism that will allow the entire condenser to be removed easily, or swung completely clear of the optical axis of the microscope when desired.

THE MIRROR

When a microscope is not equipped with built-in illumination, it should be fitted with a double-sided mirror that is mounted in a gimbal and located below the condenser. One side of the mirror should be plane (flat), while the opposite side should be concave (indented). Its function is to direct the light rays from the light source through the optical systems of the microscope (Fig. 7).

The *plane side of the mirror* is always employed in conjunction with a condenser as it reflects parallel rays of light.

When *no condenser* is utilized then the *concave side of the mirror* is employed because it will cause the parallel rays of light to converge to an approximate point of focus at the plane (level) of the surface of the stage. Only low-powered objectives should be used in this instance. The source of light for the concave mirror should be low powered, and the most common source of this is daylight, preferably from a northerly direction.

A *convex mirror is not employed* because this will scatter the parallel rays of light.

THE FOCUSING MECHANISMS

The Coarse Adjustment

Works on a rack-and-pinion movement in which smoothness of action is secured by accurately fitting dovetailed bearings and precise

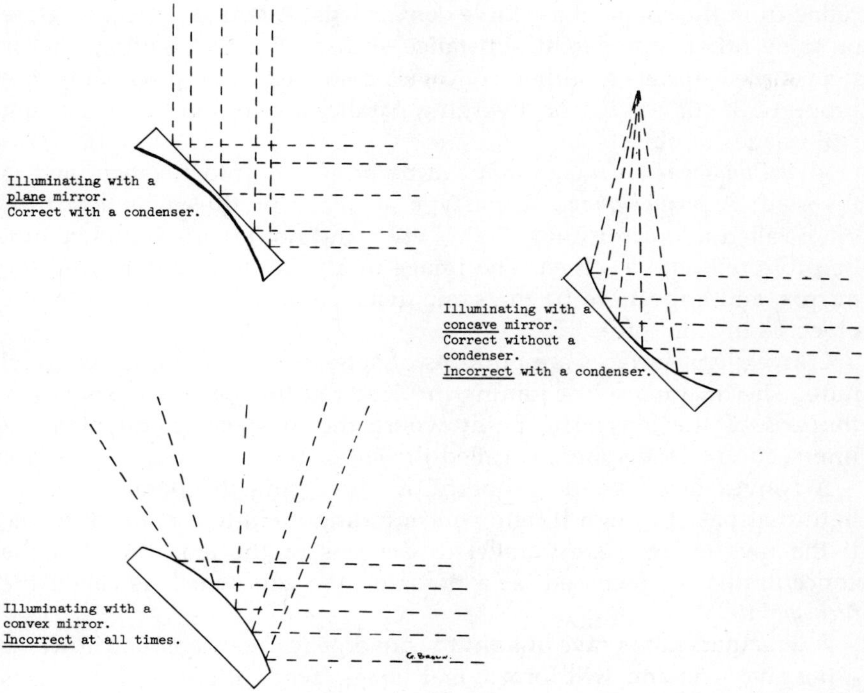

Figure 7-7. Diagram showing the correct way to use the mirror.

correspondence between the teeth of the rack and the leaves of the pinion. Provision is usually made for adjustment of clearance by means of locking screws.

The Fine Adjustment

This should be of the vertical lever type and should not depend upon the direct action of springs. The unequal length of the arms of the lever ensures very delicate movement, and only a small portion of the weight of the body tube (or the stage if this is raised and lowered to secure focus), is transmitted to the thread of the vertical screws actuating the movement.

THE OPTICAL SYSTEMS

The optical systems of the compound microscope consists of three separate series of lenses, each having a specific purpose.

The word "lens" is derived from the Latin word for lentil, and is so called from the shape of a double convex lens. A lens is a piece of glass or some other transparent substance such as fluorite, having one or two curved surfaces, either concave or convex, and possessing the property of converging or diverging parallel rays of light and forming real images of objects.

A *real image* is an image that can be projected onto a screen, and is inverted. A *virtual image* is the type of image produced by a mirror, often called a "mirror image." It is erect and not inverted, and cannot be projected onto a screen. The image in a plane mirror is behind the mirror, and appears to be the same distance behind the mirror as the object is in front of it.

Convex lens surfaces are portions of spheres of approximately equal radii. The imaginary line joining the center of the spheres is known as the *axis* of the lens. The point where the axis meets the plane of intersection of the sphere is called the *pole*.

A convex lens has the property of converging the parallel rays of light that pass through it, and concentrating them to a point of focus. If the rays of light are parallel to the axis of the lens they will be concentrated, or focussed, at a point on the axis which is called the *focal point*.

A lens that causes rays of light to converge (convex lens) is known as a positive lens and will form a real image, while the lens that causes rays of light to diverge or scatter (concave lens) is known as a negative lens and it will not form a real image (Fig. 8).

All lenses that have a greater thickness in the middle than at the periphery are positive lenses, while the opposite is true of the negative lenses. By employing various combinations of positive and negative lenses many optical faults may be corrected (Fig. 9).

Common Defects In Lenses

The lens systems in the microscope must not only produce a magnified image, but also ensure that this image is sharp and well defined. Lenses have certain faults inherent to them (Fig. 10) because of (1) their shape and (2) because white light is composed of a series of vibrations of differing wavelength, each producing the effect of a single color in the human eye. These are the colors of the primary spectrum which may be seen in a rainbow: they are red, orange, yellow, green, blue, indigo, and violet.

Spherical Aberration. This defect in a lens is due entirely to its shape. When the central and peripheral rays of light are parallel to the axis and passed through a lens they are refracted at slightly differing degrees to each other, due both to the curved surface and the varying

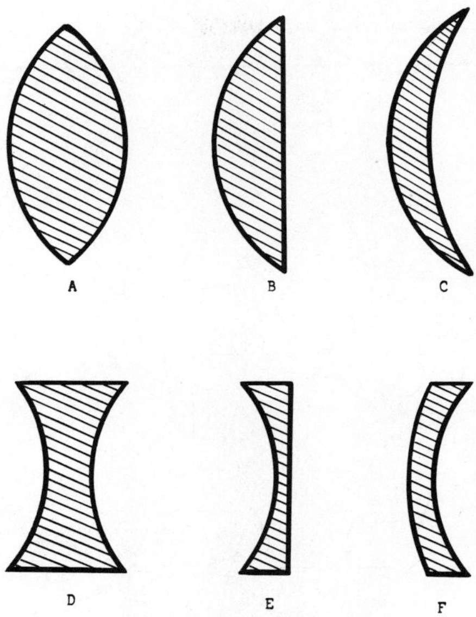

Figure 7-8. Diagram of positive and negative lenses. A, B, and C: Positive lenses. D, E, and F: Negative lenses.

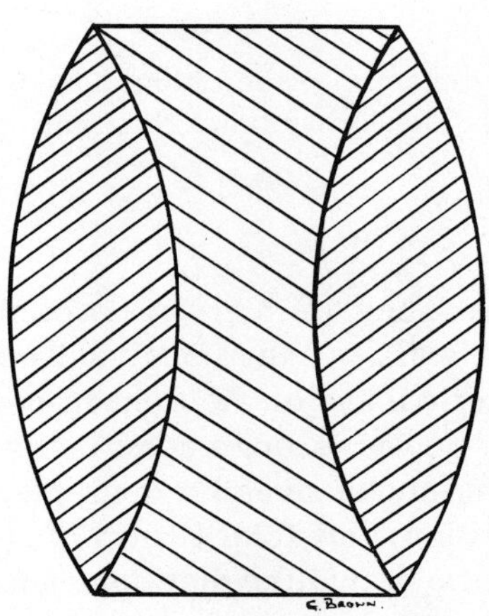

Figure 7-9. Diagram showing a typical arrangement of positive and negative lenses.

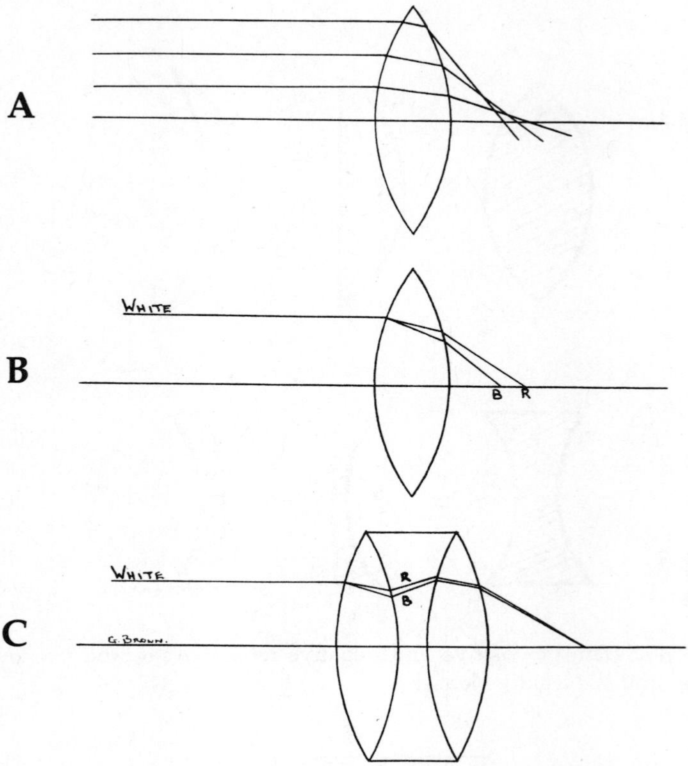

Figure 7-10. Diagram illustrating aberrations. A: Spherical aberration. B: Chromatic aberration. C: The correction of chromatic aberration.

thicknesses of the lens. They are therefore brought to focus at slightly different points on the axis, and the image will appear to be fuzzy and ill-defined in the outer fringes of the field in view. Spherical aberration can be corrected to some degree by using a combination of a powerful positive lens and a negative lens made of glass having a greater relative aberration, but total correction is extremely difficult. The intelligent use of the draw tube may also partially correct spherical aberration.

Chromatic Aberration. When white light is passed from a rare medium (air) through a dense medium (glass) it cannot vibrate as easily in the dense medium. The spectral colors with the shorter wavelengths, such as blue (wavelength 0.45μ), will be affected to a greater degree than those with longer wavelengths, such as red (wavelength

0.7μ). White light entering a lens is refracted to differing degrees, and on emerging forms a different point of focus for each of the component colors. Blue comes to a point of focus closer to the lens than does red. This gives rise to a colored fringe or halo around the edges of the image.

Chromatic aberration can be corrected by employing different types of glass, each possessing different optical properties, and by combining a positive lens with a negative lens, thus reducing the aberration to within useful and acceptable limits. The negative lens should be made of glass possessing a greater chromatic aberration than that of the positive lens, but have the same refractive index. Such a lens will correct the chromatic aberration of the positive lens while only partially reducing its magnifying power.

Most of the optics in general microscopy are corrected to two colors of the spectrum (red and blue) and are known as *achromatic lenses*.

Lenses that have been corrected to three colors of the spectrum are used for critical work, and are known as *apochromatic lenses*. If apochromatic objectives are employed then a *compensating occular* is required. In the apochromatic objective the internal positive or convex lenses are made of *fluorite* and the negative or concave lenses are made of *barium flint*. These lenses are usually reserved for the high-power or oil-immersion objectives. Because they are very expensive *semi-apochromatic* lenses are often used instead.

Numerical Aperture and Resolving Power

The numerical aperture (N.A.) and the resolving power of a lens bear a direct relationship to each other. Resolving power is the ability of a lens to define detail, and it is measured by the number of lines to the inch, or by the distance apart of two lines or dots, that can be visually separated from each other. It follows therefore, that a lens which will resolve 30,000 lines to the inch has a greater resolving power than one defining only 20,000 lines to the inch. It can also be seen that the definition of detail is of far more importance than great magnification. For example, if an object is magnified fifty times and appears as a single line, and further magnification still shows it as a single line when in fact it is three separate lines set closely together, the definition or resolving power of that lens is poor. Actual magnification is, within limits, of less value than clear definition and high resolving power, for the knowledge of the detailed structure of objects examined is dependent upon these properties. Continued magnification which reveals no further detail is termed *empty magnification*.

Resolution is restricted by two factors: (1) the wavelength of the light employed and (2) the numerical aperture of the lens. It may be defined as follows:

$$\text{Resolution} = \frac{1.2 \times \text{Wavelength}}{2 \times \text{Numerical Aperture}}$$

The numerical aperture of an objective is dependent upon the cone of light entering the front lens of the objective. The wider the cone of light the higher the numerical aperture.

Numerical aperture may be defined as *half of the diameter of the lens over the distance from the periphery of the lens to the object, times the refractive index of the medium between the lens and the object* (Fig. 11). This may be expressed as N.A. = N sin$U$, where N is the refractive index of the medium between the lens and the objective (the refractive index of air is 1.0 and the refractive index of immersion oil is 1.5, which is the same as glass), and sin$U$ is the sine of one-half the angle of aperture. Since the sine of an angle is opposite over hypotenuse, sin$U$ may be expressed as O/H. Therefore, N.A. = $N \times O/H$.

The resolving power of the objective is directly proportional to the numerical aperture. The higher the numerical aperture the greater number of lines are resolved to the inch. As a rough guide, the following will hold true:

N.A. 0.25 = 25,000 lines resolved to the inch.

N.A. 0.95 = 95,000 lines resolved to the inch.

However, a very high numerical aperture does have some disadvantages. It can (1) reduce the depth of focus, that is, the ability to focus at more than one level of an object at the same time; or (2) it reduces the flatness of the field, so that when the center is in focus the edges are out of focus and vice versa.

The ideal visual field would be large and flat, where objects at the periphery would be in as sharp a focus as those in the center of the field. This is however an optical impossibility, and the field is always slightly spherical in shape. Some objectives do give a larger area that is in common focus and are referred to as flat-field or planachromatic objectives. In theory this does cause a slight sacrifice of other qualities, but is often more desirable.

It can be seen that depth of focus and flatness of field are very important, and further magnification should, in theory, be obtained by changing to a higher-powered eyepiece. However, as a general rule, changing to a higher-powered objective will give both increased resolution and greater magnification which is to be preferred.

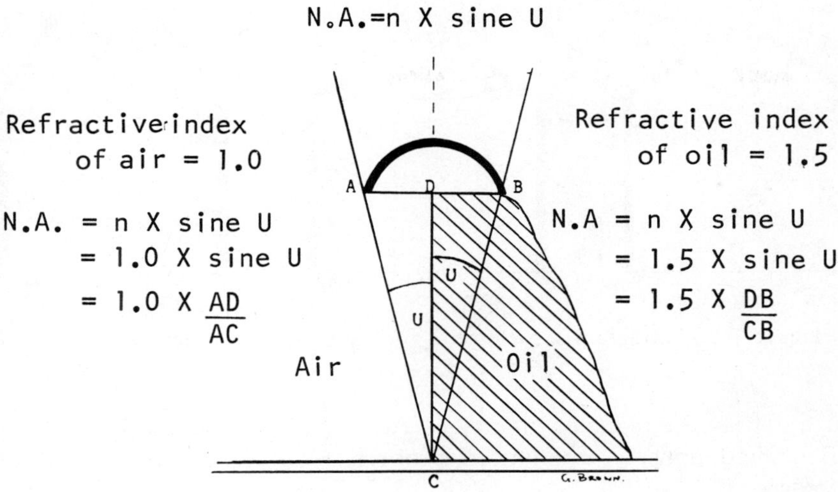

Figure 7-11. Diagram illustrating how the numerical aperture is calculated.

Optical Components

As stated previously the optical system of the compound microscope consists of a series of three lens systems, each having a very specific purpose. They are:

1. The condenser which brings the parallel rays of light to a point of focus in the plane of the object;
2. the objective which magnifies the object and forms a real image in the upper part of the body tube; and
3. the occular which further magnifies the image formed by the objective.

THE CONDENSER

The condenser (Fig. 12) is mounted in the substage directly beneath the stage of the microscope. The type in general use for routine microscopy is the Abbé condenser, designed by Professor Ernst Abbé, a German Physicist, in 1872. This two-lens condenser consists of a planoconvex lens mounted immediately above a biconvex lens. By means of these lenses the parallel rays of light reflected by the *plane mirror*, or from the built-in illumination system, are collected and brought into a cone of large aperture, which can then be focussed

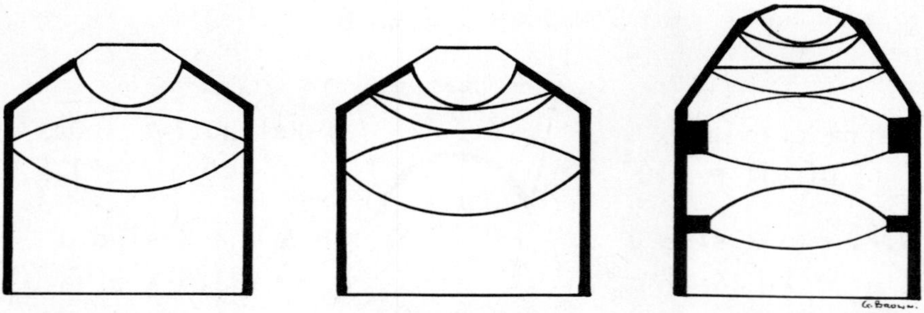

Figure 7-12. Diagram showing the general construction of condensers.

accurately in the plane of the object. Although this is not a particularly efficient condenser, when used properly it is adequate for routine microscopy.

The Abbé condenser should not be employed in conjunction with fluorite or apochromatic objectives. A three-lens aplanatic condenser or the more highly corrected achromatic condenser will give a sharp image and good resolution with these objectives. It is good practice to have the numerical aperture of the condenser matching that of the objective being used, but not always feasible.

Directly below the lenses there should be an *iris diaphragm*, and below this a holder of the swing-out type to carry filters. There is sometimes an additional auxiliary lens located below this filter holder, also in a swing out holder.

When examining unstained specimens a haziness may be noticed around the image. This is due to the counteracting effects of parallel and peripheral rays of light which give respectively, a dark image on a light ground, and a light image on a dark ground. This is easily eliminated by closing the iris diaphragm slightly to block the peripheral rays of light. Close the diaphragm slowly until the image is clearly visible.

This phenomenon is not so noticeable with stained preparations. When examining stained preparations the diaphragm should be so adjusted as to limit the angle of the cone of light passing through the object so that it will just fill the front lens of the objective. Light that passes through the object but does not enter the lens is unnecessary and should be eliminated by the correct use of the iris diaphragm.

If it should become necessary or desirable to reduce the intensity of the illumination, this may be achieved by inserting light-absorbing filters into the filter holder, or by using a variable resistance on the light source. *Under no circumstances* should the diaphragm be closed down, or the condenser lowered, to achieve reduced intensity of light.

To obtain optimum uniformity of illumination the condenser must be properly centered and set for *critical* or *Köhler* illumination. It is advisable to have the microscope *and* its light source in a fixed, stable position, as the slightest movement of either will disrupt the setting.

The following procedure will give a properly centered condenser and critical or Köhler illumination:

1. If the microscope is not equipped with built-in illumination, position the lamp above twelve inches in front of the microscope and adjust the mirror (plane side) so that it directs the light upwards into the condenser. *Remove the filters*.
2. Open the iris diaphragm of the substage condenser.
3. With the 10× objective in position, adjust the mirror, and focus on a stained preparation.
4. a. *Critical illumination*: Close the diaphragm of the lamp and focus the *condenser* until a sharp image of the diaphragm is seen superimposed on the slide. Center this image (Fig. 13). If

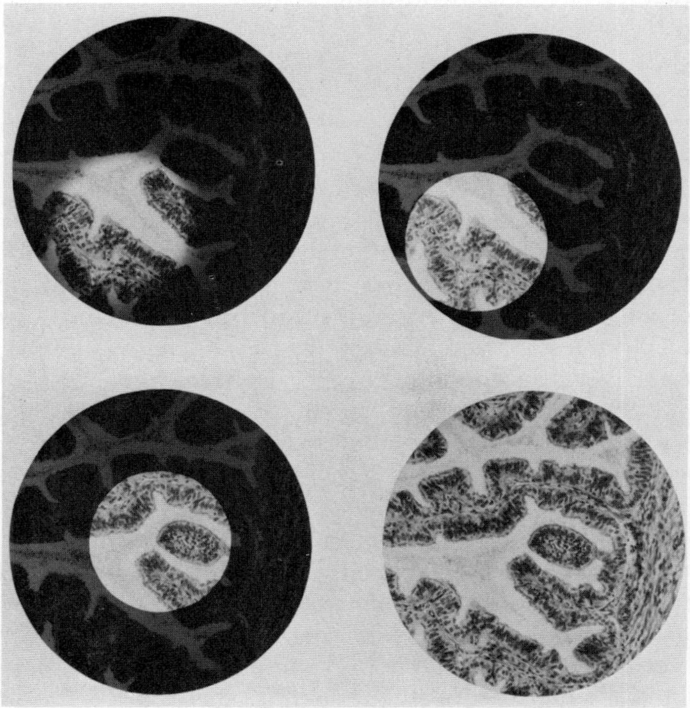

Figure 7-13. Illustration showing the focussing and centering of the iris diaphragm. (*From* Microscopy From The Very Beginning. *Courtesy of Carl Zeiss Inc., Oberkochen, West Germany.*)

the lamp has no diaphragm, focus the condenser on an ink spot made on the light bulb or the front lens of the lamp, or the tip of a pencil held against the front of the lamp. A frosted white bulb is best.

b. *Köhler illumination*: Close the diaphragm of the lamp until the field is just filled with light. Focus the condenser as above. Now focus the *light source* so that the image of the filament is sharply defined at the level of the substage diaphragm. Use a mirror to check this. With built-in illumination the condenser must be focussed to produce this image.

5. Open the diaphragm of the lamp.
6. Remove an occular and close the iris diaphragm of the substage condenser. By means of the centering screws, if present, adjust the circle of light until it is in the center of the field.
7. Open the iris diaphragm until two-thirds of the area of the back lens of the objective is evenly filled with light. Check that it is central. Replace the occular.
8. Open the iris diaphragm until the field is just filled evenly with light.

The microscope is now set with either critical or Köhler illumination and is ready for use (Fig. 14).

THE OBJECTIVES

The majority of modern microscopes are fitted with either triple or quadruple nosepieces, and carry the corresponding number of objectives. These objectives are used to form a real, enlarged, inverted image of the object (specimen) in the upper part of the body tube.

Three objectives are necessary, having focal lengths of 16, 4, and 2 mm, respectively, and giving primary magnifications of 10×, 40× or 45×, and 90× or 100×. The fourth objective for the quadruple nosepiece is usually a low-powered scanning lens having a magnifying power varying from 2.5× to 4.5×. Magnifying power is measured in diameters.

The highest-powered objectives, 90× or more, require the use of an immersion oil that has the same refractive index as glass (Fig. 15).

The focal length of the objective should not be confused with the working distance, ie, the distance from the front lens of the objective to the specimen. This is relative to the numerical aperture. The higher the numerical aperture of the objective the shorter the working distance.

Objectives are manufactured in three qualities. They are achromatic, fluorite or semi-apochromatic, and apochromatic (Fig. 16).

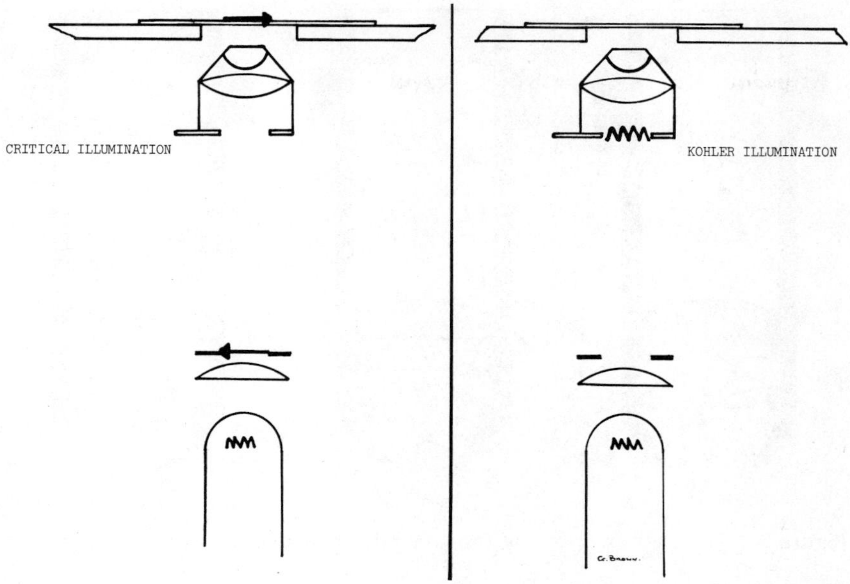

Figure 7-14. Diagram illustrating the difference between critical and Köhler illumination.

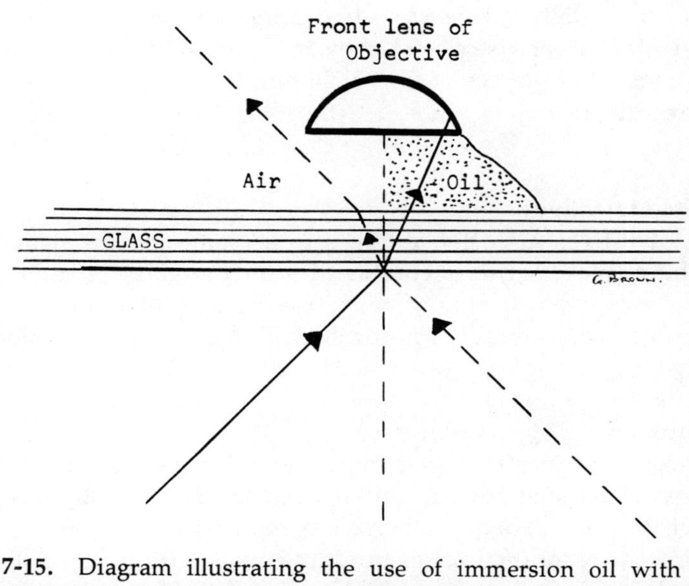

Figure 7-15. Diagram illustrating the use of immersion oil with a high-powered objective. Notice that the left-hand side is without oil and that the light is refracted away from the front lens of the objective.

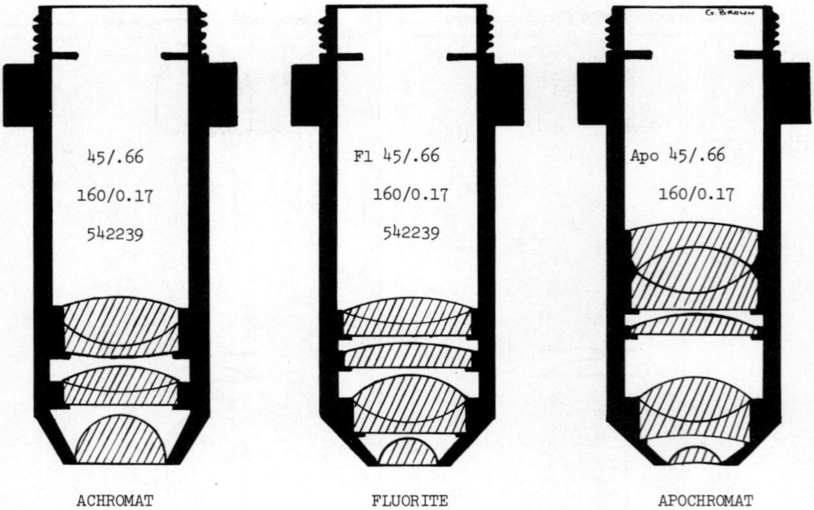

Figure 7-16. Diagram showing the general construction of the 45× objective.

Achromatic Objectives

This objective is suitable for most general microscopic work, but should not be employed for high-quality photography. Chromatic aberration is usually corrected to two colors and spherical aberration for one. Unless otherwise stated, they are corrected for a tube length of 160 mm and cover glasses of 0.13–0.16 mm in thickness, the standard No. 1 coverglass.

Fluorite Objectives

These objectives are often referred to as semi-apochromatic objectives. The crystal *fluorite* is combined with the glass, a combination that, because of its dissimilar refractive index and dispersion, produces an image of a quality approaching that of the apochromats.

Apochromatic Objectives

Apochromatic objectives are superior to either achromatic or fluorite objectives. Chromatic aberration has been corrected to three colors of the spectrum and spherical aberration for two colors, which means that practically all of the images produced by the different colors of the spectrum lie in the same plane and are all equally sharp. The result is a higher efficiency for apochromats.

Engravings on Objectives

Objectives are engraved with several numbers that indicate far more than the initial magnification. These may vary slightly with the country of origin and the manufacturer, or even with the age of the microscope. Let us look at some examples:

4 mm 0.65

45×

This means the focal length is 4 mm, the N.A. is 0.65 (resolving 65,000 lines to the inch), and the initial magnification is 45 times or diameters.

HOM 0.1 mm–1.8 mm-N.A.1.25–95×

542239

This means Homogenous Immersion Oil, working distance is 0.1 mm, the focal length is 1.8 mm, the N.A. is 1.25, and the initial magnification is 95×. The number below this is the serial number of the objective.

A-0.65

PhA 30:1

This means that the N.A. is 0.65, it is a phase-contrast objective for use with the A diaphragm of the phase-contrast condenser, and the initial magnification is 30×.

Fl Oil 95/1.32

This means that it is a fluorite objective for use with immersion oil, has an initial magnification of 95×, and that the N.A. is 1.32.

Plan 40/0.65

160/0.17

This means that the objective is a planachromat, flat-field achromat, the initial magnification is 40×, the N.A. is 0.65, and that it is corrected for a tube length of 160 mm and cover glasses of 0.17 mm thick. Some of the more frequently found engravings are:

PLAN = planachromat, ie, flat-field achromat.
NEOFLUAR = high-aperture objective with improved color rendition.
FL = fluorite objective.
APO = apochromatic objective.

PLANAPO = planapochromatic, ie, flat-field apochromat.
POL = Strain-free objective for polarized-light microscopy.
PH = phase-contrast objective. Usually has either a letter or a number following the initials designating which diaphragm of the phase-contrast condenser it should be used with.

THE OCCULARS

The purpose of the occular (Fig. 17) is to magnify the image produced by the objective, and transmit it to the eye. The most commonly used occular is of the *Huygenian* type consisting of two planoconvex lenses of differing size. The front, or field lens, has a focal length of two to three times that of the eye lens. A diaphragm is situated inside the eyepiece at the focal plane of the eye lens. The Huygenian eyepiece is named after its inventor, Christian Huygens, a Dutch scientist of the seventeenth century.

The *compensating* eyepiece or a *periplanatic* eyepiece should be used when either apochromatic or fluorite objectives are employed. These are over compensated to rectify the undercorrected lenses of the objectives.

Occulars usually magnify 5×, 6×, 10×, and 12×.

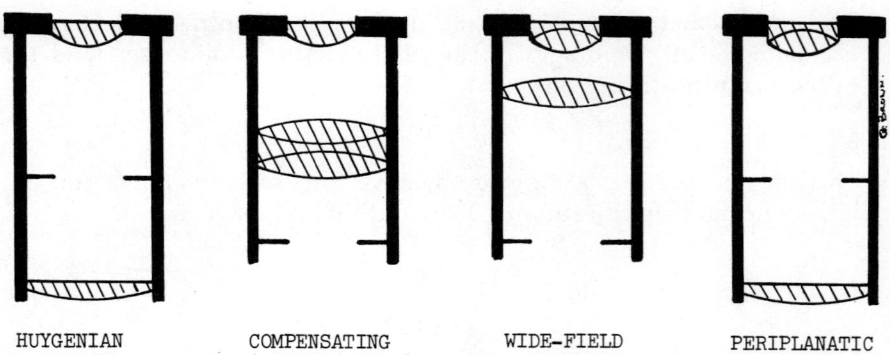

Figure 7-17. Diagram showing the general construction of occulars.

MAGNIFICATION

Magnification is the process of increasing the apparent size of an object, as with a lens. In microscopy this increase in size is measured in diameters, and with certain known facts magnifying power can be calculated.

At the normal tube-length of 160 mm, the total magnifying power is the product of the magnifying power of the objective and the eyepiece. For example, the objective is 40× and the eyepiece is 10×. Thus we have

$$40 \times 10 = 400\times$$

If only the focal length of the objective is known, as opposed to its magnifying power, plus the magnifying power of the occular, then the total magnification is:

$$\frac{\text{Working tube-length}}{\text{Focal length of objective}} \times \text{Magnification of eyepiece}$$

or

$$\frac{160}{4} \times 10 = 400\times$$

If the microscope is fitted with a draw tube that has been extended, the magnification will be increased, and is calculated as follows:

$$\begin{matrix}\text{Magnification} \\ \text{of objective}\end{matrix} \times \begin{matrix}\text{Magnification of} \\ \text{the eyepiece}\end{matrix} \times \frac{\text{Working tube-length}}{\text{Normal tube-length}}$$

or

$$\frac{40 \times 10 \times 180}{160} = 450\times$$

Micrometry

Micrometry uses the micron (abbreviated μ) as a linear unit of measurement. It is equal to 0.001 mm (1/1000 mm or 1/25,000 inch).

The occular micrometer is used to make these measurements. An occular micrometer consists of a glass disc upon which is engraved a graduated scale, usually consisting of 100 divisions that may be subdivided into groups of 5, 10, and 50. These divisions have no particular linear value, and must be standardized against a stage micrometer of known value. As the occular micrometer is used to take all measurements, it must be standardized with each of the objectives in turn, and a record kept as to its value with each objective.

The stage micrometer (Fig. 18) is a 3 × 1 inch slide upon which is engraved a scale, usually 2 mm in length. This scale is graduated in small divisions, each being equal to 0.01 mm. (1/100 mm or 10μ). The scale is marked with a larger division marker at each tenth division or 0.1 mm (1/10 mm or 100μ) (Fig. 19).

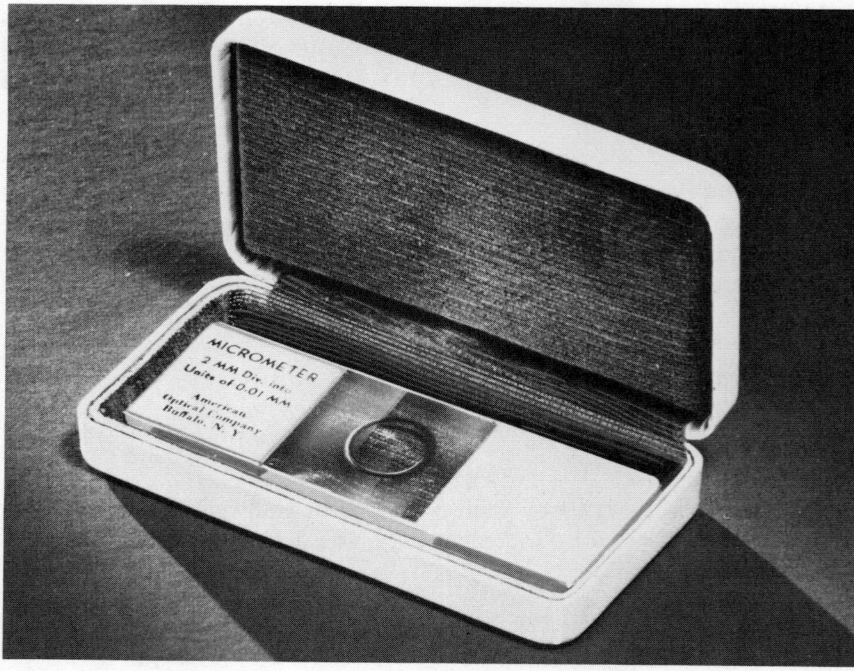

Figure 7-18. The stage micrometer. (*Courtesy of American Optical Corp., Buffalo, N.Y.*)

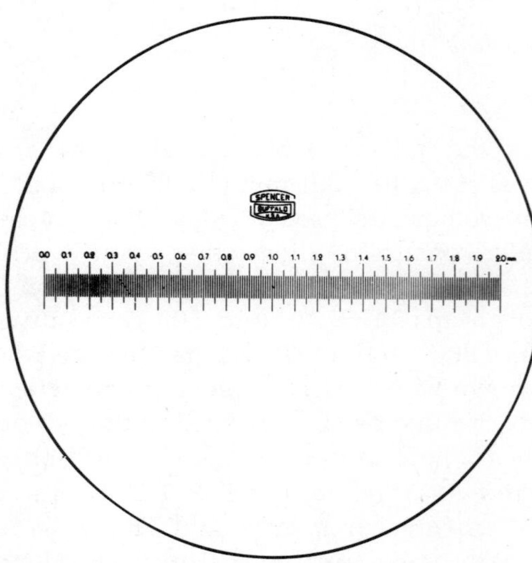

Figure 7-19. A magnified view of the engraving of the stage micrometer. (*Courtesy of American Optical Corp., Buffalo, N.Y.*)

STANDARDIZATION

The older monocular microscopes with a draw tube must be adjusted so that the tube length is exactly 160 mm. Modern microscopes have a standard tube-length of 160 mm and no adjustment is necessary.

Place the occular micrometer in the eyepiece, resting on the diaphragm, with the engraved side facing down. Focus on the stage micrometer. The occular divisions will be seen superimposed over the graduations of the stage micrometer. Move the stage micrometer until the zero mark corresponds to the zero mark on the occular micrometer, and determine the number of occular divisions that correspond to a definite number of stage divisions. For this example we will say that 50 occular divisions are equal to 9 stage divisions.

Calculation

Given: 1 stage division is equal to 0.01 mm. (10μ).

Known: 50 occular divisions equal 9 stage divisions (0.09 mm); therefore,

$$1 \text{ occular division} = \frac{0.09}{50} = 0.0018 \text{ mm} = 1.8\mu$$

The occular micrometer is now standardized and the stage micrometer is removed and replaced with the specimen to be examined and measured.

Example of Measuring

Six divisions on the occular scale cover the diameter of the cell being measured. Therefore, since

$$1 \text{ occular division} = 1.8\mu$$

then

$$6 \text{ occular divisions} = 6 \times 1.8 = 10.8$$

Therefore, the diameter of the cell is 10.8μ.

Note. If you have an occular micrometer but do not have a stage micrometer, a hemacytometer may be employed to standardize the occular micrometer. Each of the small squares engraved in the central portion of the hemacytometer is 1/20 mm (50μ) square. To calculate the value of one occular division, determine how many small squares are covered by the entire occular scale and multiply by 50. This will give the micron value of the full occular scale. Now divide by the number of graduations on the occular scale to obtain the micron value of one division.

For example, 100 occular divisions covers 15 small squares. Therefore,

$$100 \text{ occular divisions} = 15 \times 50 = 750\mu.$$

Therefore,

$$1 \text{ occular division} = \tfrac{750}{100} = 7.5\mu.$$

Proceed as before to measure the object.

Care of the Microscope

DO keep the microscope covered when not in use, or store in a dust-free box.

DO clean the lens surfaces daily (Fig. 20). Clean with distilled water (breathe on the lens surface) and lens paper or well-laundered (fluff-free) cotton sheeting or silk. The pieces of polystrene foam (styrofoam) used for packing are excellent for cleaning the front lenses of objectives. Break a piece in half. Press the freshly fractured surface lightly against the lens and rotate it coaxially. The lens will be cleaned to the recess of its mount. Avoid using xylol or other solvents when doing this or the styrofoam will dissolve.

DO remove slides from the stage when not in use.

DO remove immersion oil immediately after use. If a solvent is required use *very little* xylene on a lens paper or preferably ether. Remove this from the lens *immediately*.

DO focus upwards—NEVER downwards.

DO ensure that the condenser is properly centered.

DO support the microscope properly when carrying it. CRADLE IT.

DON'T touch the lens surfaces with fingers (Fig. 21).

DON'T clean the lens surfaces with anything else but lens paper or thoroughly laundered cotton or silk. Kimwipes and Kleenex are a very effective fine sandpaper on coated lenses.

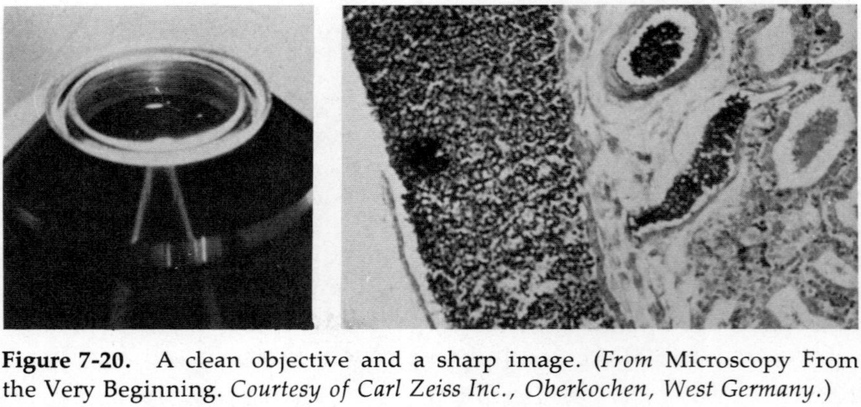

Figure 7-20. A clean objective and a sharp image. (*From* Microscopy From the Very Beginning. *Courtesy of Carl Zeiss Inc., Oberkochen, West Germany.*)

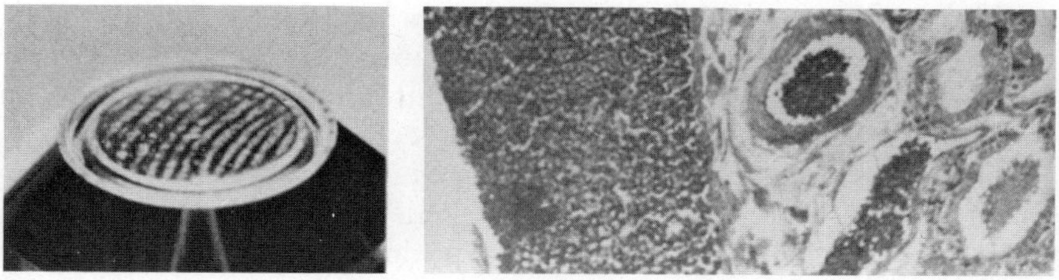

Figure 7-21. A dirty objective and a fuzzy image. (*From* Microscopy From the Very Beginning. *Courtesy of Carl Zeiss Inc., Oberkochen, West Germany.*)

DON'T dismantle the objectives. The centering may be ruined.

DON'T use a concave mirror with the condenser.

DON'T use a higher-powered objective than necessary.

DON'T close the diaphragm or lower the condenser to reduce the brightness of the illumination. Use a filter or a variable resistance transformer.

DON'T leave a high-powered objective in the optical axis when not in use. Swing the scanning lens into place.

DON'T clean objectives with a lot of solvent (xylene). It may dissolve the cement holding the lenses in place.

DON'T MEDDLE.

The Polarizing Microscope

Normal light rays may be said to be composed of waves of energy vibrating in all planes. Generally speaking this vibration will be in any direction at right angles to the direction of transmission.

Polarization is the process of excluding all rays except those vibrating in a single plane, and is accomplished by the use of *Nicol prisms*. The Nicol prism was devised just over 100 years ago, and is composed of a crystal of transparent calcite (Iceland Spar), cut into a rhomboid and bisected. The cut surfaces are polished and then cemented together with Canada Balsam. Light rays entering the prism from below are, for the most part, refracted by the balsam. Only the rays that penetrate the balsam and emerge at the upper surface are those vibrating in a single plane.

In the polarizing microscope, one prism is fitted below the substage condenser (the polarizer) and a second prism is located above the specimen, usually in the occular (the analyzer). They may be so arranged that the plane of light emerging from the analyzer is at right angles to the plane of light emerging from the polarizer. Thus when the two Nicol prisms are crossed in the path of light the field is dark.

An effective and inexpensive substitute for Nicol prisms is a substance called "Polaroid." It is employed in the same way as the Nicol prisms, and is crossed by rotating the analyzer.

The polarizing microscope is used in histopathology and chemical pathology in the identification of certain doubly refractile substances with specific characteristics, one of the most important of these being cholesterol. Substances with a single index of refraction (*isotropic*) do not interfere with the polarized light and are invisible on the dark field. Crystalline substances, other than iso-axial crystals, are doubly refractile (*anisotropic*), and when introduced between crossed Nicol prisms or Polaroids break the polarization and are visible as brightly illuminated bodies on the dark field. For example, cholesterol crystals are seen as bright tetrodlike spherical bodies with very distinctive maltese-cross markings.

The Dark-Ground Condenser

For any object to be examined, either microscopically or macroscopically, it must be visible. Visibility depends upon the object being in contrast to its surroundings and not blending into the background. This is why we employ a multitude of stains to color our sections, thus enabling us to optically differentiate the various cell and tissue components from each other by contrasting colors.

Most unstained objects, when examined microscopically, are naturally transparant, but in general they reflect or scatter light rays. If oblique light is thrown on them, and that light does not enter the objective, they will be seen as luminous objects on a dark background.

The dark-ground condenser (Fig. 22) is a paraboloid immersion substage condenser of high aperture. The central rays of light are blocked out by means of an opaque stop, while the peripheral rays are reflected from the sides of the condenser and refracted by the object being viewed, which is then seen as brightly luminous against a dark ground. The Abbé condenser may be used for dark ground examination of specimens by the insertion of an opaque stop in the filter holder, but only with low-powered objectives. For work with high-powered objectives a proper dark-ground condenser must be employed.

High-power objectives have a high N.A. which must be reduced to at least 0.9. This is achieved by inserting a funnel stop into the objective. The low-power objectives do not require this.

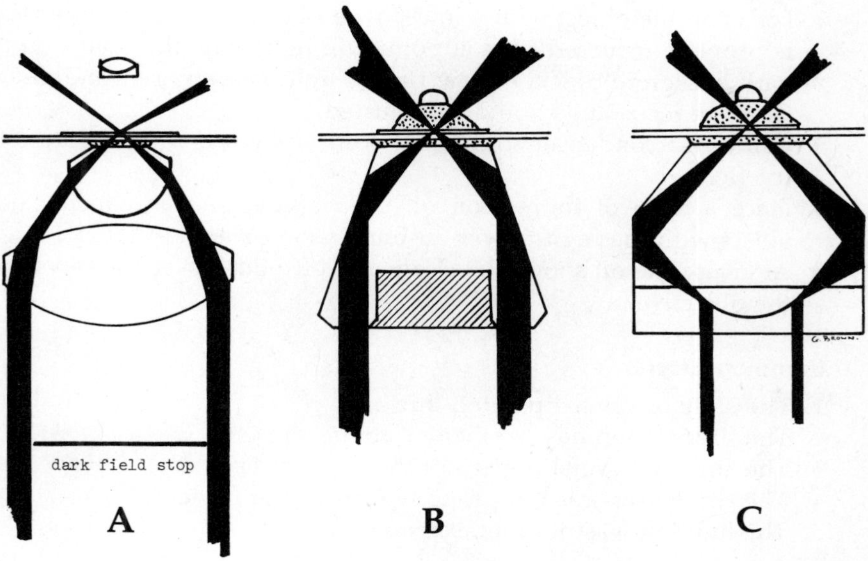

Figure 7-22. Diagram showing the different types of dark-ground condensers. A. Abbe Condenser with a dark field stop, B. Paraboloid Condenser, C. Cardinoid Condenser.

To obtain the best results a powerful illuminant must be used. A tungsten Pointolite arc lamp is probably the best, although any modern high-intensity lamp will give very acceptable results. The light is directed to the condenser with the plane side of the mirror and the rays should be parallel. It is also essential that the condenser is accurately centered. Adjustments may have to be made with different objectives as it is possible that they are not par-central.

DARK-GROUND MICROSCOPY

1. Make thin preparations on thoroughly clean, extra-thin slides and coverslips, ensuring that there are no bubbles present.
2. Focus the image of the light source on the plane side of the mirror and direct the light up through the condenser so that it is evenly distributed.
3. Rack the condenser down and place a drop of immersion oil on the top lens. Place another drop of oil on the bottom of the slide and rack the condenser back up until the two drops of oil meet. Do not form bubbles.

4. Focus on the object with a low-power objective. If the condenser is properly focussed a small point will illuminate the object on a dark background. If a hollow ring of light is seen, the condenser is not in focus and should be adjusted.
5. Center the condenser so that the point of light is in the center of the field.
6. Place a drop of immersion oil on the coverslip and focus the object with the high-power oil-immersion objective.
7. After use the oil should be cleaned of off both the condenser and the objective.

Common Errors

1. The slide or coverslip is too thick.
2. The preparation has too many bubbles present.
3. The slide or coverslip was not thoroughly clean.
4. The condenser was not properly focussed or centered.
5. The lighting was not intense enough.

Definitions

Chromatic Aberration: The inability to bring a source of white light to focus.

Spherical Aberration: The inability to bring all rays to a point of common focus.

Optical Tube-Length: Distance from the upper focal plane of the objective to the lower focal plane of the eyepiece.

Mechanical Tube-Length: Distance from the eye lens of the eyepiece to the point where the objective screws into the nosepiece, usually 160 mm.

Magnification: The process of increasing the apparent size of an object, as with a lens.

(1) Magnifying power of the eyepiece × the magnifying power of the objective.

(2) $$\frac{\text{Mechanical tube-length} \times \text{eyepiece}}{\text{Focal length of objective}}$$

Empty Magnification: Magnification that does not reveal any more detail.

Focal Length: Distance from the object to a point that is approximately midway between the component lenses of the objective. Usually stated in mm.

Working Distance: Distance from the front lens of the objective to the object.

Depth of Focus: The ability to focus at more than one level. This varies inversely with the N.A.

Defining Power: The capacity to render the outline of an object distinct. This varies directly with the N.A.

Resolving Power: The ability to show as separate and distinct two points that are extremely close together.

Numerical Aperture (N.A.): Measured as half of the diameter of the lens over the distance from the periphery of the lens to the center of the object. It is expressed as N.A. = $N \sin U$, where N = the refractive index of the medium between the object and the lens (air = 1.0 and immersion oil = 1.5). Since the sine of an angle is the opposite over the hypotenuse, the equation may be expressed as

$$\text{N.A.} = N \times O/H$$

The resolving power depends largely upon the N.A. The higher the N.A., the higher the resolving power. For example:
N.A. 0.25 = 25,000 lines per inch resolved.
N.A. 0.45 = 45,000 lines per inch resolved.

BIBLIOGRAPHY

Leitz (T.M.) Tech. Information Bull. Vol. XIV (No. 1) April 1976.

Mollring FK: *Microscopy from the Very Beginning*. Carl Zeiss, Oberkochen, West Germany.

Richards OW: *The Effective Use And Proper Care Of The Microscope*. American Optical Company, Instrument Division, Buffalo, New York. 1958.

EIGHT

Microtomes and Microtome Knives

The Microtome

The microtome is the machine or instrument on which sections are cut. These machines are available in a variety of models, each one having its own special use. The main types of microtomes available for routine histologic sectioning methods are:

1. Rocking microtomes
2. Rotary (Minot) microtomes
3. Sliding or base sledge microtomes
4. Freezing microtomes

All of these microtomes work on the same basic principle: *A pawl is brought into contact with a ratchet wheel that is connected to a millhead micrometer screw. This action turns the ratchet wheel which in turn rotates the screw. By these means the block is moved towards the knife at a predetermined thickness.*

It is possible to see these parts in the diagrams of the microtomes, which were drawn for this specific purpose. In the photographs, as in the microtomes themselves, these parts are often out of sight.

THE CAMBRIDGE ROCKING MICROTOME

The Cambridge rocking microtome (Figs. 1 and 2) is manufactured in two sizes, and can therefore be used to cut both small and large blocks of paraffin-embedded tissue. It is not recommended for serial sections

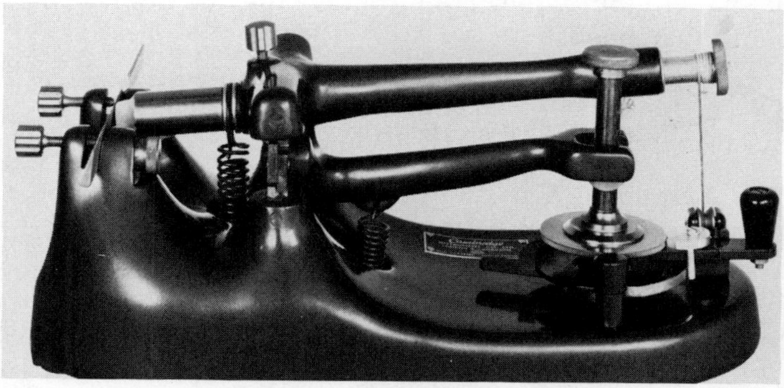

Figure 8-1. The Cambridge rocking microtome. (*Courtesy of Cambridge Medical Instruments Ltd., Cambridge, England.*)

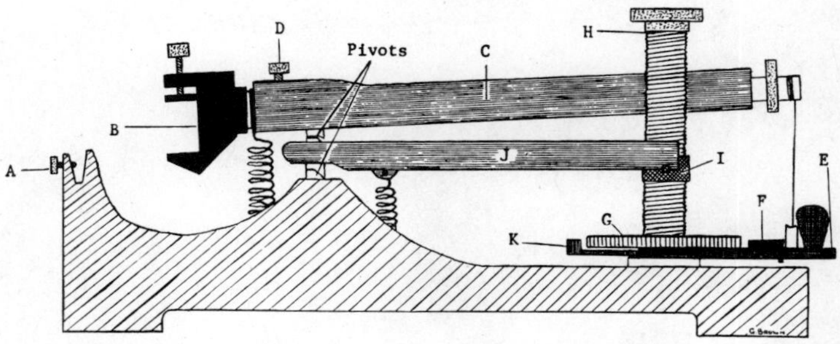

Figure 8-2. Diagram of the Cambridge rocking microtome. A is the knife holder. The block holder (chuck) B, is clamped onto the arm C by means of a screw, D. A length of nylon thread or catgut passes from the end of this arm, under a pulley wheel, to the lever E. By pulling this lever forward and allowing it to return to rest the upper arm C is moved up and down; the chuck passes the knife in the arc of a circle with the radius at right angles to the knife edge. On the forward movement of the lever E, the pawl F is brought into contact with the ratchet wheel G (to which is attached the millhead micrometer screw H), turning the ratchet wheel and the attached micrometer screw. This movement causes the sleeve I and the lower arm J to raise slightly. This lower arm has one end resting on a pivot and the other on the sleeve. The raising of this arm causes the upper arm (which is also resting on a pivot) to be advanced towards the knife. The rate of advance is controlled and is normally between 4μ and 6μ. K is the gauge or scale by which the thickness of the section is set. This is graduated in 2μ divisions.

because the sections are cut in a slightly curved plane, although in practice they cut well. There is a modified version of this machine available for use in cryostats.

The special merits of this microtome are its relatively low cost, and the cheapness of the knives. These are of one piece construction of the "Heiffor" pattern. Since they are biconcave they do not require a back when being sharpened.

THE ROTARY (MINOT) MICROTOME

The rotary microtome (Figs. 3-7) is probably the machine that is in most common use in routine laboratories and research establishments today.

In contrast to the rocking microtomes the block holder moves up and down vertically in front of the knife. On turning the flywheel a system of cams activates this movement. Towards the top of the upward stroke the pawl is caused to come into contact with the ratchet

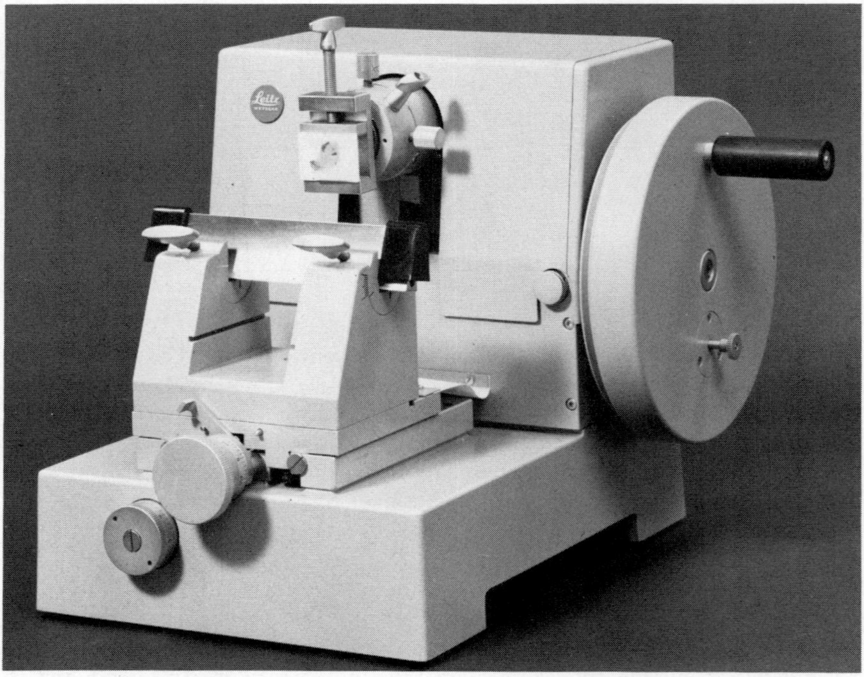

Figure 8-3. The Leitz 1512 rotary microtome. (*Courtesy of Ernst Leitz Inc., Wetzlar, Germany.*)

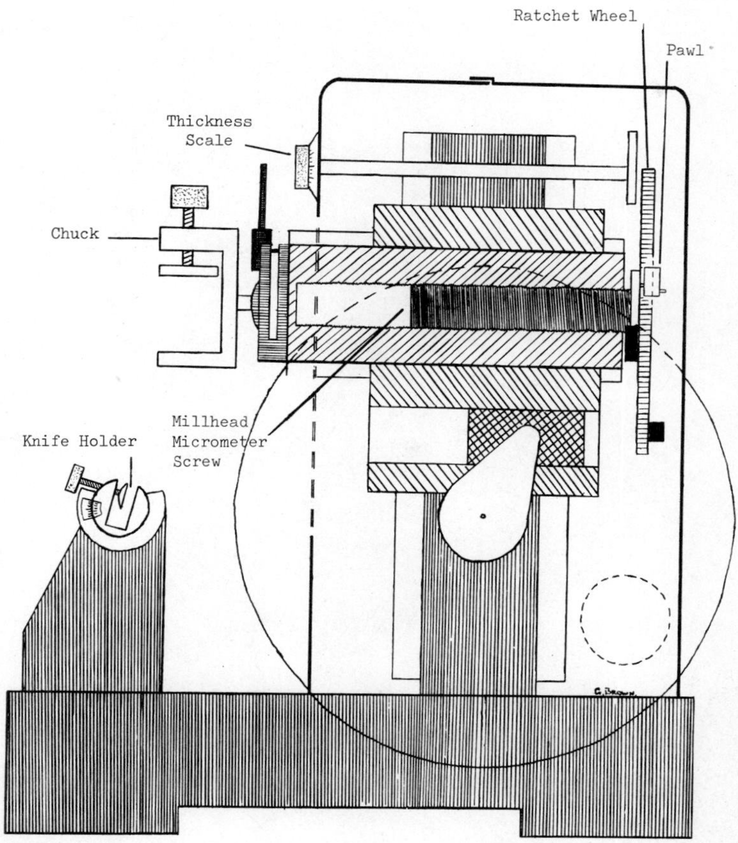

Figure 8-4. Diagram of the mechanism of the Leitz rotary microtome.

wheel which in turn rotates the micrometer screw, thus making the block move towards the knife at a predetermined rate.

Rotary microtomes are heavier and more stable than the rocking models and can be used to cut larger blocks of tissue. Sections are cut in a perfectly flat plane, and the machine will cut excellent serial sections. Modified models are available for cutting ultra-thin sections and for use in the cryostat.

Although fairly expensive, and with knives costing considerably more than those of the "Heiffor" pattern, this machine is thoroughly recommended for both routine and research histology. With some modifications of the knife holder it is possible to cut celloidin sections on a rotary microtome.

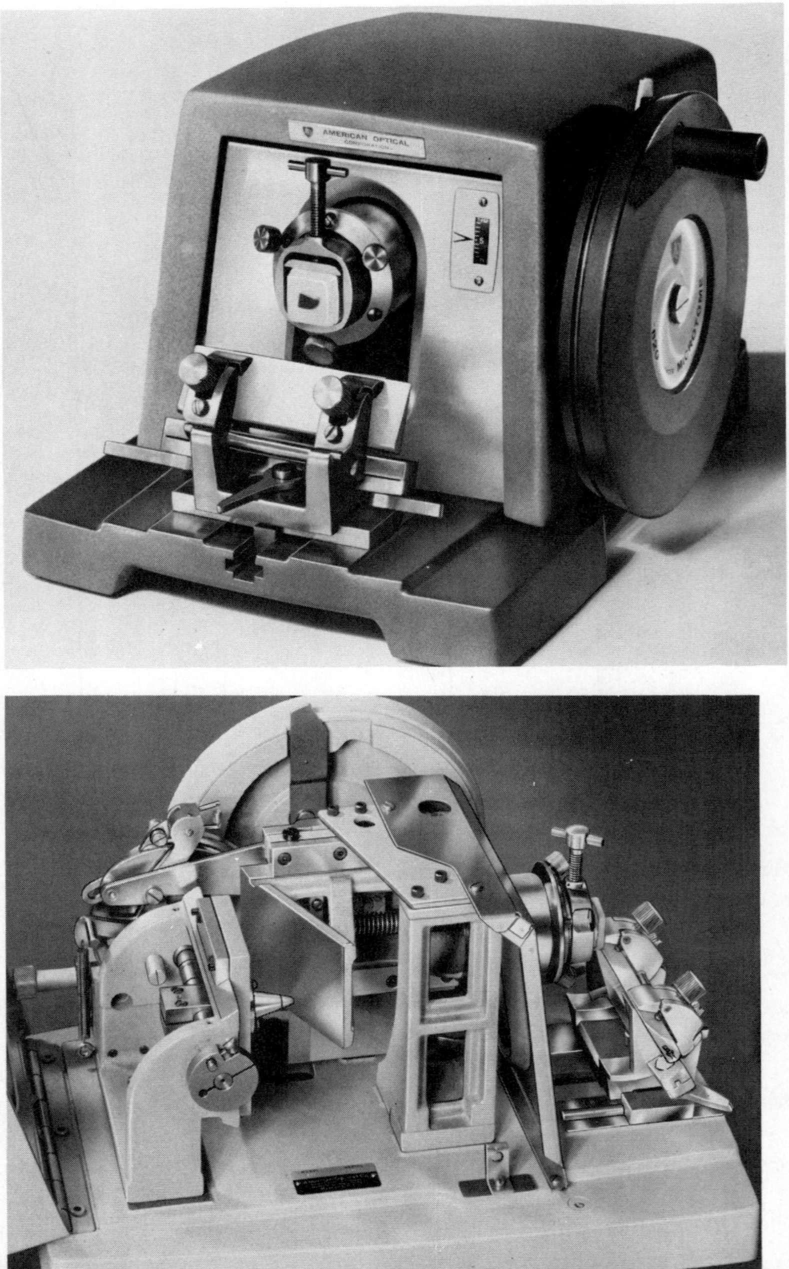

A

B

Figure 8-5. A. The AO 820 rotary microtome. B. View of the mechanism of the AO 820 rotary microtome. (*Courtesy of Amercan Optical Corp., Buffalo, N.Y.*)

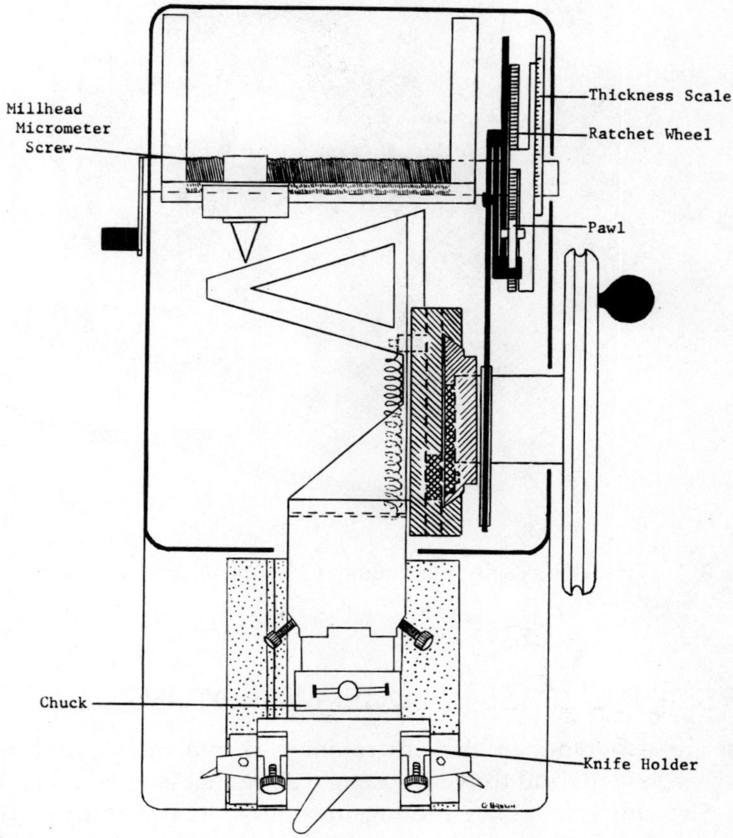

Figure 8-6. Diagram of the mechanism of the AO 820 rotary microtome.

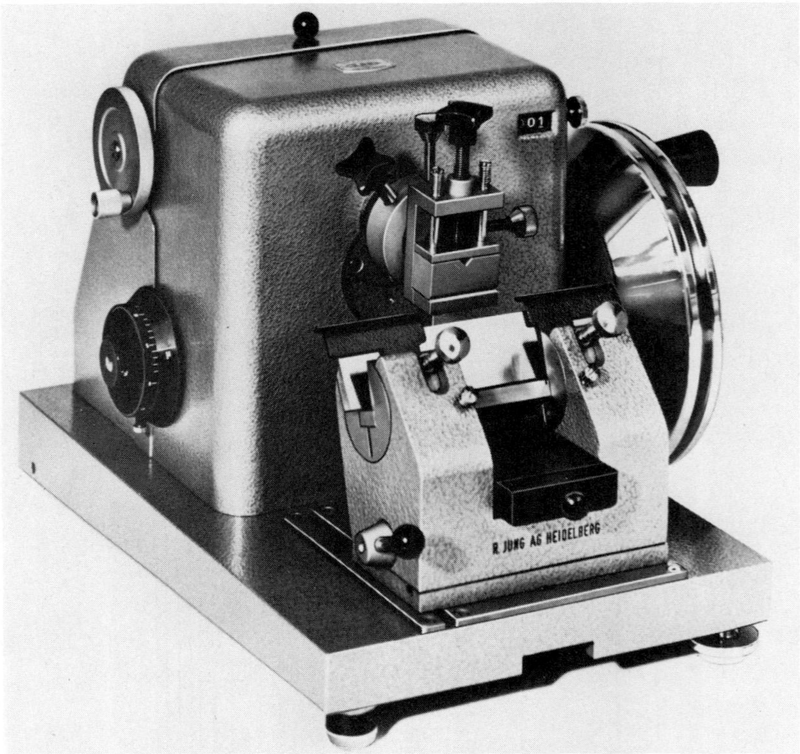

Figure 8-7. The JUNG rotary microtome. (*Courtesy of American Optical Corp., Buffalo, N.Y.*)

THE SLIDING (BASE SLEDGE) MICROTOME

There are two types of this microtome. In one model the knife is moved backwards and forwards along a slide that is affixed to a heavy base. The chuck is situated alongside the slide and is fitted onto a micrometer screw, at the lower end of which the ratchet wheel is fixed. As the knife is pulled back a lever makes contact with another lever and causes the pawl to activate the ratchet wheel and so turn the micrometer screw. Thus the block is raised towards the knife at a predetermined thickness. The scale for setting the thickness of the sections is situated below the ratchet wheel.

The second of this type of microtome (Figs. 8 and 9) is a more stable machine than the one described above. Both ends of the knife are held in the knife holders which are supported on two pillars. One of these pillars is movable, allowing the knife to be set at an angle for cutting

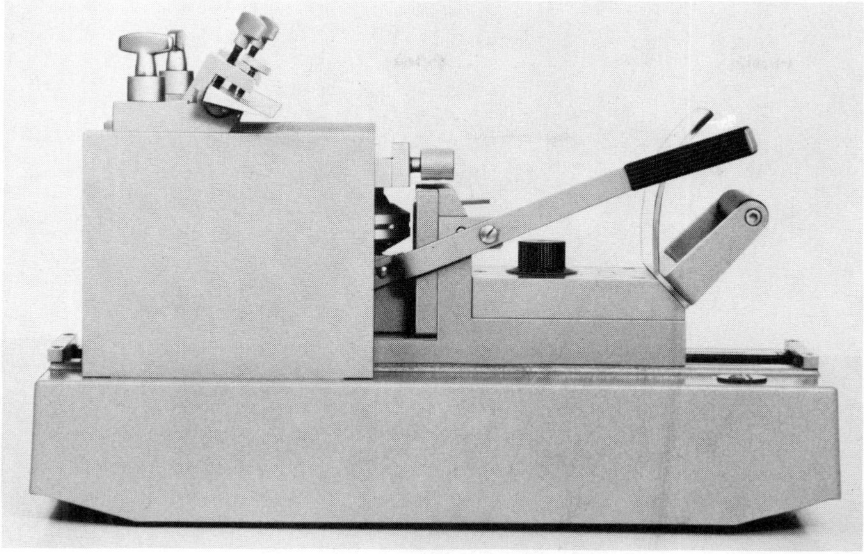

Figure 8-8. The Leitz 1400 base sledge microtome. (*Courtesy of Ernst Leitz Inc., Wetzlar, Germany.*)

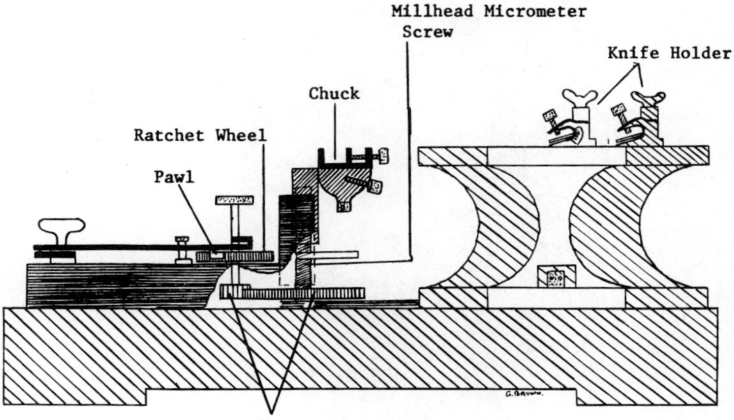

Figure 8-9. Diagram of the mechanism of the Leitz 1300 base sledge microtome.

celloidin sections. The chuck, set on a heavy sliding base, is moved backwards and forwards under the knife. On the backward stroke the handle is given a twist and a series of levers cause the pawl to come into contact with the ratchet wheel, which in turn activates the micrometer screw and raises the block towards the knife.

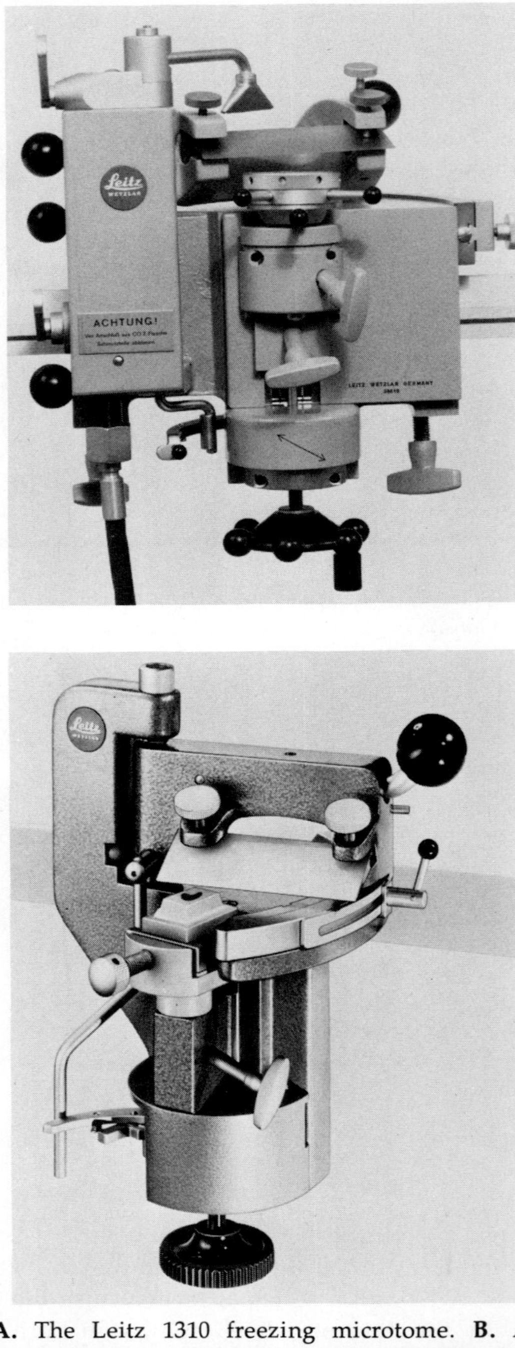

A

B

Figure 8-10. **A.** The Leitz 1310 freezing microtome. **B.** A smaller Leitz freezing microtome. (Courtesy of Ernst Leitz Inc., Wetzlar, Germany.)

On both of these machines the knife can be set obliquely for celloidin sections, or square for paraffin blocks. Both large and small blocks can be cut with equal ease, and because of the rigidity of the microtome it is this type that is recommended for cutting extremely hard blocks. With some small modifications to the block holder, whole organs may be sectioned, and with various attachments, frozen sections can be cut in addition to paraffin and celloidin blocks. Sections are cut in a perfectly flat plane.

THE FREEZING MICROTOME

The freezing microtome (Figs. 10 and 11) is used to cut undehydrated tissue in a frozen state. This is necessary for the demonstration of fat, for tissue constituents that may be damaged or destroyed by heat, for histochemical methods, and for sections required for rapid diagnosis.

The knife holder swings out over the chuck, immediately beneath which is a tap to allow carbon dioxide gas to be turned on and off, keeping the tissue frozen to the correct degree for sectioning. Below this is the micrometer screw and ratchet wheel.

Attached to the knife holder is a long lever. As the knife is returned

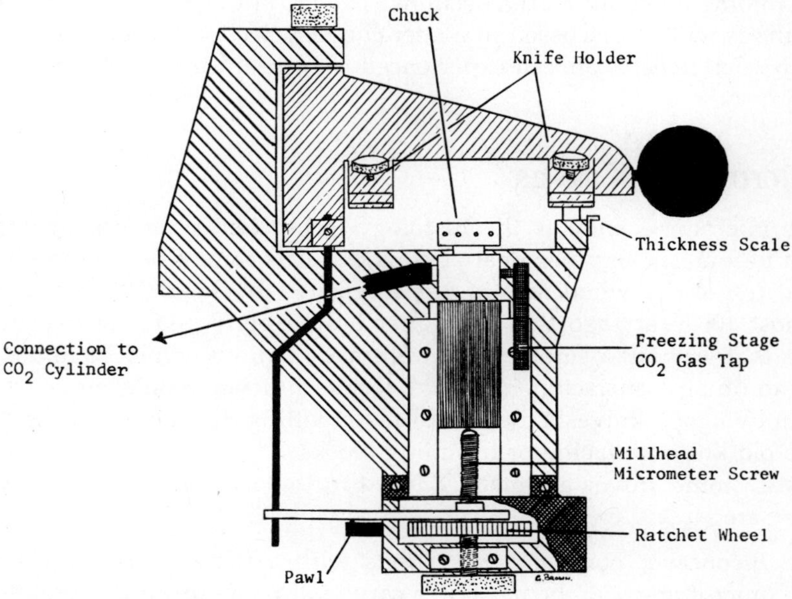

Figure 8-11. Diagram of the mechanism of the Leitz freezing microtome.

to its starting position this lever connects with a shorter lever which has the pawl attached to it. The pawl is thus moved to make contact with the ratchet wheel and thereby turn the micrometer screw. By this means the block is raised towards the knife.

This microtome is firmly clamped onto the edge of the bench for use, or it may be mounted on a specially constructed cart with the cylinder of carbon dioxide lying on the shelf below. This is a convenient arrangement if the microtome has to be moved from the laboratory to the operating rooms for rapid frozen sections.

THE CRYOSTAT

The cryostat is a cold chamber that is kept at a temperature of −20 C. There are several models available, but the ones which prove most useful are those incorporating a microtome in the construction (Figs. 12 and 13). These contain a rotary (Minot) microtome that has been specially manufactured to operate and remain rust-free at low temperatures. On one side of the chamber is a rapid freezing block that will freeze the tissue onto the block holder, and to the correct degree of hardness for sectioning, in 2–3 minutes.

The cryostat is used to cut fresh-frozen tissue for many histochemical techniques and has totally replaced the carbon dioxide freezing microtome for rapid frozen sections. The techniques for both of these methods will be discussed in a later chapter. Sections of 4μ can be cut with relative ease, and an experienced technician can section at 1μ.

Microtome Knives

The microtome knife is the histology technicians's professional tool and becomes a very personal possession. This cannot be overemphasized, *especially* when knives are sharpened by hand. It was stated almost 100 years ago that no matter how experienced a microtomist was that without a suitable and well-made knife it would be impossible to obtain satisfactory results. Every technician should be given at least two good knives, an older knife for cutting decalcified blocks and one old knife for facing or trimming blocks.

Microtome knives are manufactured in three basic shapes (Fig. 14). They are:

1. Biconcave: For paraffin sections with a rocking or rotary type microtome. Can be used on a carbon dioxide freezing microtome.
2. Planoconcave: One side of this knife is flat and the other is

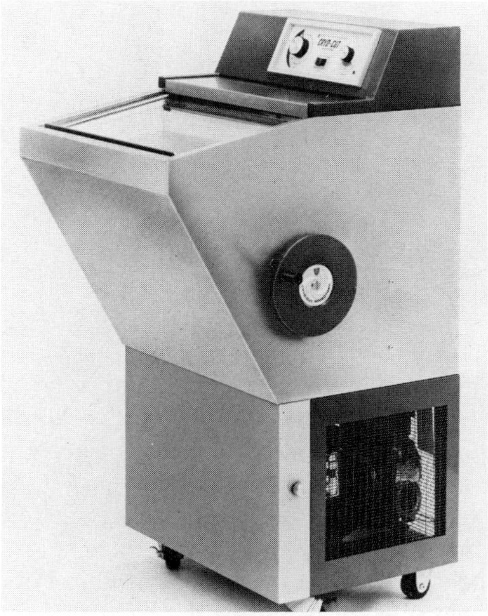

Figure 8-12. The AO 840C CRYO-CUT Cryostat. (*Courtesy of American Optical Corp., Buffalo, N.Y.*)

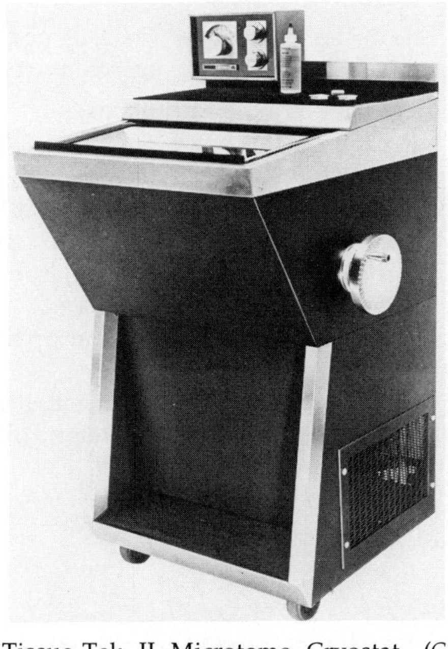

Figure 8-13. The Tissue-Tek II Microtome Cryostat. (*Courtesy of Lab-Tek Products, Division of Miles Laboratories, Inc., Naperville, Ill.*)

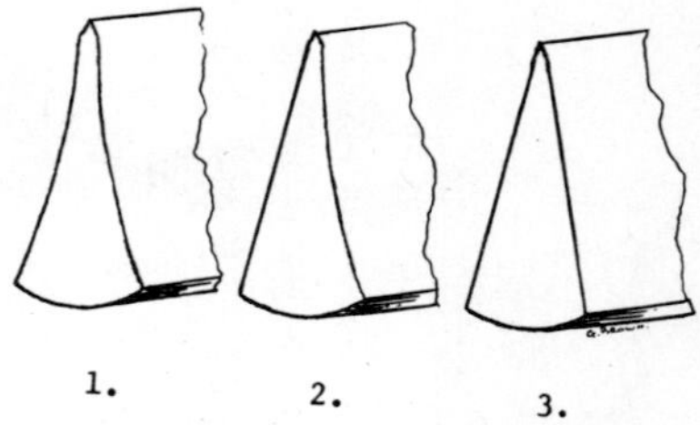

Figure 8-14. Cross-sectional views of microtome knives: (1) Biconcave. (2) Planoconcave. (3) Plane-wedge.

concave. There are two degrees of concavity available; the one with the lesser concavity is used for celloidin sections. The second type of knife is used for paraffin sections on the sledge, rotary, or rocking microtome.

3. Plane wedge: Routinely used for frozen sections and extremely hard specimens embedded in paraffin wax. It is also used for paraffin blocks cut on the rotary microtome. Personally, I prefer a planoconcave knife for use with the rotary microtome.

CARE OF MICROTOME KNIVES

The microtome knife is an expensive piece of equipment and great care must be taken of it. The following points must be observed:

1. Store the knife in its box when not in use.
2. Never lay a knife flat on the bench.
3. Never allow an edge to become badly "nicked." It is advisable to have a second knife for cutting bone and hard tissues.
4. The edge of the knife should be "touched up" daily before use.
5. Always use a back, when required, for sharpening (see Fig. 23). This is not necessary with biconcave knives.
6. The knife should be cleaned with xylene or toluene before and after use. Never allow it to become rusty.
7. When being stored for any length of time, the knife should be smeared with a good grade of a light weight oil.
8. *Never lend or borrow a knife.*

SHARPENING MICROTOME KNIVES

Types of Hone

There are several types of hone (sharpening stone) available for sharpening microtome knives in addition to the mechanical sharpe-

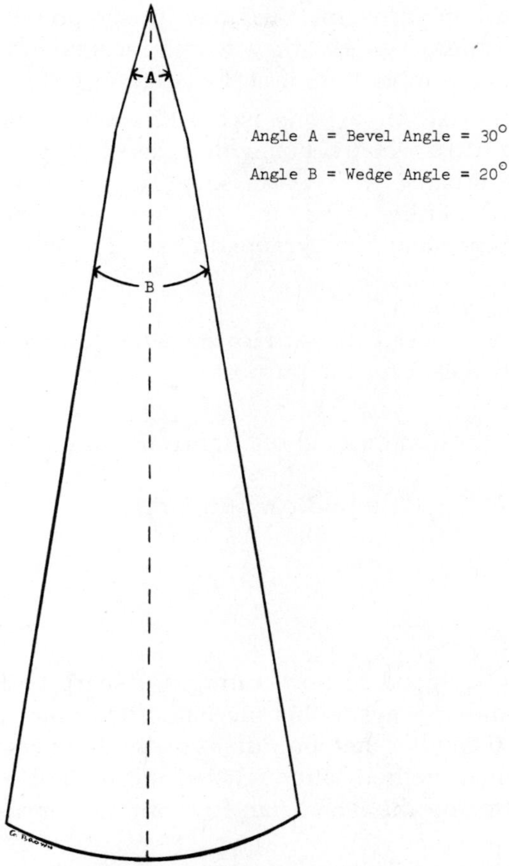

Figure 8-15. Diagram showing the wedge angle and bevel angle of the plane-wedge microtome knife.

ners. Those that are most recommended are:

Belgium Yellow. A natural sandstone set into a slate backing. This is the best hone for manual sharpening.

Arkansas. An artificial stone with more of a polishing effect than the Belgium yellow.

Fine Carborundum. An artificial stone with a much coarser bite than either the Belgium yellow or the Arkansas. It should only be used for badly "nicked" knives, which should then be finished on one of the other hones.

Plate Glass. A piece of plate glass measuring 8 × 3 × 1 inches and with bevelled edges is an excellent substitute for a stone. An abrasive must be used on this, and finely powdered aluminum oxide made into a paste with water is recommended. The "bite" given by this is similar to that of the Belgium yellow.

A convenient size for a hone is 8 × 3 inches, and it should be purchased in a fitted wooden box with a close fitting lid. After use the hone must be washed with warm soapy water to remove all metal particles from the knife, dried, and put away in its box. If no box is available the hone should be wrapped in soft lint-free cloth.

Lubricants for Hones

Before a hone is used the surface must be lubricated. Any of the following are excellent for the purpose:

1. Soapy water
2. 3-in-1 oil (a mixture of three light oils, animal, vegetable, and mineral)
3. Mineral oil U.S.P. (liquid paraffin B.P.)
4. Castor oil
5. Clove oil
6. Xylene

Honing

The criterion for good section cutting is a sharp knife. Knives may be sharpened in two ways, either mechanically or manually. Opinions as to which is the better method differ greatly. My personal preference is for the manual method, although the mechanical method has the advantage of freeing the technician from a time-consuming chore for other duties.

Of the machines available for mechanical knife sharpening there are five types which must be mentioned. The first type (Fig. 16) has a large flat circular plate which revolves in a horizontal plane. The knife edge is held against this plate at the correct angle by means of a special knife holder. At regular intervals of time the knife is turned over automatically in order that both sides of the blade are honed evenly.

The second type of machine (Fig. 17) has a wheel which rotates in a vertical position. Abrasive is added to the wheel and the knife, which is held manually, is passed across the wheel with a slow steady movement so that the entire length of the blade is honed. The knife must be turned over periodically to hone both sides of the blade evenly. This machine is no longer in production but is mentioned because many are still in use.

The third type of machine (Fig. 18) has an oblong glass plate in a horizontal plane. Abrasive is added to the plate along which the knife

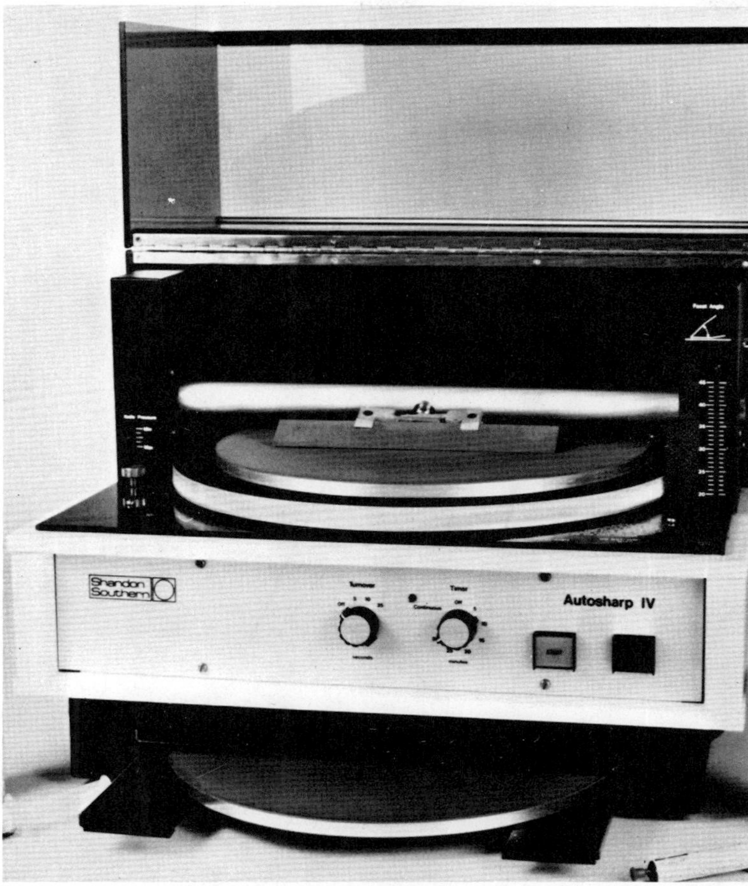

Figure 8-16. The AUTOSHARP IV automatic microtome knife-sharpener. (*Courtesy of Shandon Southern Instruments Inc., Sewickley, Pa.*)

is pushed, edge first, held at the correct angle by the knife holder. Every four strokes the knife is automatically turned for even sharpening on both sides of the blade. Some of these machines have a system for resurfacing the glass plates by mechanical means.

The fourth type of machine (Fig. 19) does not require an abrasive as the plate is a hone in the true sense. The knife is turned automatically for even honing on both sides of the blade. Knives that have been honed on this machine must be stropped before use.

The fifth type of mechanical knife sharpener (Figs. 20 and 21) has a matched pair of honing wheels at one end of the machine and a matched pair of stropping wheels at the other end. The wheels rotate

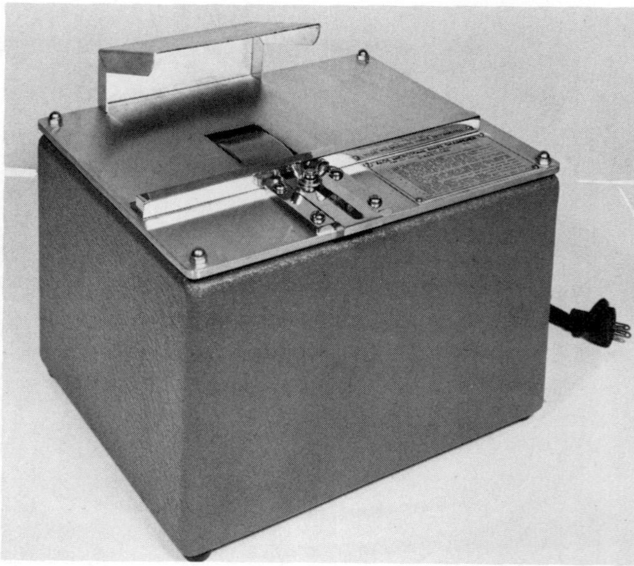

Figure 8-17. The HT automatic microtome knife-sharpener. (*Courtesy of Curtin Matheson Scientific Inc., Houston, Tx.*)

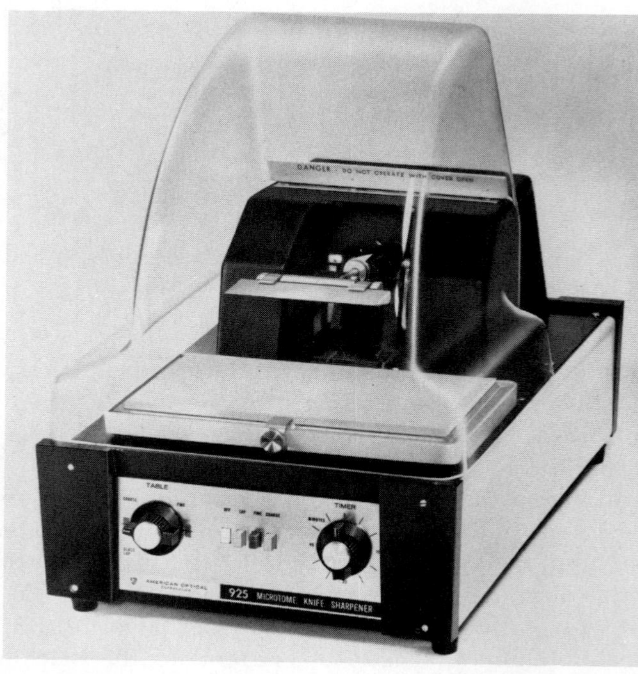

Figure 8-18. The AO 925 automatic microtome knife-sharpener. (*Courtesy of American Optical Corp., Buffalo, N.Y.*)

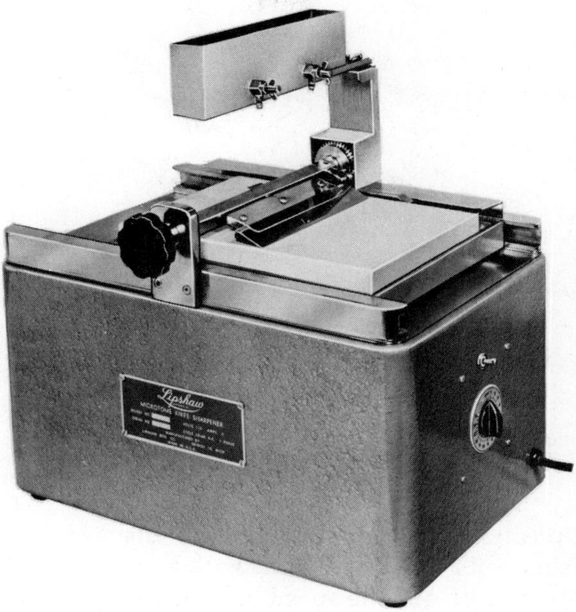

Figure 8-19. The Lipshaw 775 automatic microtome knife-sharpener. (*Courtesy of Lipshaw Manufacturing Co., Detroit, Mich.*)

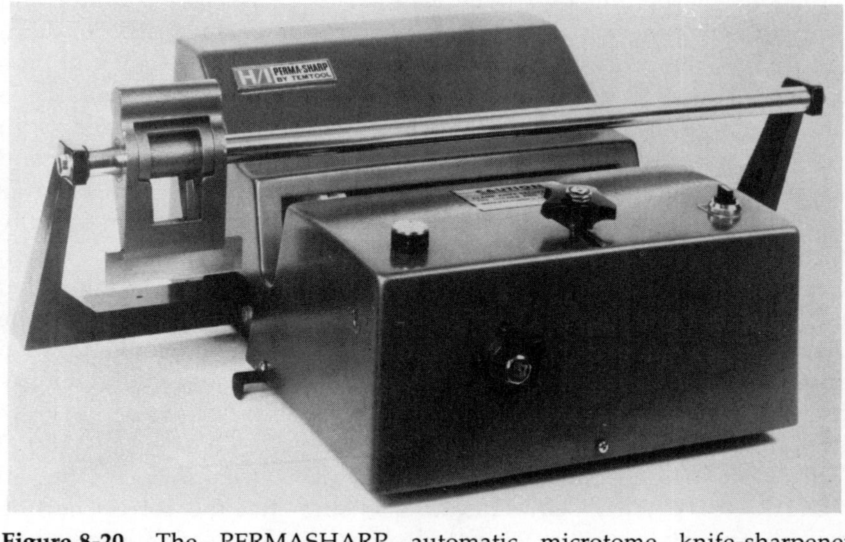

Figure 8-20. The PERMASHARP automatic microtome knife-sharpener. (*Courtesy of Hacker Instruments Inc., Fairfield, N.J.*)

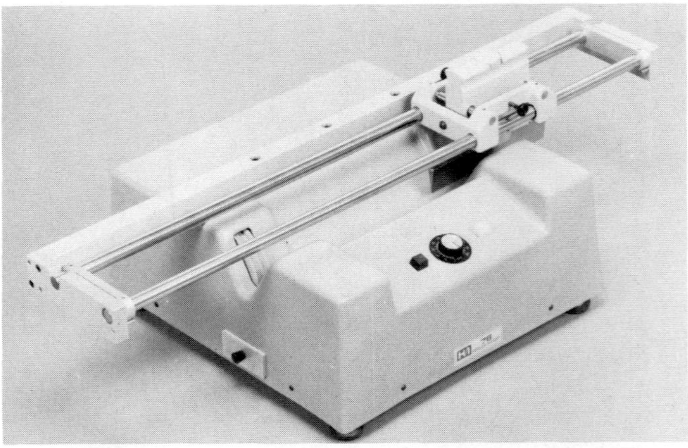

Figure 8-21. The H/I-76 automatic microtome knife-sharpener. (*Courtesy of Hacker Instruments Inc., Fairfield, N.J.*)

in a vertical position and the knife, which is attached to a knife holder on a slide, is passed across the wheels with an equal number of passes for each side of the blade. The speed of rotation may be controlled and a slower speed used for stropping. This type of knife sharpener hones the edge very rapidly, the entire operation taking less than three minutes, but also wears the knives quickly so that they have to be replaced more frequently.

Manual sharpening of knives is done in two stages, honing and stropping. Honing which can be of two grades, coarse (carborundum) and fine, is the process of grinding the cutting edge of the knife on a stone to acquire an even edge, free from nicks or bumps. The knife is laid flat across the stone and pushed up the hone, cutting edge first in a heel-to-toe movement (Fig. 22). The heel of the knife is the end nearest the handle. On reaching the end of the stone, the knife is turned over on its back, never leaving the stone, and drawn steadily back towards the operator. Ten to twenty strokes in each direction should be sufficient for a knife that is in good condition. Knives that are badly nicked should be honed on a fine carborundum stone (coarse honing) until the blemishes have been removed and then finished on the normal hone. At no time during honing should any pressure, other than the slight amount necessary to hold the knife steady on the hone, be applied.

Plane-wedge and planoconcave knives always require a back when being honed or stropped. This is to ensure that the correct cutting bevel be maintained (Fig. 23; see also Fig. 15). Backs should never be

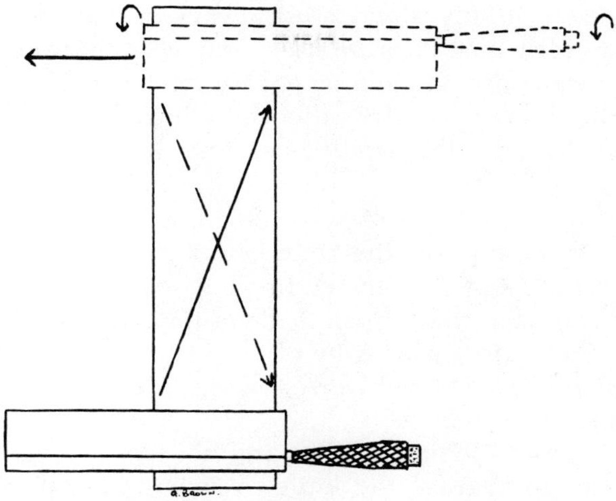

Figure 8-22. The action of honing (see text).

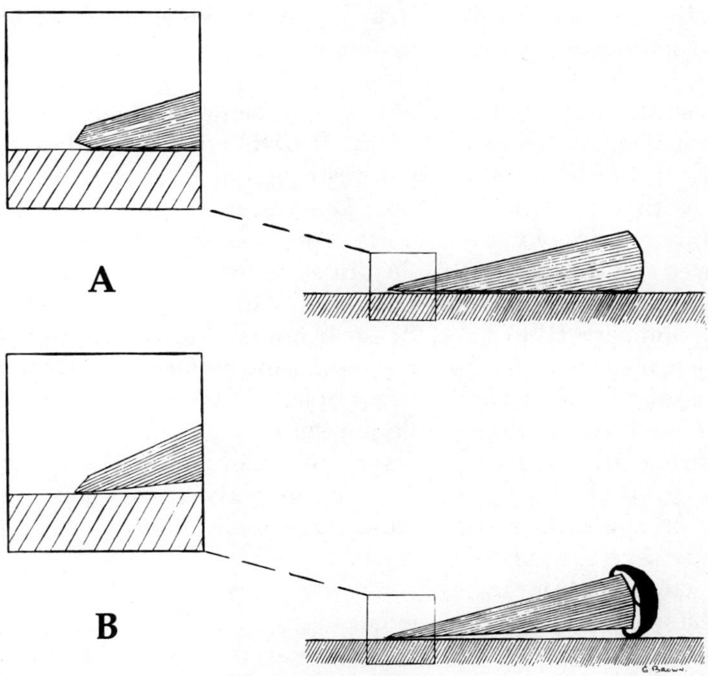

Figure 8-23. Diagram illustrating the need for a back on plane-wedge or planoconcave microtome knives when honing and stropping. **A.** Knife with no back. Notice that the cutting edge is not being honed. **B.** Knife with a back. Notice that the cutting edge is being honed.

exchanged between knives and must always be put onto the knives the same way each time they are used. It is wise to mark the back in order to identify which end will be nearest the handle. One end of the back is slightly curved, and it is this end which normally goes to the end of the blade where the handle is affixed.

Stropping

The purpose of stropping the knife is to remove the "burr" formed during honing and to polish the cutting edge. There are a great many designs of strops, but they are all made of the same materials, canvas and leather. The leather should be of the finest quality. Good leather strops are often labeled "Shell Horse," which indicates that the skin is from the rump of the animal.

Stropping surfaces should be firm and not loose or springy as this tends to turn the edge of the knife. Many firms will manufacture strops to the customer's specifications, and in this way it is possible to obtain exactly what is required. A good design is to mount the leather, or canvas, over a felt pad on a solid block of wood. This is screwed securely to the bench. Strops that are stretched between two points with no solid backing are not recommended as they tend to sag during use.

The canvas strop should always be used before the leather surface. It is normally ready for use when purchased, with the surface already dressed. If the canvas strop requires dressing, it should be smeared lightly with carborundum paste. Leather strops are often dry and frequently require oiling before use. This is fairly common with newly purchased or stored strops. A little castor oil or mineral oil is thoroughly worked into the *back* of the strop, never the stropping surface, and allowed to stand for 24–48 hours. If too much oil has been applied it may be removed by scraping the *surface* of the strop with the back of a knife or similar blunt object. The surface of the strop is then dressed by rubbing a little jeweler's rouge over the entire area. Some strops are purchased dressed with diamond dust. When not in use the strop should be kept covered to prevent dust and grit from settling on the surface. This could quite easily damage a knife edge and undo several hours of work.

The action of stropping is the exact reverse of honing. The knife is drawn along the strop with the cutting edge trailing and in a toe-to-heel direction (Fig. 24). Care should be taken, as any slip could easily sever the strop and damage the knife. The knife is turned over on its back (Fig. 25) at the end of each stroke in the same manner as when honing. No pressure should be applied other than that necessary to hold the knife level and steady on the stropping surface.

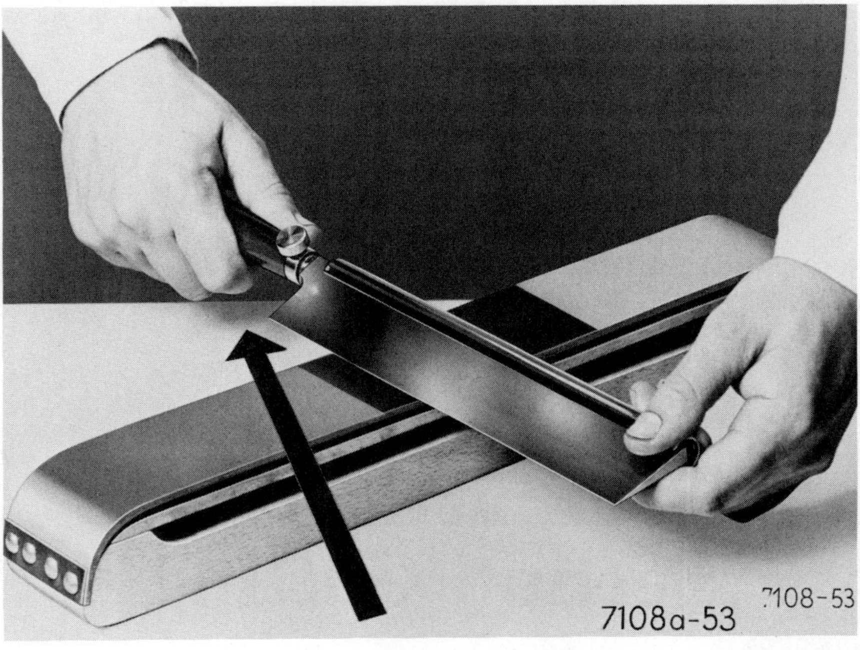

Figure 8-24. The action of stropping. (*From* The Microtome. *Courtesy of Ernst Leitz Inc., Wetzlar, Germany.*)

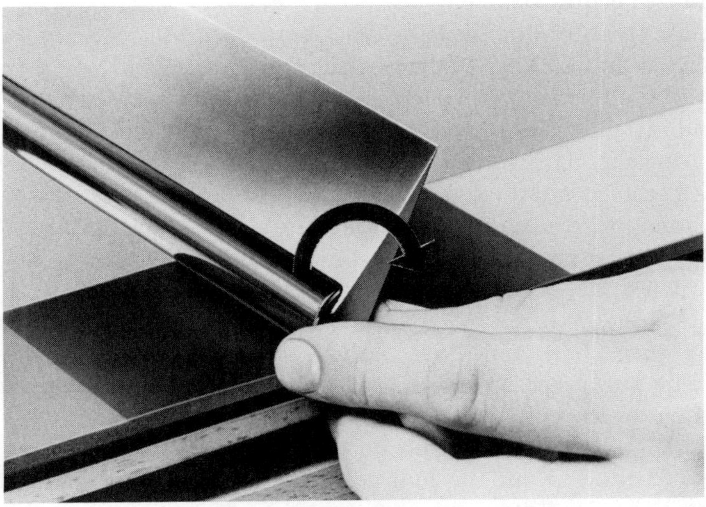

Figure 8-25. Turning the knife over without leaving the strop. (*From* The Microtome. *Courtesy of Ernst Leitz Inc., Wetzlar, Germany.*)

NINE

Practical Section Cutting

Paraffin Sections

When the tissue has been completely processed; fixed, decalcified if necessary, dehydrated, cleared, impregnated, and embedded; it is ready to be sectioned.

In most institutions today the laboratory will use one of the commercial embedding systems such as Tissue-Tek,* Lab-Tek,* or Tims,† which form a base to support the block, or they will cast blocks that will fit into the chuck (block holder) of the microtome. These blocks do not require any further mounting prior to sectioning. However, this is not always possible, and sometimes a block of larger dimensions must be cast to accommodate a large piece of tissue. Such a block must be mounted onto an object holder that will fit the chuck of the microtome before it can be sectioned.

Object holders (Fig. 1) may be metal discs of varying diameter attached to a shaft, vulcanite blocks, or homemade from blocks of wood. The surface of the blocks made from vulcanite or wood should be crosscut to improve adhesion.

The sides of the block should be trimmed, almost to the edge of the tissue, and the top and bottom edges to within 3 mm of the tissue.

* Miles Laboratories, Inc.

† Lab-Line Biomedical Products, Inc.

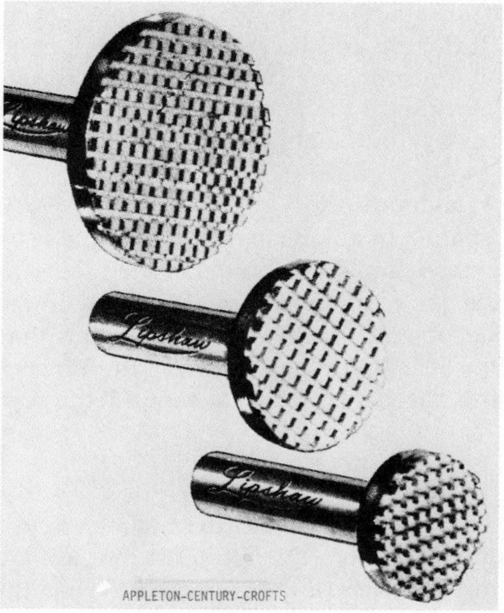

A

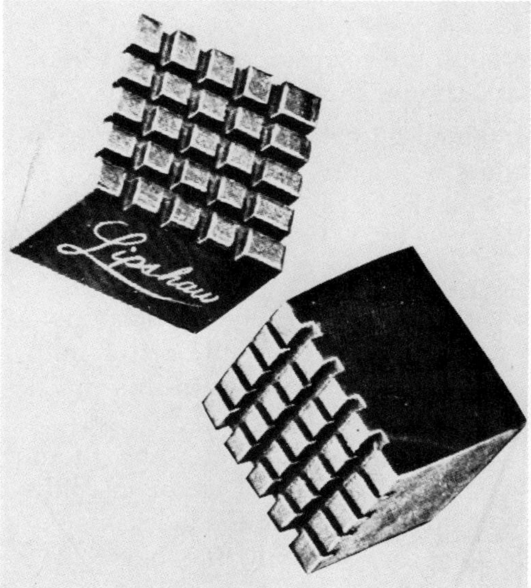

B

Figure 9-1. **A.** Metal object-holders. **B.** Vulcanite object-holders. (*Courtesy of Lipshaw Manufacturing Co., Detroit, Mich.*)

Make sure that all sides of the block are parallel and square. The margin of wax at the top and bottom of the block is necessary to form a ribbon when the sections are cut. Surface wax is now trimmed from the face of the block until the tissue is just exposed. The block is now ready for mounting onto the object holder.

Vulcanite or Wooden Blocks

Heat a metal spatula in a bunsen flame and hold it between the back of the wax block and the object holder. When the wax starts to melt, the heated blade is withdrawn and the block is gently but firmly pressed onto the object holder, and held in position until the wax starts to solidify. Seal the edges between the object holder and the block by running the heated spatula around the joint and allow to harden.

Metal Object Holders

With a pair of large forceps, hold the metal disc in a bunsen flame until it is thoroughly heated. Do not get it too hot. Gently but firmly press the disc onto the back of the wax block. When the wax begins to solidify plunge the block into cool water to set the disc firmly in position.

SECTIONING

The art of microtomy, the correct terminology for section cutting, has four fundamental requirements. They are

1. A well-maintained microtome
2. A sharp knife
3. Properly processed blocks
4. Experience

All of the tuition in the world will not, in itself, produce a skilled technician. The manner in which the technician obtains this skill and expertise is by constant practice in the art of microtomy. It is also inevitable that each technician will, with this practice, develop their own personal "tricks of the trade."

Prior to sectioning the blocks should be thoroughly cooled by placing them face down on a pan of ice or in cold water. I prefer to trim the excess wax from the face of the blocks before placing them on the ice. This is done by clamping the block in the chuck of the microtome, and with an old knife, trimming away the surface wax until the tissue is fully exposed. The block is advanced manually during this procedure. After being trimmed, the two top corners of the block are cut off at an angle. This gives instant identification of which way up the block should be placed on the microtome for sectioning, and a clear mark for dividing sections from the ribbon. By trimming with an old knife before cooling, calcium deposits or foreign objects such as sutures or metal clips are located, and damage to a good knife is prevented. If this procedure is not followed, and as stated, this is my preference, the blocks are chilled on the ice and then trimmed immediately before sectioning, exposing the full surface of the tissue in the block. The sides of the block should always be trimmed close to the tissue. This helps in the flattening of the section when it is floated out on the water bath.

Sections are normally cut in the range of 4μ–6μ in thickness, but there are exceptions. Tissue from the central nervous system, brain, and spinal cord, is sectioned in the range of 10μ–20μ, depending upon the staining techniques to be employed, and renal biopsies should be sectioned as thinly as possible—preferably in the range of 1μ–2μ in thickness.

The technique for section cutting is as follows:

1. Place the block in the chuck of the microtome and orientate it so that the top, bottom, and face of the block are parallel to the knife edge.
2. Clamp the block firmly in position.
3. Check that the knife (Fig. 2), knife holder, and chuck are clamped firmly in position.
4. If the block has not been trimmed of excess wax on the face of the block, trim away the wax until the entire surface of the tissue is exposed. The block may require further cooling with a block of ice before any sections are cut.
5. Start cutting until full sections start to come off of the block. Discard the incomplete sections.
6. Cut with a slow, smooth rhythm and gently draw off the ribbon of sections. The sections may be supported with either a blunt pair of forceps, a camel hair brush, or the fingers. Sections being cut in the range of 1μ–2μ must be cut very slowly and very smoothly.

   Tissue that has a tendency to crumble or fragment during cutting (this is fairly common with blood clots, bone marrow, and spleen) can be sectioned with ease using the following procedure. With the mouth open, and sounding a soft, long-drawn "H" thus, "hhhhhhhh," exhale gently onto the section as it leaves the knife and cut very slowly. This also helps to reduce the effects of static electricity. Some tissue, such as a lens, can be sectioned with ease after the surface of the tissue has been

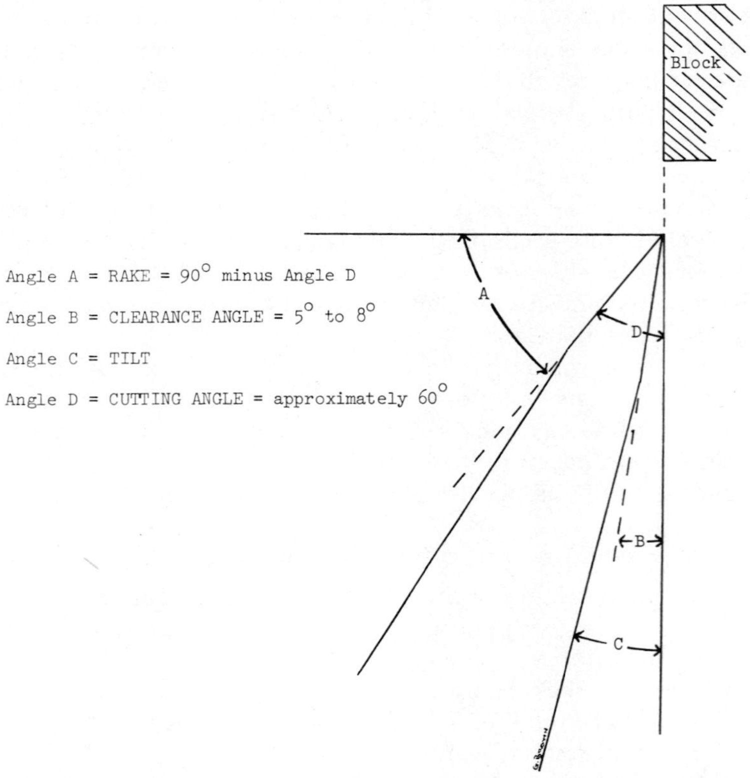

Figure 9-2. Diagram showing the cutting angle and tilt of a microtome knife.

soaked with warm water applied to the block with a small piece of wet cloth.

7. Sections should be removed from the knife in ribbons of ten. This enables easy location during serial sectioning.
8. Selected sections or a ribbon of sections are floated out on a waterbath that is set at 45–50 C. This is to flatten the sections, readying them for mounting onto slides (Fig. 3). Any folds or creases may be removed by gently stretching the sections with a pair of forceps or with a pair of dissecting needles, one of which should be bent to resemble a hockey stick. Bubbles which have been trapped beneath the section may be removed with the edge of a slide or teased out with the bent dissecting needle (Fig. 4). Care must be taken not to tear or puncture the section as this will produce an artifact.

Sections may also be flattened by placing them on a large slide

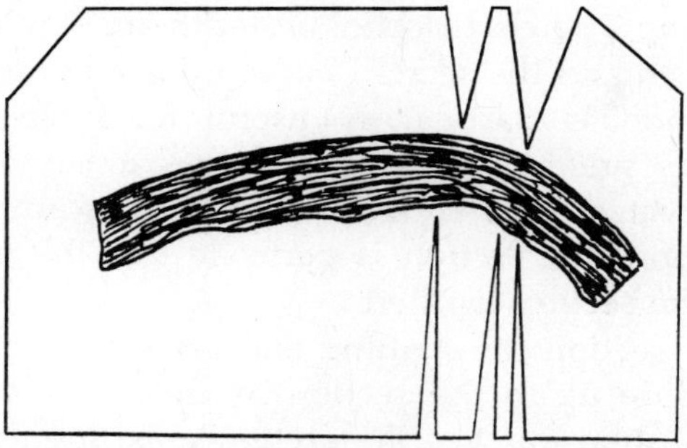

Figure 9-3. Diagram showing how a curved or "elastic" specimen can be flattened by "nicking" the section. This is often applicable to blood vessels.

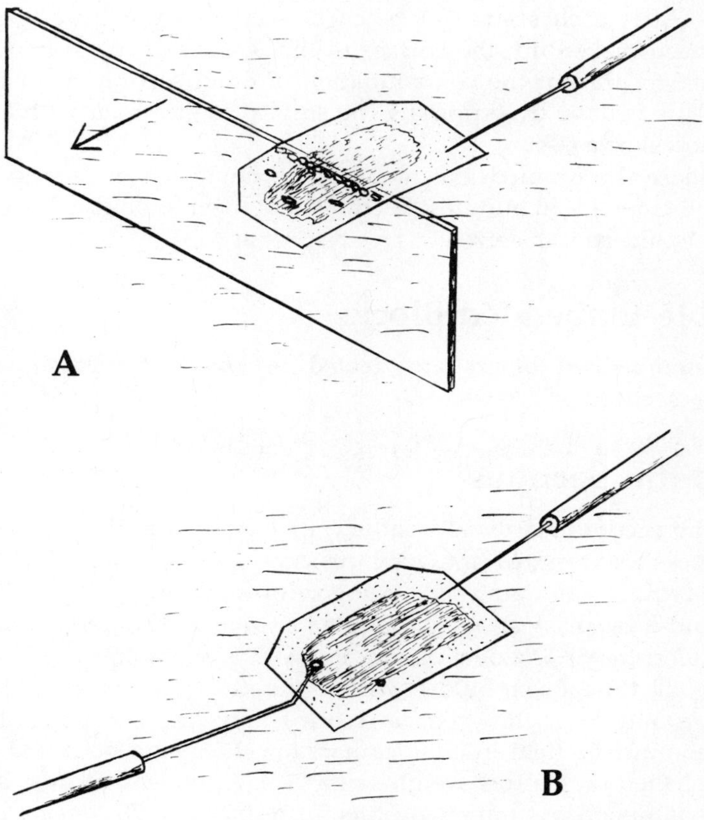

Figure 9-4. Two methods for teasing bubbles from under a section. A. Removing bubbles with a slide. B. Removing bubbles with a dissecting needle.

and running 2 percent alcohol under them. Any folds or bubbles are removed and the section is then floated onto the waterbath. This method is particularly useful for large sections. Some technicians prefer to float out the section on a few drops of distilled water on a slide. This is then warmed gently on a hotplate until the section is perfectly flat, the water is drained off, and the section is dried.

9. Select the section for staining and separate it from the ribbon. Bring a slide up to the section in an almost vertical position. When the slide touches the section it is lifted vertically out of the water and drained (Fig. 5). If necessary the section can easily be orientated at this stage, and it should be positioned so that the center of the section is about one third of the way up the slide. This allows ample space for a label after staining.

   After each section or batch of sections from the ribbon has been picked up, the surface of the water bath must be cleaned off to prevent the contamination of other sections with debris. This is done by skimming the surface of the water with a paper towel or a tissue.
10. Place the drained and mounted sections in the oven to dry at 60 C for 20–30 minutes. Sections that need to be dried overnight should be transferred to an oven set at 45 C.

Double-Embedded Blocks

Double-embedded blocks are treated in exactly the same way as paraffin sections.

Celloidin Sections

Celloidin sections are usually cut in the range of 10μ–15μ in thickness. The blocks are trimmed in exactly the same way as paraffin blocks, but do not require hardening by chilling prior to cutting.

Celloidin blocks need to be mounted onto object holders for sectioning. Vulcanite or wooden blocks are normally employed. Cover the surface of the object holder with a liberal quantity of 2 percent celloidin and press the celloidin block firmly into position. The two surfaces must be held in close contact for at least an hour and this is accomplished with either weights or a vise. At the end of this time the seal is hardened by immersing the entire block in 70 percent alcohol and leaving it for at least 30 minutes before sectioning.

The blocks are clamped securely onto the chuck of the sledge (sliding) microtome in exactly the same way as for paraffin blocks, and

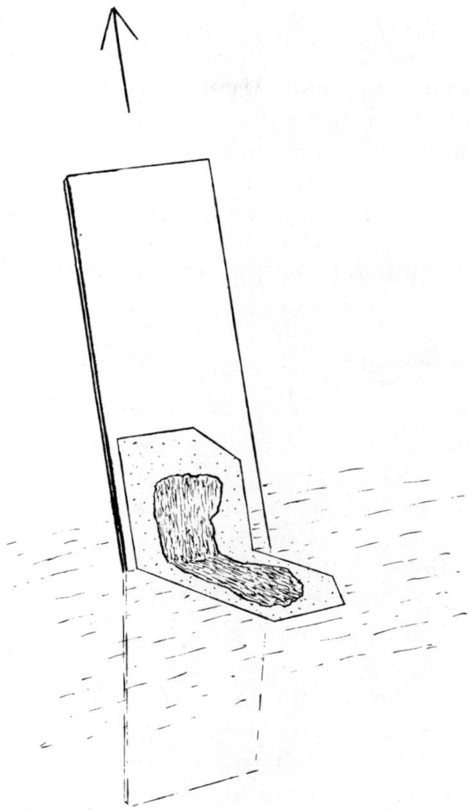

Figure 9-5. Picking a section up onto a slide.

the same precautions are taken. Sections do not come off in ribbons and must be collected individually. Celloidin sections tend to roll up during cutting, but they can easily be flattened on the knife with a camel hair brush moistened with 70 percent alcohol. Both the block and the sections must be kept moistened with 70 percent alcohol during cutting and the sections are collected into 70 percent alcohol for storage until they are stained. Celloidin sections are usually floated through the staining reagents and mounted onto slides after they are stained.

Blocks of LVN are treated in the same manner as celloidin blocks.

Frozen Sections

Frozen sections may be cut from tissue that has been fixed and frozen with carbon dioxide, or from fresh or fixed tissue frozen in the cryostat. Both methods will be discussed, including the methods for rapid frozen sections (both the carbon dioxide method and the cryostat method) for emergency diagnosis while the patient is still in the operating room. Frozen sections are most commonly used for the demonstration of fat, although most staining methods may be performed.

CARBON DIOXIDE (CO_2) TECHNIQUES

Routine Frozen Sections

Frozen sections are normally cut at 10μ with this method.

1. Place the block of fixed tissue on a piece of moistened filter paper and position it on the chuck of the microtome. Freeze with short bursts of carbon dioxide. A small beaker held over the tissue will assist in accelerating the freezing.
2. Raise the tissue up to the knife manually, and trim the tissue until a flat surface is obtained. If the tissue is frozen too solid it will not cut, but will chip into fragments. Warm the block slightly by rubbing it with a finger. If the tissue is not frozen sufficiently it will crumble and come off of the chuck. Refreeze.
3. Cut sections at 10μ. Sections should be cut at the "dew line." This is the point where the hard-frozen tissue is just starting to thaw and is easily visible to the naked eye.
4. Sections do not ribbon, but collect on the knife blade. They are removed with either a camel hair brush or with a finger moistened with water.
5. The sections are collected into distilled water where they will separate and are easy to pick up with a glass hockey stick.
6. Sections may be mounted onto slides from the water and then stained, or they may be stained and then mounted onto slides.

Frozen Sections for Rapid Diagnosis

Frozen sections are normally cut at 10μ with this method.

1. Fix a selected portion of tissue* by dropping it into boiling 10 percent formalin for 2 minutes.
2. Wash rapidly in tap water.
3. Cut sections at 10μ as previously described.

* *Note*. This portion of tissue must be kept for routine processing. Paraffin sections are made for comparison with the frozen section and confirmation of the diagnosis.

4. Mount sections onto albuminized slides and blot gently with filter paper moistened with alcohol. Dry and fix in a bunsen flame (or on a hot plate) as for bacteriological smears.

   Sections may be stained loose and then mounted onto slides, but my personal preference is to mount before staining.
5. Rinse rapidly in distilled water.
6. Harris' hematoxylin for 30–45 seconds.
7. Rinse in distilled water.
8. Blue in ammonia water for 5 seconds.
9. Rinse thoroughly in distilled water.
10. Eosin of choice for 30–60 seconds.
11. Dehydrate, clear, and mount.
12. Take the section to the pathologist for reporting.

Note. Although this method is considered outmoded and was replaced by the cryostat a long time ago, it is still an extremely useful method for use as a backup in cases of breakdown of equipment. Most laboratories still have a clinical microtome and access to a cylinder of carbon dioxide, and the method is included in this text for this specific reason.

Another alternative in cases of mechanical breakdown is the touch preparation. These can be very informative, but in some instances only a section will suffice.

THE CRYOSTAT TECHNIQUE

Routine Frozen Sections

Frozen sections may be cut at 2μ, but are normally cut at 5μ–6μ by this method. Sections may be cut from either fresh or fixed tissue, but when fat is to be demonstrated fixed tissue is preferred.

1. The selected block of fresh or fixed tissue is positioned on the object holder and placed in the cryostat on the rapid heat extractor. Adhesion of the tissue to the object holder is obtained by either placing a few drops of water, or a little Ames O.C.T. compound* on the face of the object holder. O.C.T. compound may also be used to form a base for small pieces of tissue which must be raised away from the face of the object holder to allow sufficient clearance for sectioning without hitting the object holder with the knife. It can also be used as an embedding medium for friable tissue and small fragments of tissue.

* Miles laboratories, Inc.

Rapid freezing of the tissue can be assisted by spraying the block with one of the commercial freon sprays, although it should be remembered that this can be a health hazard in confined and poorly ventilated areas.

2. Place the object holder in the chuck of the microtome and manually advance towards the knife, trimming the block until the full surface of the tissue is flat.
3. Cut sections at the desired thickness. Fixed tissue sections may be removed with a camel-hair brush and collected in distilled water. Sections of unfixed tissue are picked up on a microscope slide and placed into a fixative. The antiroll plate is swung out of the way and a slide (at room temperature) is gently lowered onto the section which will immediately become attached to the slide.
4. Stain as desired.

Frozen Sections of Fresh Tissue for Rapid Diagnosis

1. Place the selected block of fresh tissue on the object holder and freeze as rapidly as possible. The remainder of this tissue should be processed routinely as a paraffin block for later comparison with the frozen section and confirmation of the diagnosis.
2. Cut sections at 6μ, or as thinly as possible in the same way as for routine frozen sections. Fatty tissue, such as breast, may require repeated bursts of freon to keep the block really hard. The knife must be kept free of grease.
3. Pick up the sections onto a slide.
4. Place the mounted sections into either 10 percent formalin, absolute methyl or ethyl alcohol, or ether/alcohol for 30–60 seconds to fix. The coagulation of the protein will cause the section to adhere firmly to the slide.
5. Wash briefly in distilled water for 15–30 seconds.
6. Harris' hematoxylin for 30 seconds.
7. Rinse in distilled water.
8. Blue in ammonia water for 5 seconds.
9. Wash thoroughly in distilled water for 30 seconds.
10. Eosin of choice for 30–60 seconds.
11. Rinse in 70 percent alcohol.
12. Dehydrate, clear, mount, and label.*
13. Hand to the pathologist for reporting.

* The section should be labeled with the patient's name and the accession number for filing with the permanent sections.

STAINING OF UNMOUNTED FROZEN SECTIONS

Unmounted frozen sections of fixed tissue can be stained using the identical methods as those employed for paraffin or celloidin sections. The stains, differentiating reagents, and washing fluids are assembled and dispensed into Stender dishes of a suitable size. These are set out in the sequence of the staining procedure being used, finishing with the dish from which the sections will be mounted onto slides. This is usually distilled water.

The sections are picked up and passed from jar to jar by means of a glass rod. These rods are made by heating a six-inch length of glass rod with a diameter of from 2 to 3 mm until it is soft. It is then gently pulled out so that the center portion tapers to a thin rod of approximately 1 mm in diameter. While pulling, the rod is removed from the flame. When cool, cut the rod to a suitable length and round off both ends to remove all sharp edges. One rod should have its end bent to resemble a hockey stick, the angled portion being about 1 cm in length. Great care should be taken while handling the sections as they are very friable, and any sharp edges on the glass rod (there should not be any if it is made properly) will tear the sections.

Sections that are to be dehydrated and cleared should be mounted onto slides and gently blotted with filter paper moistened with alcohol. Proceed with care to complete the dehydration, clearing, and mounting of the section. Sections that are to be mounted in an aqueous medium do not, and often should not, require blotting in this manner. If glycerin jelly is used as the mountant, it is advisable to mount from warm distilled water. This helps to keep the mountant fluid and prevent the formation of bubbles.

Faults in Section Cutting

Although the majority of blocks of tissue are easily sectioned with excellent results, there are occasions when poor quality sections will be cut. Apart from this being caused by a very difficult tissue specimen, which can happen, the three major causes of poor sections are:

1. Faulty equipment.
2. Poor technique.
3. Faulty processing of the tissue.

The first two faults may be grouped together under the heading of faults during sectioning, while the third fault should come under the separate heading of faults due to poor processing. These faults are not caused during sectioning, but they are often not apparent until the block is being trimmed or sectioned. The primary cause of faults that occur during processing is that the block of tissue was too thick for the time allowed to process it. The blame for this is given to the person who examined the specimen grossly and selected the tissue blocks, but it is also the responsibility of the technologist who is assisting in the grossing to ensure that the tissue is correctly trimmed to blocks of a manageable size, and to bring this to the attention of the pathologist when they are too large.

It is important that the technologist learn these faults, their causes, and their remedies, and learn to distinguish which faults occur during sectioning and which are due to poor processing.

FAULTS OCCURRING DURING SECTION CUTTING

1. Fault: Tear or scratch across the section, or splitting of the ribbon (Fig. 6).
   Cause: a. A jagged knife edge.
   b. Dirt or hair on the knife edge.
   Remedy: a. Hone the knife to remove the nicks.
   b. Clean the knife edge.
2. Fault: Tear or scratch across part of the section.
   Cause: Grit, calcium, carbon, or sutures, etc. in the tissue or wax.
   Remedy: Examine the block under a magnifying glass. If calcium is present; decalcify the block. Remove sutures or grit from the tissue with a scalpel point. If the grit is in the wax, re-embed in clean filtered wax.
3. Fault: Holes in the section.
   Cause: a. Air bubbles in the tissue or wax.
   b. A piece of hard material in the tissue.
   c. A soft piece of tissue in the block.
   Remedy: a. Re-embed the specimen.
   b. Remove the hard material if possible.
   c. Reprocess the specimen.
4. Fault: Cracks across the section parallel to the knife (Fig. 7).
   Cause: a. A blunt knife.
   b. Knife tilt too small.
   c. Block too hard for the thickness of section.
   Remedy: a. Sharpen the knife.
   b. Adjust the tilt.
   c. Warm the block slightly, or re-embed in a softer wax.

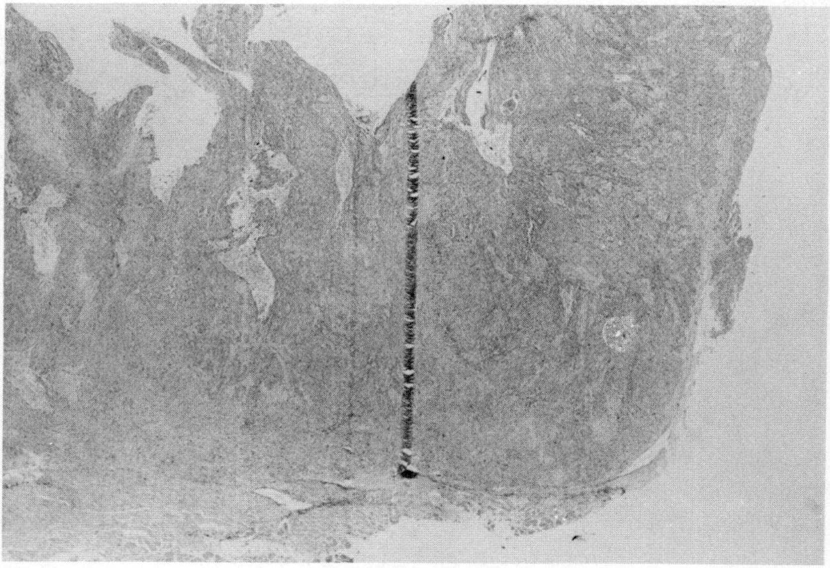

Figure 9-6. "Scores" in a section. Notice that the heavier tear does not start at the edge of the tissue. This is due to a foreign body. The lighter score to the left is caused by a nick in the knife.

5. Fault: Section shows thick and thin horizontal lines (chatters) (Fig. 8, p. 154).
   Cause: a. A loose knife.
   b. A loose block.
   c. A blunt knife.
   d. Extremely hard tissue.
   Remedy: a. Tighten the knife clamps and knife holder.
   b. Tighten the chuck.
   c. Sharpen the knife.
   d. Soften the tissue if possible or embed in a harder wax.
6. Fault: Sections cut thick and thin alternatively.
   Cause: Knife tilt is too great and is compressing the block.
   Remedy: Adjust the tilt.
7. Fault: Sections compress at one end.
   Cause: a. A blunt spot on the knife.
   b. A soft spot in the wax due to presence of clearing agent.
   Remedy: a. Move block along the knife or sharpen the knife.
   b. Reinfiltrate the tissue and re-embed.

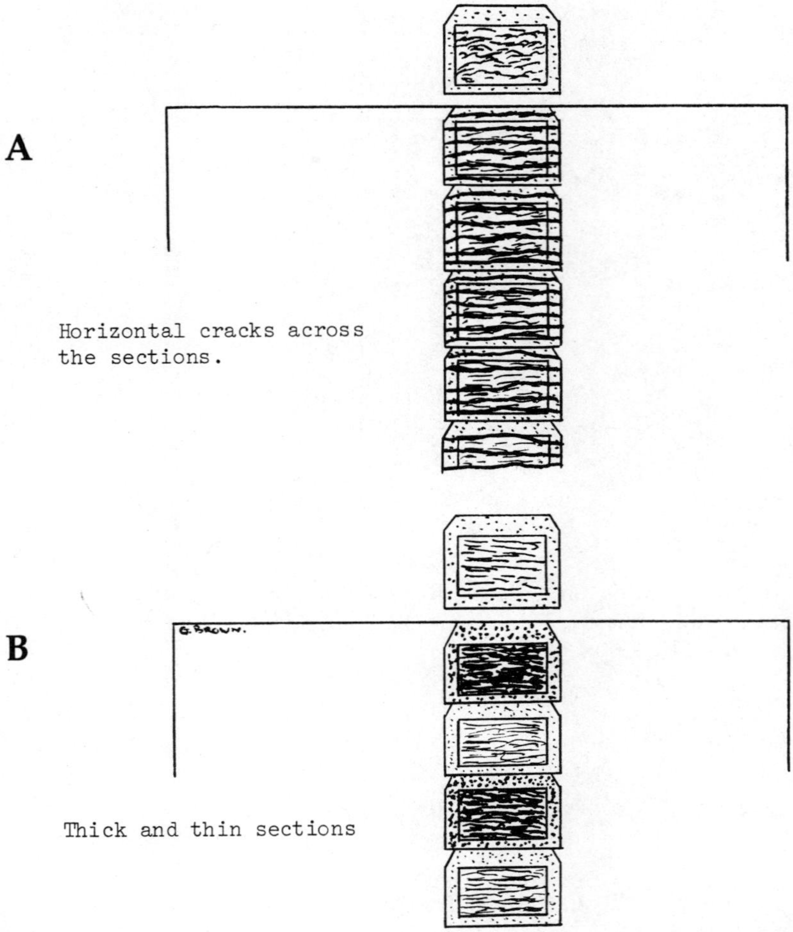

Figure 9-7. Faults in section cutting. **A.** Horizontal cracks across the sections. **B.** Thick and thin sections.

8. Fault: Ribbon curves to one side.
   Cause: a. Edges of block are not parallel to the knife.
   b. A dull spot on the knife.
   Remedy: a. Trim the edges so that they are parallel.
   b. Move block along knife or sharpen knife.
9. Fault: Sections curl as they are cut.
   Cause: a. A blunt knife.
   b. Sections too thick.
   c. Too much tilt on knife.

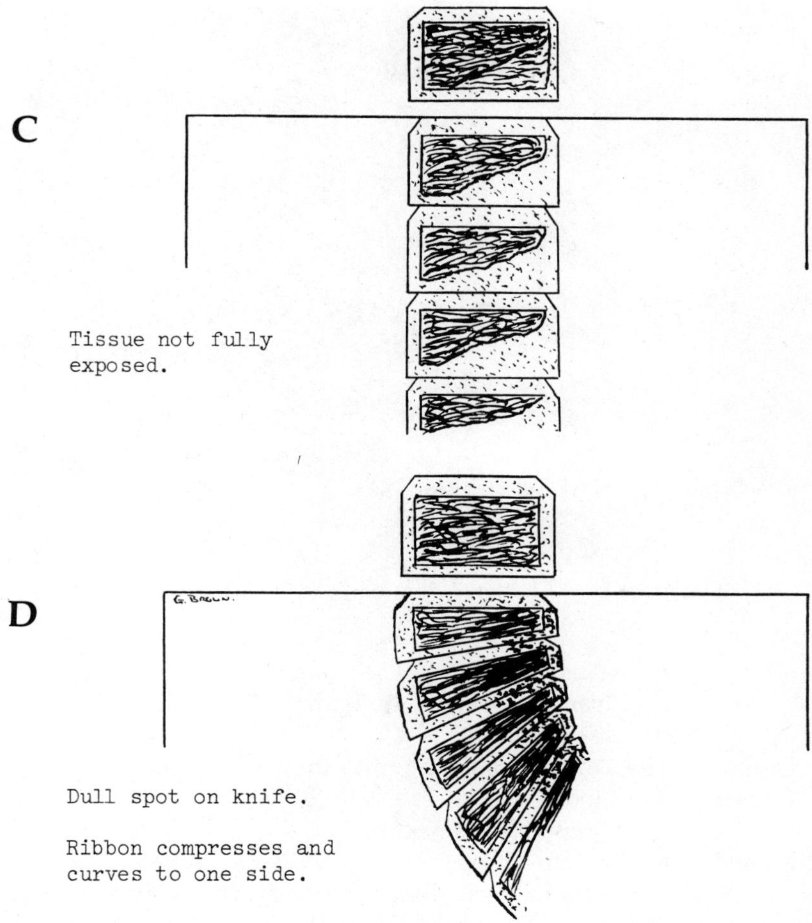

Figure 9-7. **C.** Tissue not fully exposed. **D.** Dull spot on knife. The ribbon is compressed at one end and curves to one side.

Remedy: a. Sharpen the knife.
b. Cut thinner sections.
c. Adjust the tilt.

10. Fault: Section lifts from knife on upward travel of block.
Cause: a. A blunt knife.
b. Too much tilt on knife.
c. A build-up of wax debris behind the knife.
d. A greasy knife.
Remedy: a. Sharpen the knife.

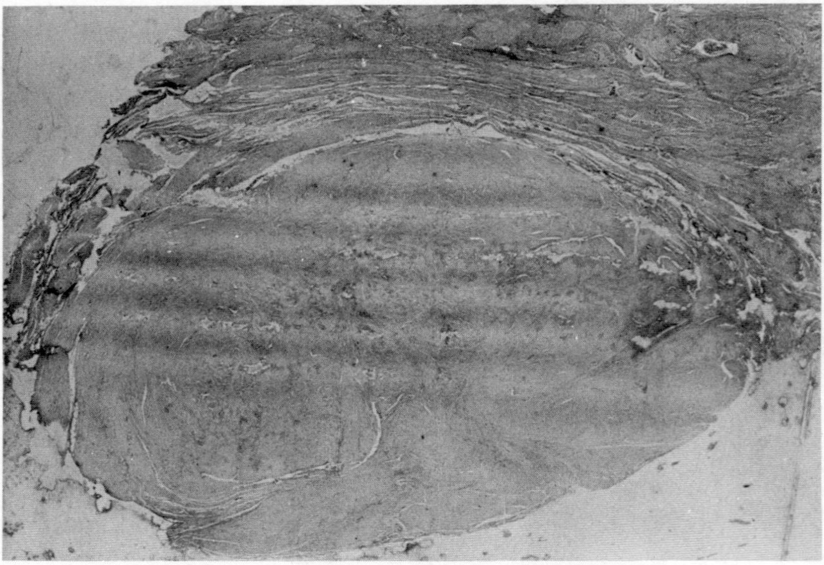

Figure 9-8. "Chatters" due to a loose block or knife.

b. Adjust the tilt.
c. Clean the back of the knife.
d. Clean the knife.

11. Fault: The knife bites deeply into the block.
    Cause: a. A loose knife.
    b. A loose block.
    Remedy: a. Tighten knife.
    b. Tighten block. Block may be coming free of object holder. Remount. If badly gouged the tissue may require reorientating and re-embedding.
12. Fault: The block no longer feeds towards the knife.
    Cause: The forward feed mechanism has expired.
    Remedy: Release the safety locking catch. Manually back off the feed mechanism and readjust the knife holder.

FAULTS DUE TO POOR PROCESSING

1. Fault: On trimming, the tissue smells of clearing agent.
   Cause: The clearing agent has not been completely removed from the tissue due to insufficient time for complete infiltration.
   Remedy: Reinfiltrate and re-embed.

2. Fault: The tissue is shrunken away from the wax.
   Cause: Insufficient dehydration.
   Remedy: Reprocess the tissue.
3. Fault: The tissue is quite soft when the block is trimmed.
   Cause: Insufficient fixation.
   Remedy: Reprocess the tissue.
4. Fault: The tissue appears full of holes.
   Cause: Insufficient infiltration.
   Remedy: Reinfiltrate and re-embed the tissue.
5. Fault: On trimming, the wax appears crystalline.
   Cause: a. Contaminated wax.
   b. Block not cooled rapidly enough.
   Remedy: a. Reinfiltrate and re-embed in fresh wax.
   b. Re-embed and cool rapidly.
6. Fault: On sectioning, the tissue compresses but the wax does not.
   Cause: Insufficient infiltration.
   Remedy: Reinfiltrate the tissue and re-embed.
7. Fault: Specimen crumbles and drops out of the wax leaving a rim of wax as a section.
   Cause: a. Insufficient infiltration.
   b. Overheated paraffin bath causing tissue to become hard and brittle.
   Remedy: a. Reinfiltrate and re-embed.
   b. Service the paraffin bath and replace if necessary. Reprocess the tissue or embed in a harder wax.
8. Fault: Sections crumple instead of flattening on the waterbath.
   Cause: Insufficient infiltration.
   Remedy: Reinfiltrate and re-embed.
9. Fault: Tissue is dried out and mummified.
   Cause: Mechanical failure of the tissue processing machine or a basket was out of balance and hung up.
   Remedy[1]: Place the specimens in the following rehydration solution for 18–24 hours:

Sodium carbonate*	1.0 g
Distilled water	70.0 ml
Absolute ethyl alcohol	30.0 ml

The rehydrated tissue can then be reprocessed in the same manner as normal fixed tissue. There is minimal loss of nuclear detail and slight tissue distortion.

* The original formula called for 5 g of sodium carbonate.

Adhesives

Properly dried sections will normally adhere to slides securely, but when they do not, it is usually because the slide was not clean and grease free, or there were air bubbles trapped under the section. Some staining techniques employ reagents, usually strong alkalis, which will cause the sections to lift off of the slide. It is advisable therefore, to employ some form of adhesive to ensure that the section will be securely attached to the slide. These adhesives are used either as additives to the water bath or smeared thinly on the surface of the slide. Sections are picked up, drained, and dried in the normal way.

A few of the more common adhesives are:

Agar

Agar, granular	5 g
Distilled water	2000 ml

Dissolve with heat and add a few crystals of thymol to prevent the growth of molds.

For use: Add 50 ml of melted agar to the water bath.

Gelatin

Solution A

Gelatin	1 g
Distilled water	100 ml
Glycerol	15 ml
Phenol crystals	2 g

Dissolve the gelatin in the distilled water and add the glycerol and phenol crystals. The phenol is added to prevent the growth of molds.

For use: Smear thinly onto slides and dip into 2 percent formalin. Mount sections in the usual way and dry.

Solution B

Gelatin	5 g
Distilled water	100 ml

Dissolve the gelatin in the water and add a few crystals of thymol to prevent the growth of molds.

For use: Add approximately 30 ml of melted gelatin to the water bath. Mount sections in the usual way and dry.

Glycerin and Albumen

This is probably the most popular of the adhesives in routine use. It is easy to make (but more convenient and relatively inexpensive if purchased from commercial sources):

Fresh egg whites	50 ml
Glycerol	50 ml

Beat and stir the egg whites and add the glycerol. Filter, in a moist atmosphere, through coarse filter paper or several thicknesses of butter muslin. Add a few crystals of thymol to prevent the growth of molds.

For use: Smear thinly on slides. Mount sections in the usual way and dry. Do not apply too much to the slide.

Plasma

Sterile plasma is an excellent adhesive and is readily available from out-of-date bottles of blood in the blood bank. It should be dispensed into sterile tubes in amounts of 0.5 ml.

For use: Smear thinly onto slides. Mount sections in the usual way and dry. Do not apply too heavily to the slide as it is readily eosinophilic and will leave a messy smear on the slide.

Starch Paste

Powdered starch	1 g
Distilled water	30 ml
N/1 Hydrochloric acid	2 drops

Mix the starch into a smooth paste in 10 ml of distilled water and add to 20 ml of boiling water. Add the hydrochloric acid and boil for 5 minutes with continued stirring. Cool and add a crystal of thymol to prevent the growth of molds.

For use: Smear thinly onto slides. Mount and dry in the usual way.

Tissue Bond*

For use: Smear thinly onto slides. Mount and dry in the usual way.

Tissue-Tac†

For use: Smear thinly onto slides. Mount and dry in the usual way.

REFERENCE

1. Zimmerman MR: Rehydration of accidentally desiccated pathology specimens. Lab Med 7:13–17, 1976.

BIBLIOGRAPHY

Culling CFA: Handbook of Histopathological and Histochemical Techniques, 3rd ed., Butterworth, London, 1974

Steedman, HF: Section Cutting in Microscopy. Blackwell, Oxford, 1960

* Harleco.

† Dade.

TEN

Special Procedures and Techniques

Certain procedures and tissue specimens need to be handled with extra care and separated from the general run of processing and sectioning, regardless of whether they be surgical specimens, autopsy tissues, or research material. Specimens and requests falling into this category are:

1. Serial sections
2. Step sections
3. Bone marrow biopsies
4. Muscle biopsies
5. Rectal biopsies
6. Renal biopsies
7. Eyes
8. Tissue for electron microscopy

Serial Sections

Serial sections are requested when it is desired to study each section through the block. This may be to study the track of a nerve or to locate and study the extent of a minute lesion in the tissue.

In serial sectioning, every section through the entire block must be saved and mounted. If the request for serial sections is made prior to any sections having been cut, then the surface of the block is not trimmed. Sections are collected from the very first cut that includes any tissue, no matter how small it may be, and continued through the block until no more tissue is left.

Often the request for serial sections is made after a section has been cut and examined. When this happens, the block is carefully placed in the chuck and reorientated to match as closely as possible its original cutting position. All of the sections cut from this point are collected, no matter if they are not complete, and the sectioning is continued through the entire block.

Sections should be collected in ribbons of ten and laid out in strict sequence: 1–10, 11–20, 21–30, until the entire block has been cut. If possible the sections should be laid out on sheets of matt black paper, obtainable from art supply stores or the x-ray department, and covered to protect them from dust and drafts. Cardboard lids from empty boxes are suitable for this purpose. Alternatively they may be collected into empty slide boxes.

After sectioning, the ribbon is divided and mounted onto slides in the same sequence. The number of sections per slide depends on how large the sections are. Care must be taken to ensure that the sections run in the same direction on each slide. If a section is lost a space must be left where it should have been.

When stained, the sections should be labeled clearly, care being taken to ensure that the correct sequence is maintained. The numbers may be written on the coverglass with India ink if a series of sections are mounted on a single slide.

Step Sections

Step sections may be requested as an alternative to serial sections, and for the same reasons. This means that sections are taken at periodic levels through the block. The request is usually made for every nth section for a total of o sections, or for sections at $x\mu$ levels for a total of y sections. The request may also ask that the intermediate sections be saved for further studies. If the intermediate sections are not saved, it is advisable to collect and save the section on either side of each of the step sections for possible requests for special stains at that level.

The level of each step section should be noted on the slide as it is mounted, but care must be taken to ensure that the exact sequence of the steps is maintained. Small sections can be mounted in series on a single slide with the same precautions against disruption of the series.

Bone Marrow Biopsies

Bone marrow biopsies are small plugs of bone approximately 1 cm in length and 2 mm in diameter, consisting of both cortical and cancellous bone. They should be placed into 10 percent neutralized or buffered formalin immediately and left for a minimum of 2–4 hours to fix. There is usually some urgency in getting the sections completed for reporting, and the subsequent procedures are determined by the suspected diagnosis and which special stains may be required. The cooperation of the attending physician in making a notation of the time that the biopsy was taken can prove to be extremely helpful to the laboratory. Specimens taken before 10 A.M. can often be processed that same evening with the routine surgical blocks.

If the specimen is taken early in the morning and delivered promptly to the laboratory, processing of the biopsy can be started almost immediately. Fixation should be complete within 4 hours, although this may be accelerated by warming the container with the fixative and specimen in it in an oven or water bath at 37–45 C. After fixation the specimen is transferred to a decalcifying agent. It can be very advantageous if the decalcifying agent selected is one that does not require washing out of the specimen prior to processing. This will save time. Decalcification of such a small specimen should be complete in 2–3 hours, and it will be ready to process with the surgical specimens on the overnight schedule.

Specimens taken later in the day must be left in fixative overnight and processed the following day. First thing in the morning the biopsies are transferred to the decalcifying agent for 2–3 hours. This should be enough time for complete decalcification, but it must be remembered that this could be dependent upon the amount of dense cortical bone present in the plug.

After decalcification is complete the biopsy is processed on the two-hour schedule of the Ultra-Technicon, or by hand, using the following times:

Hand Processing		**Ultra-Technicon**	
1. 50% Ethyl alcohol	15 min	1. 50% Ethyl alcohol	10 min
2. 70% Ethyl alcohol	15 min	2. 70% Ethyl alcohol	10 min
3. 80% Ethyl alcohol	15 min	3. 80% Ethyl alcohol	10 min
4. 95% Ethyl alcohol	15 min	4. 95% Ethyl alcohol	10 min
5. Absolute alcohol	15 min	5. Absolute alcohol	10 min
6. Absolute alcohol	15 min	6. Absolute alcohol	10 min
7. Absolute alcohol	15 min	7. Absolute alcohol	10 min
8. Xylene	10 min	8. Xylene	10 min
9. Xylene	10 min	9. Xylene	10 min

10. Xylene	10 min	10. Xylene	10 min
11. Paraplast	15 min	11. Paraplast	10 min
12. Paraplast	15 min	12. Paraplast	15 min

Embed in filtered Paraplast and cool the block rapidly.

Sections should be taken at 4μ and stained by the following techniques:

1. Hematoxylin and eosin
2. Giemsa
3. Perls' method for hemosiderin
4. Reticulin
5. Periodic acid Schiff reaction (PAS)
6. Trichrome (sometimes requested)

If the suspected diagnosis is such that a request for the Naphthol ASD Chloroacetate-Esterase technique is made, then the biopsy cannot be decalcified with the usual acid decalcifying agents. Decalcification is achieved by using the EDTA (ethylene-diamine-tetra-acetic acid) technique. This is very effective for cancellous bone, but is not as effective on the cortical bone. The well-fixed biopsy is placed into a 7 percent solution of EDTA with the pH adjusted to 7.2. The pH may be raised to 7.2 by adding ammonium hydroxide a few drops at a time, or lowered to 7.2 by adding a few drops of 0.1 percent hydrochloric acid a few drops at a time. Complete decalcification of the biopsy will take from 1–2 days, depending upon the amount of dense cortical bone present. Upon completion of decalcification, the biopsy is processed on the Ultra-Technicon using the two-hour schedule.

Bone marrow aspirations may also be blocked and sectioned. These are especially useful for the NASD method, as no decalcification is required.

After the required smears have been made, the remainder of the marrow aspirate should be squirted from the syringe into a small bottle containing 10 percent neutral buffered formalin. Upon reaching the laboratory it is filtered through an embedding bag.* The blood and formalin will pass through leaving the marrow aspirate inside the bag, which is folded and placed in a tissue cassette and processed with the regular surgical specimens or on the Ultra-Technicon with the bone marrow biopsy.

The residue in the bottom of the embedding bag is scraped out and embedded in the usual manner.

* Obtainable from Curtin Matheson Scientific Co.

Muscle Biopsies

Muscle biopsies should be transported to the laboratory in a muscle biopsy clamp (Isometric clamp) to prevent the artifactual contraction of the muscle when it is placed into a fixative. If a clamp is not available the biopsy may be placed onto a cotton-gauze sponge moistened with saline, laid on a piece of white card and covered with a moist sponge, or pinned onto a piece of tongue depressor and covered with a moist sponge. The specimen should be left for 15–30 minutes at room temperature before it is placed into fixative.

Suitable fixatives for normal histological procedures are:

1. 10 percent neutral formalin
2. Bouin's fluid
3. Zenker's fluid

A portion of the biopsy is cut transversely from one end of the biopsy and the two portions are processed on the Ultra-Technicon using the two-hour cycle. Both portions of tissue are embedded in the same block and orientated so that on sectioning both a longitudinal and a transverse section are obtained. They should be stained by:

1. Hematoxylin and eosin
2. A trichrome method
3. Phosphotungstic acid hematoxylin (PTAH)

Specimens for electron microscopy should be placed into 3 percent buffered glutaraldehyde for overnight fixation, and those for enzyme studies should be frozen immediately on removal. Rapid freezing in isopentane and liquid nitrogen is recommended.

Rectal Biopsies

The major problems in the handling of rectal biopsies are due to the contraction or shrinkage of the specimen during fixation and processing, and in the correct orientation of the specimen during embedding. When a specimen as small as a rectal biopsy is distorted due to shrinkage and completely saturated and covered with molten paraffin, it is almost impossible to orientate it with complete accuracy. It is imperative that these specimens be orientated correctly so that sections will be cut in a longitudinal plain through the villi and include the mucosa, sub-mucosa, and muscle.

We have found that if the biopsy is orientated correctly on a small portion of absorbable gelatin sponge (Gelfoam) by the physician performing the biopsy prior to fixation and processing, then the desired sections may be obtained with ease. The foam with the specimen on it is embedded on edge and sectioned with the tissue. Gelfoam does not cause the technical problems in sectioning that are associated with paper or cotton gauze.

Rectal biopsies, once positioned on the Gelfoam, may be processed on the overnight schedule with the regular surgical specimens or with the shorter schedules on the Ultra-Technicon.

Renal Biopsies

Renal biopsies, needle biopsies of kidney, may be handled in several ways, depending upon the preference of the pathologist. Frequently one portion is taken for electron microscopy, another is taken for immunofluorescence studies, and the remainder, or another core, is sent to the histology laboratory for thin (2μ) paraffin sections.

Fixation of the renal biopsy is a matter of choice, and several fixatives are suitable. Those most frequently employed are:

1. 10 percent neutral buffered formalin
2. Formol sublimate (formol corrosive)
3. Bouin's fluid*
4. 4 percent glutaraldehyde
5. 4 percent paraformaldehyde in 0.1M cacodylate, pH 7.3

The tissue is collected into Bouin's fluid and left for two hours. It is then transferred to 10 percent formalin in 70 percent alcohol and kept overnight for processing in the morning. Specimens may be kept over the weekend in this solution. The processing schedule is as follows[1]:

Hand Processing		**Ultra-Technicon**	
1. 70% Ethyl alcohol	15 min	1. 70% Ethyl alcohol	10 min
2. 80% Ethyl alcohol	15 min	2. 80% Ethyl alcohol	10 min
3. 95% Ethyl alcohol	15 min	3. 95% Ethyl alcohol	10 min
4. 95% Ethyl alcohol	15 min	4. 95% Ethyl alcohol	10 min
5. Absolute alcohol	15 min	5. Absolute alcohol	10 min
6. Absolute alcohol	15 min	6. Absolute alcohol	10 min
7. Absolute alcohol	15 min	7. Absolute alcohol	10 min
8. Xylene†	10 min	8. Xylene†	10 min
9. Xylene	10 min	9. Xylene	10 min
10. Xylene	10 min	10. Xylene	10 min
11. Paraplast	15 min	11. Paraplast	10 min
12. Paraplast	15 min	12. Paraplast	15 min
13. Embed in filtered paraplast.		13. Embed in filtered paraplast.	

* Although Bouin's fluid is not recommended as a fixative for kidney, it is the solution being employed in this institution for fixing renal biopsies. The slight distortion caused by this fixative is more than compensated for in the brilliant staining results.

† It has been stated that if the tissue is cleared in benzene, impregnated in molten diethylene glycol distearate (Digol distearate) overnight at 60 C, placed into fresh molten DGD at 60 C for one hour, and embedded in paraffin wax, then sections may be cut consistently at 1μ.[2]

After embedding it is advisable to trim any excess wax from around the tissue, especially at the ends of the core. The use of a shaped mold such as those supplied by PEEL-A-WAY* will help to eliminate this chore.

The essentials for cutting sections at 2μ are: an extremely sharp knife, a well-maintained microtome, technical skill, and patience. The first sections taken should be examined unstained for the presence of glomeruli, and when they are located at least fifteen sections should be taken from each block. Sections must be cut extremely slowly and with a very smooth action if consistently thin sections are to be obtained. A jerky, uneven cutting action will result in thick and thin sections. Compression of the sections should be less than 30 percent, a fault which may be equally the result of too rapid a cutting action as the use of a dull knife.

Three sections from each level should be stained by:

1. Hematoxylin and eosin
2. A trichrome method for connective tissue
3. Periodic acid—methenamine silver for basement membranes

Eyes[3]

The entire eye should be placed into 20–25 times its own volume of 10 percent neutral buffered formalin as soon as possible after its removal. Complete fixation will take from 48–72 hours. The practice of cutting windows in the globe, or of injecting the fixative into it is poor technique and should be discouraged. When fixation is complete the eye should be transferred to running water for 8–24 hours to wash out the fixative. It is then placed into 60 percent alcohol for 8–24 hours, or until ready for gross examination and cutting the portion for processing. The 60 percent alcohol will restore much of the natural color to the specimen, and besides being the first step in dehydration, is an excellent storage solution.

If calcified material is present, then the specimen (the portion taken for processing or in some cases the whole eye) must be decalcified. The decalcifying solution of choice is equal parts of 20 percent sodium citrate and 45 percent Formic acid. Following decalcification the specimen must be washed for 24 hours in running water to remove the decalcifying solution.

The eye should be cut in the horizontal plane starting several millimeters on either side of the optic nerve. The central portion taken for processing should contain the pupil, lens, optic nerve, and any site

* Available from PEEL-A-WAY Scientific, South El Monte, California.

having gross abnormalities. This portion is placed into a suitable tissue capsule, the Thomas* tissue capsule which is $1\frac{1}{8}$-inch square and 7/16-inch deep with a fitted sliding cover is ideal in most instances, and put into 80 percent alcohol to await processing. This is the second step in dehydration. The specimen may be processed either manually or on the automatic tissue processor with an overnight schedule.

The processing schedules are as follows:

Autotechnicon		Manual Processing (Small Pieces)	
1. 95% Ethyl alcohol	3 hr	1. 95% Ethyl alcohol	Overnight
2. 95% Ethyl alcohol	1 hr	2. 95% Ethyl alcohol	2 hr
3. 95% Ethyl alcohol	1 hr	3. 95% Ethyl alcohol	1 hr
4. Absolute alcohol	1 hr	4. Absolute alcohol	1 hr
5. Absolute alcohol	1 hr	5. Absolute alcohol	1 hr
6. Absolute alcohol	1 hr	6. Absolute alcohol	2 hr
7. Chloroform[a]	1 hr	7. Chloroform	1 hr
8. Chloroform	2 hr	8. Chloroform	Overnight
9. Bioloid[b]	1 hr	9. Bioloid	1 hr
10. Bioloid	1 hr	10. Bioloid	2 hr
11. Bioloid	2 hr	11. Bioloid	2 hr
12. Bioloid, under vacuum	45 min	12. Bioloid, under vacuum	45 min

Embed in Bioloid using normal embedding techniques.

[a] Toluene may be substituted for chloroform with no adverse affects.
[b] Bioloid is available from VWR Scientific.

Manual Processing (Large Pieces)	
1. 95% Ethyl alcohol	1 hr
2. 95% Ethyl alcohol	1 hr
3. 95% Ethyl alcohol	Overnight
4. Absolute alcohol	2 hr
5. Absolute alcohol	2 hr
6. Absolute alcohol	1 hr
7. Chloroform	1 hr
8. Chloroform	Overnight
9. Bioloid	2 hr
10. Bioloid	2 hr
11. Bioloid	2 hr
12. Bioloid, under vacuum	45 min

Embed in Bioloid using normal embedding techniques.

* Available from Arthur H. Thomas Co., Philadelphia, Pennsylvania.

The block should be placed in the chuck of the microtome with the cornea and optic nerve to the side, and with the sides (sclera) of the eye to the top and bottom, parallel to the knife. Start to trim the block carefully, orientating as necessary, until a full section through the pupil, optic nerve, and any suspected abnormality is obtained. With the block still on the microtome, soak the exposed tissue with a piece of cotton or other absorbent material soaked with warm water. This soaking softens the lens and vitreous, thus minimizing any tearing during sectioning. Chill both the block and the knife with an ice cube and cut sections at 8μ with a slow steady motion. Short ribbons of sections are floated onto distilled water at room temperature where they are separated. Individual sections are then picked up on a large slide and floated onto a second flotation bath maintained at 56 C and containing a gelatin adhesive; approximately 15 ml of 5 percent gelatin per 1000 ml of water. The temperature in this flotation bath is approximately ten degrees higher than that used in general histology. Each section is stretched to conform to its original shape and size, and with practice a section conforming to the exact shape of the eye can be obtained. The sections are picked up onto slides of suitable dimensions, drained of excess water, and dried overnight on a hotplate at approximately 45 C.

After use the water bath must be thoroughly cleaned with detergent to remove all traces of gelatin. This helps to prevent the growth of bacteria and thus contaminating the sections.

Sections should be stained by the following methods:

1. Hematoxylin and eosin
2. Periodic acid Schiff (P.A.S.)
3. Special stains as required

Tissue for Electron Microscopy

Tissue for electron microscopy should be collected into 4–6 percent glutaraldehyde in either a phosphate buffer of pH 7.6 or a cacodylate buffer of pH 7.2–7.4 for 2–24 hours at 4 C:

Glutaraldehyde in Phosphate Buffer

Stock glutaraldehyde (25%)*	1 volume
Phosphate buffer, pH 7.6	3 volumes

* Stock glutaraldehyde should be discarded if the pH falls to 3.5 or lower.

Glutaraldehyde in Cacodylate Buffer

Stock glutaraldehyde (25%)*	20 ml
0.2M Sodium cacodylate $(CH_3)_2AsO_2Na \cdot 3H_2O$†	33 ml
Distilled water	47 ml

Other fixatives which are suitable for electron microscopy are:

1. 10 percent formalin in cacodylate buffer, pH 7.2–7.4
2. Luft's fixative: 0.6 percent potassium permanganate in veronal acetate buffer, pH 7.2–7.4
3. Palade's fixative: 2 percent osmic acid in veronal acetate buffer, pH 7.4
4. 4 percent paraformaldehyde in cacodylate buffer, pH 7.3

Following fixation in glutaraldehyde the tissues may be washed and stored indefinitely in a sucrose cacodylate buffer (7 percent sucrose in 0.2M sodium cacodylate), or processed immediately into blocks. This tissue is frequently subjected to postosmication in Palade's fixative to fix lipids that might otherwise be removed during dehydration.

There are many variations in the methods used to process tissue for electron microscopy with many different formulas for the embedding resins, and the reader should refer to the pertinent literature on techniques for electron microscopy for more detailed information. The method given below is one that I have found to be reliable:

1. Dice a small piece of tissue into 1 mm cubes in a pool of fixative on a sheet of dental wax or a paraffin wax block. The tissue must be kept in the fixative at all times. A new, grease-free razor blade should be used to cut the tissue rather than scalpel blade, and the motion should be a slicing action rather than chopping. Chopping tends to crush the tissue.
2. Transfer the diced tissue to a bottle of fixative by lifting the cubes on strips of filter paper. Fix for 2–24 hours at 4 C.
3. Wash in several changes of buffer solution.
4. Wash in several changes of distilled water.
5. Postosmicate in Palade's fixative for 2 hours at 4 C.

Palade's Fixative

A. Veronal acetate buffer, pH 9.6		2 volumes
Sodium barbitol	14.7 g	
Sodium acetate	9.7 g	
Distilled water to make	500.0 ml	

† 42.78 g per liter of distilled water.

B. 0.1N hydrochloric acid	2 volumes
C. Distilled water	1 volume
D. 4 percent osmic acid, aq.	5 volumes

The pH of this solution should be adjusted to 7.4. Some laboratories add 0.2 g sucrose per 4 ml of solution, which is then known as Caulfield's fixative.

6. Wash in several changes of distilled water.
7. 50 percent alcohol for 15 minutes.
8. 70 percent alcohol, 2 changes of 15 minutes each.
9. 90 percent alcohol, 2 changes of 15 minutes each.
10. 95 percent alcohol for 15 minutes.
11. Absolute alcohol, 2 changes of 15 minutes each. It is very important that this last change of alcohol is absolute.
12. Propylene oxide, 2 changes of 30 minutes each.
    Note. All of the dehydrating fluids should be removed from the bottle of tissue with a pipette and not decanted off. Minute cubes of tissue are easily lost when decanting.
13. Propylene oxide and resin in equal parts, 30 minutes.

Resin

Araldite 502	5.0 ml
Epon 812	32.5 ml
DDSA (dodecenyl succinic anhydride)	67.5 ml
DMP 30 (tridimethyl amino methyl phenol)	3.0 ml

Mix thoroughly for 2–5 minutes, avoid the formation of bubbles as much as possible.

14. Resin for 30 minutes.
15. Embed in resin and polymerize overnight at 60 C. Fill a BEEM capsule,* into which the identifying label has been placed, with resin. Add one piece of tissue to each capsule and allow it to sink to the bottom. Tissue may be centered with a straightened paperclip or an applicator stick.
    Note. Do not pour resinous mixtures down the sink.

Sections for electron microscopy are cut on special microtomes (Fig. 1) which have been specifically developed for ultramicrotomy, and require the use of glass or diamond knives.

Three examples of these ultramicrotomes are:

1. The Porter-Blum Ultramicrotome
2. The LKB Ultratome
3. The Cambridge Huxley Ultramicrotome

* Available from Ladd Research Ind. Inc., Burlington, Vermont.

Sectioning in ultramicrotomy requires a great deal of skill and practice and the techniques will not be discussed. Readers are referred to the pertinent literature on the subject. However, some knowledge of the end results is desirable.

Sections are cut in two thicknesses or grades, thick sections and thin sections. The thick sections are 1μ–2μ in thickness and are used to identify tissues and blocks for thin sectioning. Thick sections may be

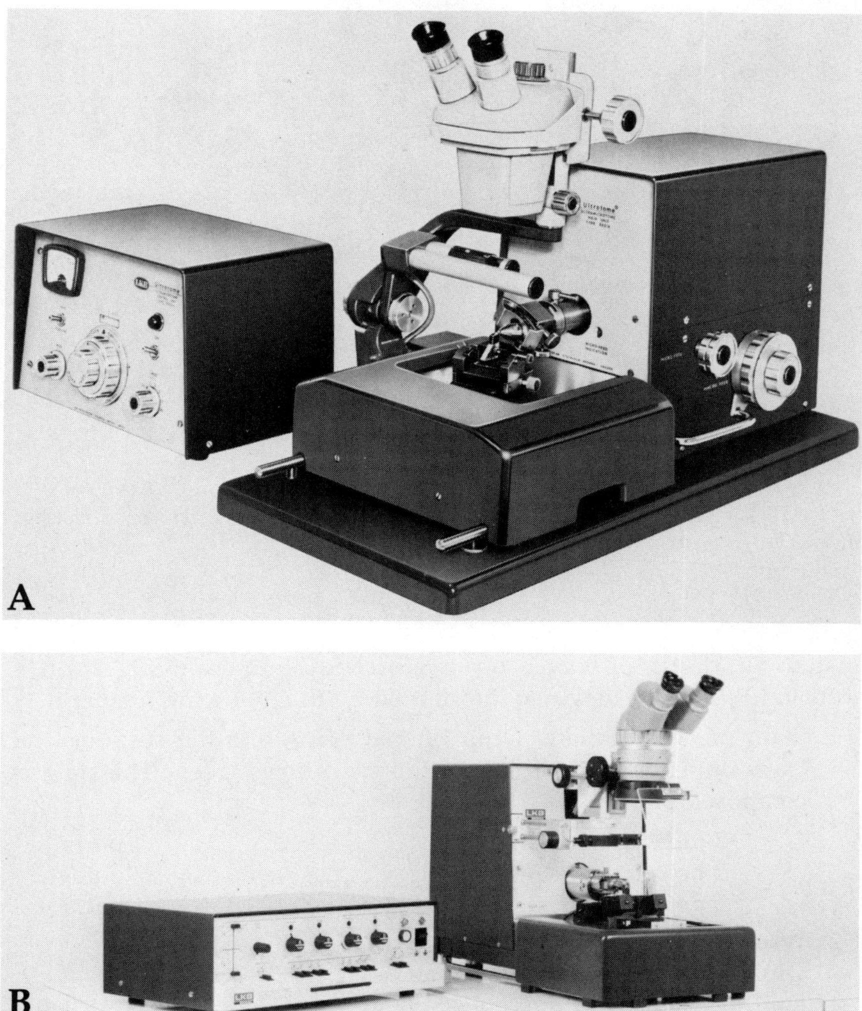

Figure 10-1. **A.** LKB ULTROTOME III. **B.** LKB ULTROTME IV. (*Courtesy of LKB Instruments Inc., Rockville, Md.*)

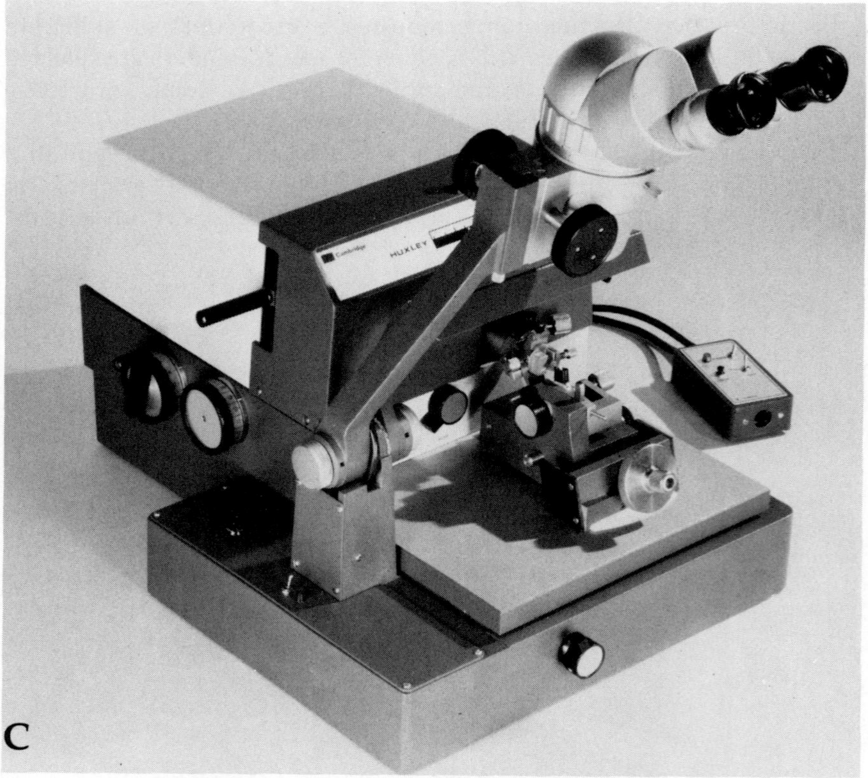

Figure 10-1. **C.** Cambridge HUXLEY Ultramicrotome. (*Courtesy of Cambridge Medical Instruments Ltd., Cambridge, England.*)

floated on drops of water on microscope slides and dried on a hotplate. When dry they may be stained by the following method:

1. Stain on the hotplate. Drop filtered stain onto the sections and leave until the edge of the pool of stain turns green. The stain is composed of:

2 percent toluidine blue	2 parts
2 percent borax	2 parts
1 percent pyronin	1 part

2. Wash by dipping into two changes of distilled water.
3. Dip into 70 percent ethyl alcohol.
4. Dip into 95 percent ethyl alcohol.
5. Dip into absolute ethyl alcohol.
6. Air dry and mount with balsam.

Thin sections are cut in the range of 500–1000 Angstroms (Å)* and may be referred to as gold or silver sections. They are picked up onto special grids for staining.

REFERENCES

1. Sugulas M: Technical procedures and staining methods for renal needle biopsies. Am J Med Technol 42:220–24, 1976
2. Moores BD: Thin histological sections from tissues impregnated with digol distearate. Med Lab Sci 33:73–77, 1976
3. Prophet E: Technique for processing eye specimens. Histo-Logic 6:1 (Lab-Tek Products, Naperville, Ill.), 1976

BIBLIOGRAPHY

Cancilla PA: Technique of muscle biopsy and staining methods with particular emphasis on commonly encountered artefacts. In Pearson CM, Mostofi FK (Eds): The Striated Muscle. Baltimore, Williams & Wilkins, 1973

Griffin RL: Ultramicrotomy. London, Bailliere Tindall, 1972

* *Note*. 1 Å = 1/10 millimicron = 1/10,000 micron; 10 Å = 1/1000 micron; 500 Å = 1/20 micron; 1000 Å = 1/10 micron.

ELEVEN

Preparing Sections for Staining and Mounting

The Staining Area

Certain essentials are required for a properly set up staining area. Ideally, a separate room should be set aside for staining, but this is all too frequently a physical impossibility. At least one bench should be kept solely for staining. Both the bench and the room must be equipped with basic plumbing and furniture requirements.

The staining bench should be at least 8-feet long, 30-inches deep, and three-feet high. Located at one end should be a large shallow sink fitted with two cold water faucets, and hopefully plumbed in deionized water from a central source. Smaller deionizers which can be tapped into the water line at the sink are available on a rental basis. Professional advice should be sought as to the size required as this is dependent upon the consumption. Deionized water is a suitable substitute for distilled water in most circumstances, but a five-gallon container (either glass or plastic) of glass distilled water should be located on a shelf immediately above the staining sink.

The sink should be large enough to accommodate a slide-washing tray and allow sufficient room for waste reagents to be poured down the drain without contaminating the slides. If the sink is too small to allow this, a hollow plug, shorter than the depth of the sink, which has been widened out at the top to form a funnel, will suffice. For laboratories with very small sinks, a bench-top slide-washer* is available which will fill from and drain back into a small sink.

The bench should also be equipped with a gas outlet for a bunsen burner and several electrical outlets. A vacuum connection is a useful accessory.

Above the bench there should be shelves and/or cabinets to hold the stock stains and working solutions, and beneath it should be cupboards and drawers for storing the necessary glassware and equipment. At least one of these cupboards should be lockable and large enough to hold large bottles of reagents such as alcohol and xylene. A small refrigerator may be fitted under the bench or located close by to hold reagents requiring refrigeration.

All stains and reagents should be stored in bottles with either ground glass stoppers or screw caps. Those reagents which must be protected from light should be stored in amber glass or dark glass bottles and kept in a dark cupboard.

The entire staining area must be well lighted.

Equipment

The most important instrument in a well-equipped staining area is the microscope. A binocular model is to be preferred over a monocular microscope. It does not have to be the latest model, but it should have excellent resolution. A 10× eyepiece, a 10× objective, and a 40× objective are essential. If the microscope is fitted with a mechanical stage, this should be removed. The result is a large stage area that allows the slides to be moved around with ease, and it is easily wiped clean and dry after use. If a proper microscope lamp is not available, the light source for the microscope may be supplied with a lamp and a 60-watt bulb.

In addition to the microscope, a water bath is a necessity. A flotation bath is suitable for this purpose. Other items that should be stored at the staining bench in adequate quantities are:

Coplin jars, preferrably with screw caps and square bases (Fig. 1).

Coverglass staining jars (Columbia jars) with screw caps.

Glass "hockey sticks" for manipulating frozen sections. These can be made in the laboratory.

Glass staining dishes, complete with fitted glass covers (Fig. 2).

* Distributed by International Histopathology Cytopathology Laboratories Inc., Middletown, New York.

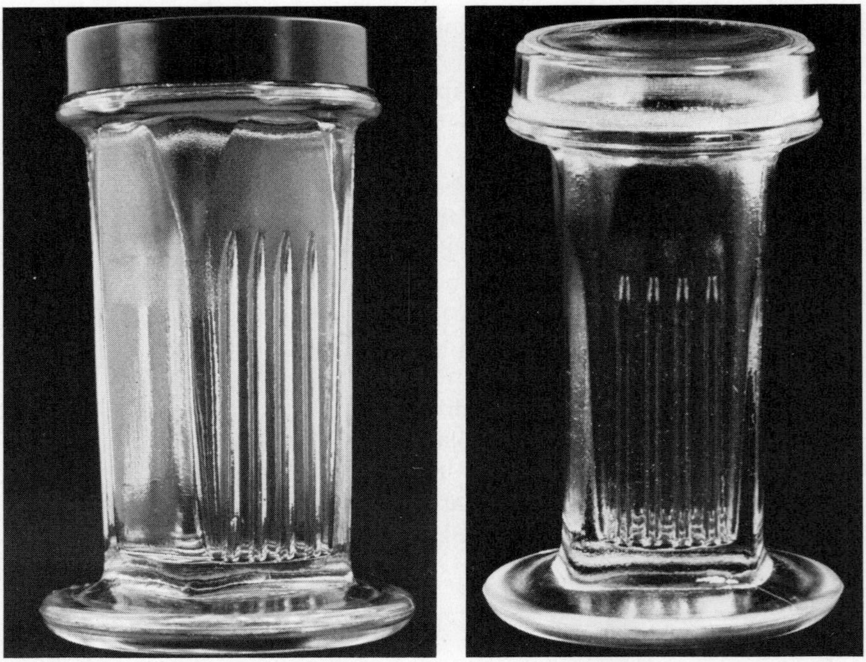

Figure 11-1. Coplin jars. (*Courtesy of Fisher Scientific Co., Pittsburgh, Pa.*)

Three sizes are necessary:
1. $3\frac{3}{4}'' \times 3'' \times 3''$
2. $5'' \times 4'' \times 3''$
3. $8\frac{1}{2}'' \times 4\frac{1}{2}'' \times 3\frac{1}{4}''$

Glass staining jars, vertical, with fitted glass covers (Fig. 3). To hold 10 or 20 slides back to back.
Slide staining racks to fit the staining dishes. Glass and metal racks to hold 10 slides, and metal racks to hold 30 and 50 slides.
Stender dishes for frozen sections (Fig. 4), in three sizes:
1. 37 × 25 mm
2. 48 × 33 mm
3. 62 × 36 mm

Staining rack to fit across the sink.
Thermometers.
Timing clocks.
Plastic forceps* for silver techniques.

* Obtainable from Ernest F. Fullam Inc., Schenectady, New York.

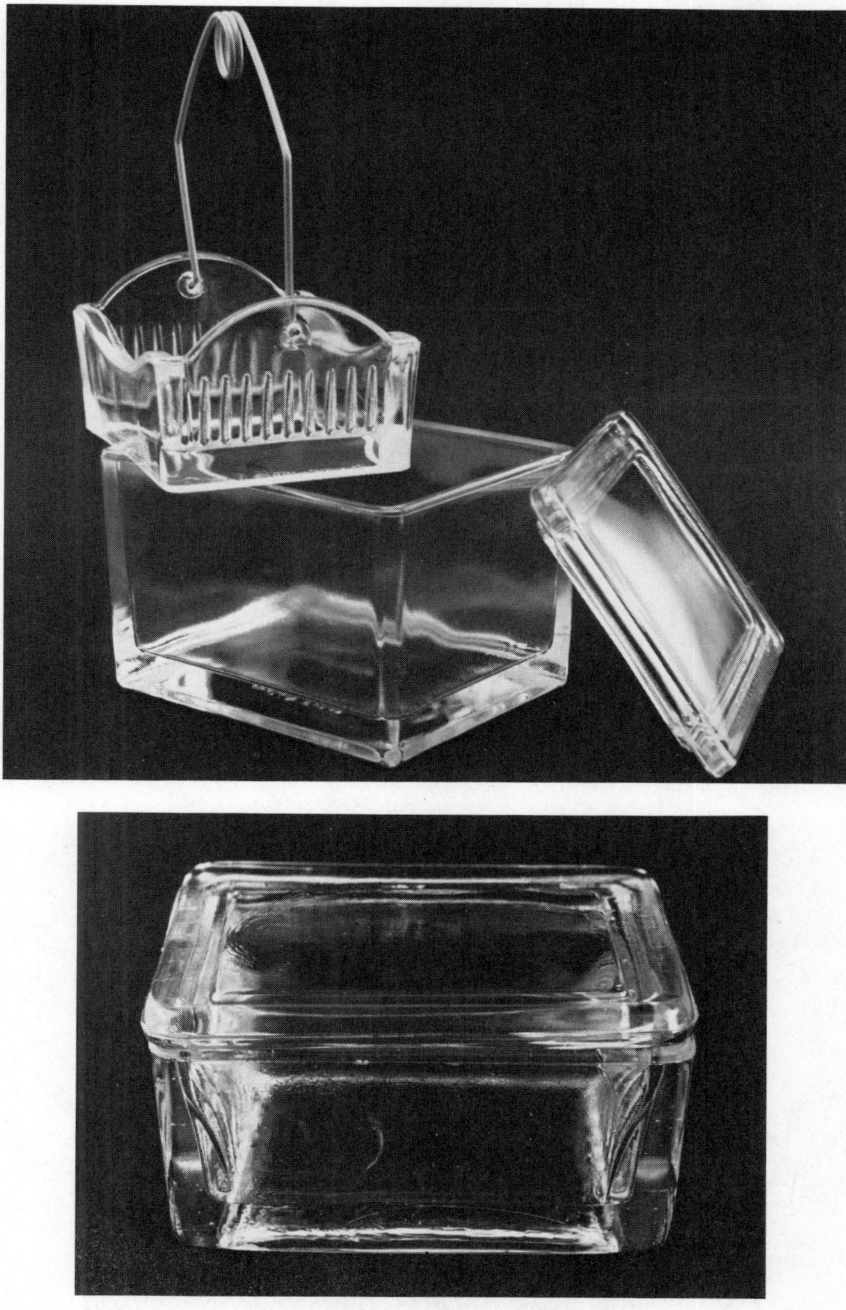

Figure 11-2. Glass staining-jars. (*Courtesy of Fisher Scientific Co., Pittsburgh, Pa.*)

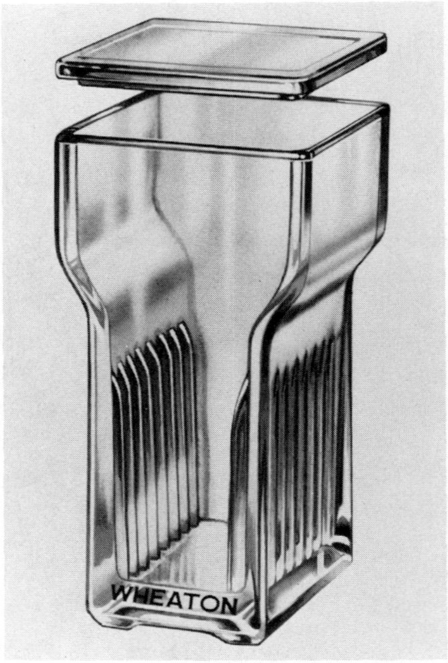

Figure 11-3. Vertical staining-jar. (*Courtesy of Fisher Scientific Co., Pittsburgh, Pa.*)

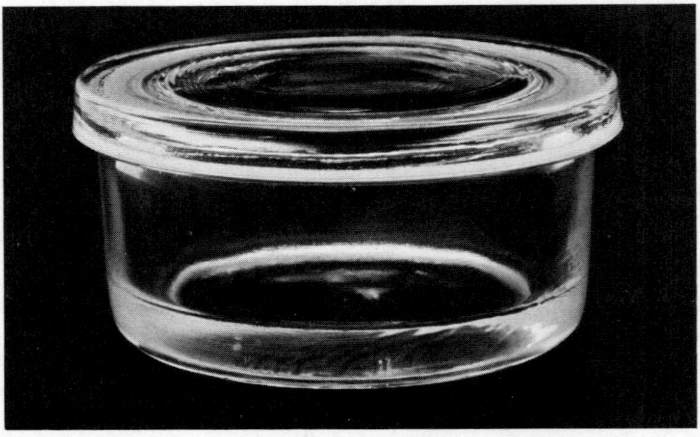

Figure 11-4. Stender dish. (*Courtesy of Fisher Scientific Co., Pittsburgh, Pa.*)

There should also be a plentiful supply of standard laboratory glassware such as beakers, flasks, filter funnels, graduated measuring cylinders, and pipettes, both graduated and dropping.

Preparing for Staining

All paraffin sections must be "deparaffinized" prior to staining, and in the majority of techniques, hydrated. The correct term for the removal of paraffin wax from sections is *decerate*. Throughout this text the phrase "sections to water" will be utilized when deceration and hydration are necessary. When an alcoholic staining solution is to be applied, the sections are decerated and taken through descending grades of alcohol to seventy percent alcohol. In these instances the phrase "sections to alcohol" will apply. These terms will be used in all staining techniques that are described.

The procedure for deceration and hydration is as follows:

1. Xylene	2 minutes
2. Xylene	2 minutes
3. Absolute alcohol	1 minute
4. Absolute alcohol	1 minute
5. 95 percent alcohol	30 seconds
6. 70 percent alcohol	30 seconds
7. Water (tap or distilled)	

Following staining, sections that are to be mounted in a resinous medium such as balsam, or one of the commercial mountants, require dehydrating and clearing. The clearing agent most commonly employed is xylene, although toluene may also be used, because most of the resinous mountants use this as a solvent. The procedure is the reverse of the hydrating process, and in the majority of cases the same times would apply. Sections can be left in the clearing agent, xylene or toluene, until it is convenient to mount them, because these reagents do not extract dyes. Under no circumstances should sections be allowed to stay for too long in alcohol as this may remove some stains.

When a different form of dehydration is to be employed, such as the use of acetone, or blotting the section dry, this will be stated in the method.

In some staining methods the dyes are readily soluble in alcohol and xylene, and the sections are mounted in an aqueous mountant such as glycerin jelly. In these instances the sections are mounted from distilled water.

Occasionally a section will lift or float off of the slide during staining for no apparent reason, and subsequent sections will continue to do this. It may possibly be the tissue, but the cause is much more likely to be that the slides are greasy, or that the sections have not been left in the oven for long enough prior to staining. Sections should be left in the oven at 60 C for 20–30 minutes after cutting, or overnight at 45 C, in order that they may fix and dry thoroughly. If this is not possible they should be fixed in a bunsen flame in the same manner as bacterial smears.

Should none of the above causes be the fault (some staining methods call for the use of a strong alkali in the reaction and this may cause sections to lift), another method must be employed to keep the sections in position during staining. The following method is recommended:

1. Sections to absolute alcohol.
2. Place into equal parts of absolute alcohol and ether for 1 minute.
3. Flood the slide with a thin layer of 0.5 percent celloidin dissolved in equal parts of absolute alcohol and ether. Drain to one end of the slide.
4. Allow the celloidin to harden until it is *just* firm enough to take a fingerprint. Place the section into 70 percent alcohol to harden completely.
5. Wash in water and stain as desired.

After staining, the procedure is reversed as follows:

1. Bring sections from water to absolute alcohol.
2. Place into equal parts of absolute alcohol and ether until the celloidin has dissolved.
3. Place into absolute alcohol for 1 minute.
4. Clear and mount.

Removal of Artifact Pigments

During fixation, tissues can become contaminated with artifact pigments that are deposited in the tissue by the reagents used for fixation. The two most common artifact pigments found in tissue sections are mercuric chloride crystals and formalin pigment. Osmium tetroxide (osmic acid) will also leave a deposit in some instances.

MERCURIC CHLORIDE

All fixatives containing mercuric chloride as a constituent will leave a deposit in the tissue. Some of the pigment may be removed during processing by the addition of iodine to the alcohols, but the remainder must be completely removed from the sections prior to staining. The treatment for the removal of artifact pigments is performed immediately following deceration and hydration. Mercuric chloride crystals are removed from sections by the following procedure:

1. Sections to water.
2. Gram's or Lugol's iodine for 5 minutes.
3. Rinse thoroughly in tap water.
4. 5 percent sodium thiosulfate for 5 minutes.
5. Wash in running water for 5 minutes.
6. Proceed with staining.

FORMALIN

Formalin will frequently leave a deposit in blood-containing and postmortem tissue, especially if fixation has been delayed or the solution is acid. Neutral or buffered formalin is to be preferred as a fixative. The deposit appears as a scattering of brown to black granules or masses throughout the tissue. It may be removed from sections by either of the following methods:

Method A

1. Sections to alcohol.
2. Saturated solution of picric acid in alcohol for 10 minutes.
3. Wash in absolute alcohol to remove the picric acid.
4. Wash in running tap water for 5 minutes.
5. Proceed with staining.

Method B

1. Sections to alcohol.
2. 1 percent sodium hydroxide in absolute alcohol for ten minutes.
3. Wash in absolute alcohol for 2 minutes.
4. Wash in running tap water for 5 minutes.
5. Proceed with staining.

OSMIUM TETROXIDE

Osmium tetroxide deposit cannot be removed from tissue sections with solvents, but it can be bleached out by either of the following methods:

Method A

1. Sections to 70 percent alcohol.
2. Place into the following solution, which should be freshly mixed for use:

Hydrogen peroxide	2 ml
70 percent alcohol	48 ml

3. Leave in bright sunlight for 15 to 30 minutes, or until bleached.
4. Wash in running tap water for 5 minutes.
5. Proceed with staining.

Method B

1. Sections to water.
2. 0.5 percent potassium permanganate for 5 minutes.
3. Wash in water.
4. Place into sulfurous acid until bleached white.
5. Wash in running tap water for 5 minutes.
6. Proceed with staining.

Bleaching Sections for Restaining

Frequently sections tend to fade after prolonged storage. It is then necessary to remove the cover glass, bleach the section, and restain in order to restore its former quality.

When sections have been stored for many years the coverglass is very difficult to remove, a procedure which should be handled very carefully as the section may be mounted on the coverglass. The following method is very effective:

> Gently heat the slide by passing it through a bunsen flame until it is evenly heated. When it is warm enough the mountant will begin to bubble. Gently insert the tip of a scalpel blade or dissecting needle under the edge of the coverglass and lift gently. If the mountant is properly melted the coverglass will lift off cleanly without breaking. Place the section in a jar of xylene to dissolve the remaining mountant.

Slides that have not hardened to this degree may have the coverglass removed by placing the slide in a jar of xylene. The coverglass will eventually slide off. In stubborn cases it is advantageous to warm the xylene in an oven to 60 C and leave the sections for an hour, or as long as may be necessary to remove the coverglass. Once the coverglass is removed the section is left in fresh xylene for 30 minutes to dissolve the residual mountant. The section may now be placed into acid alcohol to bleach or taken through the following procedure:

1. Sections to water.
2. 5 percent potassium permanganate for 5 minutes.
3. Rinse in tap water.
4. 5 percent oxalic acid for 5 minutes, or until the section is bleached white.

5. Wash in running water for 5 minutes.
6. Stain as desired.

Mounting of Sections

After staining and before examination, sections should be mounted under coverglasses (coverslips) to facilitate ease of handling and storage, and to prevent damage to the section.

An acceptable mounting medium must fulfill several criteria:

1. The medium should have a refractive index as close as possible to that of glass, ie, 1.5.
2. It should not cause stains to "bleed" or fade.
3. It should not crack or appear granular on setting.
4. It should dry to a nonsticky consistency and harden relatively quickly.
5. It should not shrink back from the edges of the coverglass.
6. It must be free flowing.
7. It must be free from bubbles.

Mounting media fall into two classifications: aqueous and resinous.

AQUEOUS MOUNTING MEDIA

The aqueous media are used for mounting sections from distilled water where the stain would be decolorized or removed by alcohol and xylene, as would be the case with most of the fat stains (Sudan methods). Some stains, namely methyl violet, tend to bleed into the medium after mounting. This can be avoided by using a potassium acetate gum syrup, Highman's medium, or a fructose syrup. Aqueous mountants require the addition of a bacteriostatic agent such as phenol to prevent the growth of molds.

When the medium has hardened, a permanent seal can be obtained by ringing the coverglass with clear nail polish.

Apathy's Medium (Refractive Index 1.52)

A very useful medium for mounting sections for fluorescent microscopy.

Gum arabic	50 g
Sucrose	50 g
Distilled water	50 ml
Thymol	1 crystal

This medium remains fluid in storage and hardens by evaporation. Store in a well-stoppered bottle.

Farrant's Medium (Refractive Index 1.43)

Gum arabic	50 g
Glycerin	50 ml
Distilled water	50 ml
Sodium merthiolate	0.025 g

This medium remains fluid in storage and is therefore more convenient than glycerin jelly, however, its disadvantage lies in the fact that it takes considerably longer to set. Store in a well-stoppered bottle.

Fructose (Levulose) Syrup (Refractive Index 1.47)

Recommended as a temporary mountant and for special techniques.

Fructose	75 g
Distilled water	25 ml

Glycerin Jelly (Refractive Index 1.47)

An excellent routine mountant for fat stains.

Gelatin	10 g
Distilled water	60 ml
Glycerin	70 ml
Phenol	0.25 g

The gelatin causes this medium to solidify and it must be melted before use. This is easily done by placing it in the oven or a water bath at 60 C some time prior to use. Do not shake or stir the medium during melting as this will produce bubbles that are difficult to remove. Mount sections from warm distilled water.

Highman's Medium (Refractive Index 1.52)

This medium is recommended for use with the metachromatic dyes, especially methyl violet.

Gum arabic	20 g
Sucrose	20 g
Potassium acetate	20 g
Sodium merthiolate	10 ml
Distilled water	40 ml

This medium remains fluid in storage and hardens by evaporation. Store in a well-stoppered bottle.

RESINOUS MOUNTING MEDIA

Resinous mountants are either natural or synthetic resins dissolved in solvents such as benzene, toluene, or xylene. It is advisable to mount sections from the same solvent as that in which the resin is dissolved. Failure to do so may result in the formation of bubbles under the coverglass.

The resinous mountants in common use are:

Canada Balsam (Refractive Index 1.52)

This may be purchased as a ready-made solution of 60 percent resin by weight in xylene, or in the dry form. If it is obtained in the dry form for preparation in the laboratory, it is made up as a 55–70 percent solution in xylene, the viscosity being dependent on personal choice. A few chips of marble in the bottom of the bottle will help reduce acidity.

Coverbond (Refractive Index 1.53)

This is Harleco Synthetic Resin (H.S.R.) dissolved as a 60 percent solution by weight in toluene. It may also be purchased as a dry resin and may be dissolved in toluene or xylene.

DePeX (Refractive Index 1.52)

Gurr's DePeX is a polystyrene resin dissolved as a 20 percent solution in xylene. Because this mountant tends to shrink on hardening it should be added to excess. Overflow is easily removed with a scalpel after drying is complete.

Gurr's Neutral Mounting Medium (Refractive Index 1.51)

This is a mixture of coumarone and other resins as a 76 percent solution in cineol. This mountant is a rather viscous solution.

Histoclad (Refractive Index 1.54)

Clay Adams' Histoclad is a 60 percent solution of a synthetic resin in toluene.

Permount (Refractive Index 1.528)

Fisher's Permount is a 60 percent solution of naphthalene polymer in toluene.

Pro-Texx (Refractive Index 1.495)

Pro-Texx from Lerner Laboratories is a mounting medium of neutral pH and with an antioxidant additive to preserve stain quality. It is soluble in both toluene and xylene.

Technicon Resin (Refractive Index 1.62)

This mountant from the Technicon Corporation is a 60 percent solution of couramone-indene polymer in benzene and xylene in equal parts. It has a tendency to form bubbles on hardening due to the high volatility of benzene.

UVinert (Refractive Index 1.517)
A patented mounting medium that is nonfluorescent from Gurr.

XAM (Refractive Index 1.52)
Gurr's XAM is a maleic polymer with a plasticizer in a 77 percent solution in xylene. It is fairly viscous in consistency. The medium should be added to excess because it tends to shrink on hardening. Any overflow can be easily removed with a scalpel blade after it has set.

A small quantity of mountant should be kept on the bench in a balsam bottle and is dispensed by means of a glass rod. A chip of marble in the bottom of the bottle will help control acidity. The bottle must be kept closed when not in use.

TECHNIQUE FOR MOUNTING SECTIONS

A properly mounted section should present a neat appearance. There should be no excess mountant on or around the coverglass, and no bubbles under it. The usual causes of a messy slide are:

1. Too much mountant.
2. Too thick a mountant that has not spread to the edges of the coverglass. If the mountant is too thick it can be diluted with either toluene or xylene.

Coverglasses used in histopathology are either square or rectangular. Four sizes are normally sufficient for routine use. They are:

22 × 22 mm
22 × 30 mm
22 × 40 mm
22 × 50 mm

Sometimes a coverglass of 24 mm in width is necessary, but it should never overlap the edge of the slide. Coverglasses should preferably be the No. 1 thickness (0.13–0.16 mm), but never more than the No. $1\frac{1}{2}$ thickness (0.16–0.19 mm).

As with many techniques, constant practice is required to become really proficient at coverslipping and in knowing just how much mountant is necessary for each size of coverglass. The technique for mounting sections is as follows:

1. Clean excess xylene (or water if the mountant is to be aqueous) from around the section. Some technologists like to blot the

section lightly with fluffless filter paper after wiping off the excess clearant from the slide.

2. Place one or two drops of the mounting media on the section or the coverglass. Allow it to run down the full length of the section or coverglass. The actual amount of mountant used will depend on the size of the section to be covered, and is gauged by experience.
3. a. Gently lower a grease-free coverglass onto the section, keeping one end supported by a dissecting needle until the glass is almost flat on the slide (Fig. 11-5A).
   b. Gently lower the section onto a grease-free coverglass. When the mountant starts to spread turn the slide right side up (Fig. 11-5B).
   c. Lay the slide on its long edge and gently lower it onto the coverglass. When the mountant starts to spread turn the slide right-side up (Fig. 11-5C).

   Any of the above methods works well. The actual method used is entirely a matter of personal preference.
4. Remove any air bubbles by gentle pressure with a dissecting needle. If this fails to dislodge them return the slide to the clearant and start again.

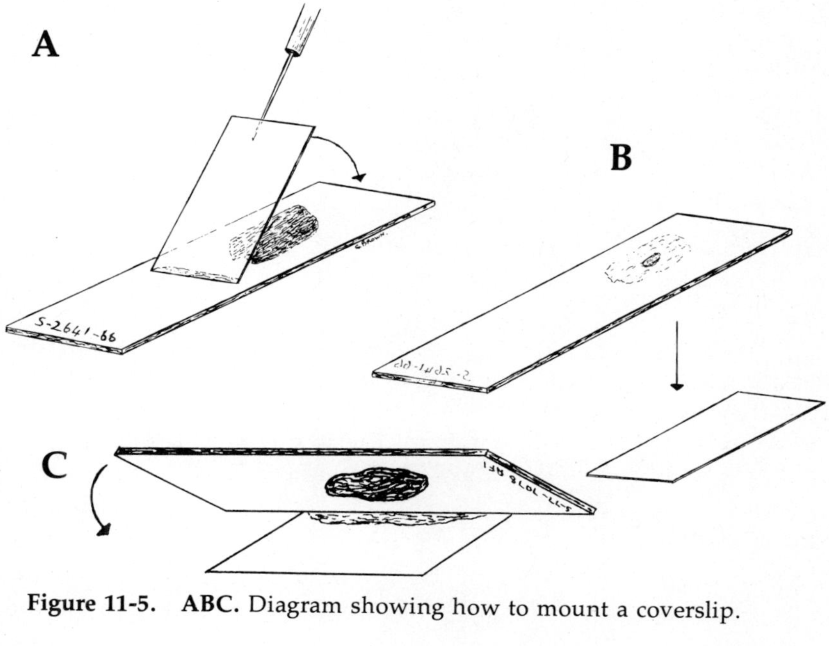

Figure 11-5. ABC. Diagram showing how to mount a coverslip.

5. Clean off any excess or smudged mountant with a little xylene (or water) and a soft lint-free cloth.

Mounted sections should be dried overnight at 60 C before they are filed for permanent records. Aqueous mountants must be air-dried. If this is not possible the sections should be placed in a temporary file with a space between each slide for one week before permanent filing.

BIBLIOGRAPHY

Lillie RD, Zirkle C, Greco JP: Final Report of the Committee on Histologic Mounting Media. Stain Technol., 28:57–80, 1953.

TWELVE

Dyes and Staining Reactions

A Short History of Stains

Up until the early eighteenth century, the pioneer microscopist had to examine his specimens and preparations in an unstained condition, an added disadvantage to the crude equipment then available to him.

In 1714 Anton Van Leeuwenhoek reported in a letter to the Royal Society that he had employed saffron (crocus extracted with wine) on sections of muscle fiber to make the structures more visible under one of his lenses. This probably makes him the first scientist to employ a biologic stain. Carmine was introduced in 1849 by Goppert and Cohn, followed with the use of hematoxylin by Waldeyer in 1863. Aniline dyes, the first "chemically produced" artificial dyes, were introduced in 1856.

Although this was a start, the demand for dyes and biologic stains by the microscopist was exceedingly small, and they had to rely on the dyes available to them from the textile industry. These were of poor quality, rather crude, and not at all constant in composition. The results obtained with them varied immensely.

A German company founded by Dr. Grübler was the first to sell dyes having some consistency to the microscopist on a commercial basis. It was said of him that, "not only did he have the best dyes, but that he also included the best impurities." Dr. Grübler did not manufacture the dyes himself, but purchased them from commercial sources. Each batch that he obtained for resale was tested, and there was, therefore, a modicum of control over the quality of the biologic stains sold under his label. During World War I this source of supply was cut off and made it imperative that other sources, preferrably domestic, be found to provide biologic stains of proven and reliable quality.

The Biological Stain Commission was established in 1922 to effect scientific standardization of biologic stains, whether from domestic or foreign manufacturers.

Sources of Dyes

Dyes are generally divided into two groups: the natural dyes and the artificial or "aniline dyes."

NATURAL DYES

As has been noted in the short history of stains, the natural dyes were of great importance to the early microscopist. Although they are few in number compared to the number of artificial dyes available to us today, some of them are still among our most valuable biologic stains.

Natural dyes are obtained from some insects and a wide variety of plants, ranging from bulbs to trees. They were employed by the textile industry for dying wool and cotton, and by the tanning industry, long before they were applied to sections of tissue as biologic stains. Many of these dyes can now be produced artificially, but some, particularly the extracts of logwood and cochineal, are still valuable biologic stains. The following are a few of the natural dyes and their sources;

Cochineal

This is extracted from the female cochineal bug (*Coccus cacti*) and has been used as a dye from as early as 1665. Carmine is produced from cochineal by treating it with alum, and because it is only slightly soluble in water at a neutral pH, solutions of carmine are either acid, alkaline, or alcoholic. It has little affinity for tissue when used alone, and is therefore employed with a salt of a metal, or to demonstrate tissues containing metal.

Hematoxylin

Obtained from the heartwood of the Logwood tree (*Hematoxylin campechianum*), which is native to Campeche, Mexico, hematoxylin is one of the most important of the natural dyes used in biologic staining methods today. The crystals, produced by extraction, digestion, soaking, and evaporation methods, do not possess any staining properties until oxidized (ripened) into hematein by either chemical or natural means. Because of its poor affinity for tissue, hematoxylin is used in conjunction with a mordant, usually the salt of a metal, either prior to the application of the stain, or as a constituent of the staining solution.

It is of interest to note that when America first tried to obtain hematoxylin from new sources, the product was very crude and inferior as a tissue stain. What they obtained was tanner's hematoxylin, spelt *hematoxylin* in the American fashion, rather than the biologic stain hematoxylin which was spelt *haematoxylin* in the British fashion.

Brazilin

Obtained from the redwood of trees and shrubs from South and Central America, this stain is closely related to hematoxylin, having one less hydroxyl group. It must also be oxidized before it can be used as a stain, and will lose two of its hydrogen atoms as does hematoxylin (Fig. 1).

Orcein

It is now possible to manufacture orcein by chemical means, and very good (sometimes better than the natural product) synthetic

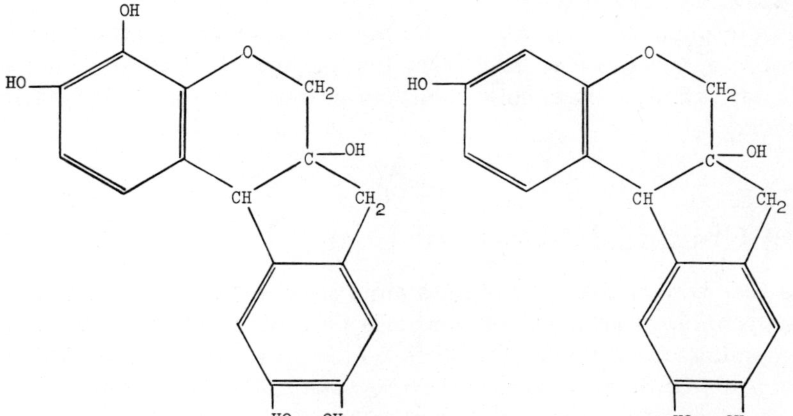

Hematoxylin ($C_{16}H_{14}O_6 \cdot 3HO$) Brazilin ($C_{16}H_{14}O_5$)

Figure 12-1. The formulas for Hematoxylin and Brazilin. Note the additional hydroxyl group on Hematoxylin.

products are now available. Natural orcein is a vegetable dye obtained from certain lichens, *Lecanora tinctoria* and *Rocella tinctoria*. Orcein is best known as a specific stain for elastic tissue.

Litmus

An indicator that turns red in acid solutions and blue in alkaline solutions. It is extracted from the same lichens as orcein.

Saffron

This is extracted from the dried stigmata of the saffron flower (*Crocus sativus*). It is a bright yellow pigment, the coloring matter of which is termed *crocin*. A similar pigment may be extracted from the fruit of *Gardinia florida*.

SYNTHETIC OR ARTIFICIAL DYES

These dyes, like the natural dyes, were being employed by the textile industry for dyeing cloth and wool. Their discovery, as is the case with so many great discoveries, was completely accidental. In 1856 a young chemist, William Perkin, accidentally discovered the first aniline dye (Perkin's Mauve) while working on an experiment at home where he was trying to synthesize quinine. Perkin was eighteen years old at the time. Since this time literally hundreds of artificial or aniline dyes have been produced by the chemical change of certain substances found in coal tar.

The term aniline is derived from the Arabic *al-nil*, meaning the blue substance, when it was discovered that aniline, the basic substance of coal tar, gave a blue coloration under the influence of bleaching powder.

The Chemical Nature of Dyes

The majority of dyes (biologic stains) used today in the practice of histotechnology are artificial, and it is becoming increasingly possible to manufacture many of the dyes which were formerly classified as natural dyes. Because there are so few natural dyes in comparison to the number of artificial dyes, and because their chemistry is not yet fully understood, they are practically disregarded in considering the chemical nature of dyes.

The earliest examples of artificial dyes were produced from aniline, and were therefore naturally classified as *aniline dyes*. This term has frequently, and mistakenly, been applied to the much larger group of artificial dyes available today, even though these dyes have no relationship to aniline. These dyes, like aniline, are derivatives of coal tar. They should therefore be called *coal-tar* dyes, which is the more correct nomenclature.

All of the coal-tar dyes are derivatives of *benzene*. For this reason a thorough knowledge of the molecular structure of benzene is very important to the understanding of dye chemistry.

BENZENE

The hydrocarbon benzene molecule, or the benzene molecule as it is more commonly known, is composed of six carbon atoms and six atoms of hydrogen (C_6H_6) that are so arranged as to form a hexagonal ring of carbon atoms, with a hydrogen atom attached to each free valency. This is known as the benzene ring.

Because carbon has a valency of *four* it forms a double bond on one side and a single bond on the other, alternatively around the ring. Hydrogen has a valency of *one*.

The double bonds in benzene are not fixed and may be rearranged. This property makes benzene very important to organic chemistry because of the infinite number of combinations it can make with other radicals and elements, forming extremely complex compounds. Figure 2 shows the construction of the benzene ring.

If two oxygen atoms, each having a double valency, replace two of the hydrogen atoms, each having a single valency, and the substitution takes place simultaneously on opposite sides of the benzene ring, a readjustment of the double bond takes place and a new compound,

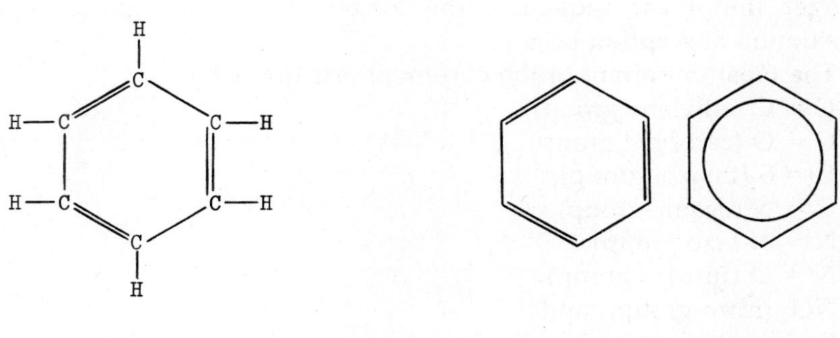

The Benzene Ring (C_6H_6). Abbreviated Forms,

Figure 12-2. The Hydrocarbon Benzene Molecule.

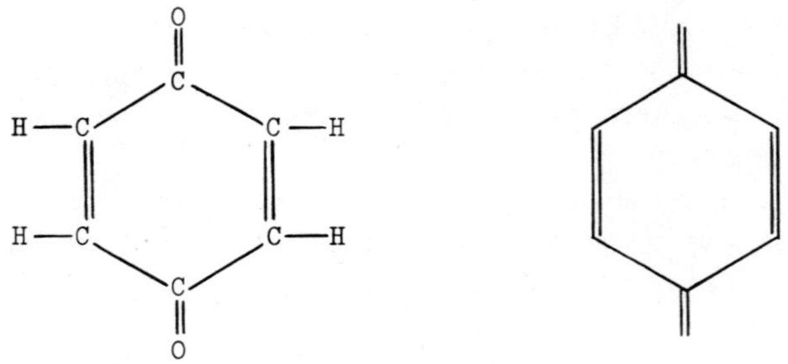

The Quinoid Molecule ($C_6H_4O_2$). Abbreviated Form.

Figure 12-3. The formula for Quinone. Note the difference between this molecule and the Benzene ring (Figure 12-2).

quinone ($C_6H_4O_2$), is formed. It is from this compound that we obtain quinoid compounds. In quinoid compounds the double bonds become fixed and are not rearrangeable as in the benzene molecule. This change is important. Figure 3 illustrates the change that has taken place.

CHROMOPHORES

In order to exhibit color, a substance must absorb light from wavelengths in the visible spectrum. Benzene and its derivatives are colorless and absorb light only in the ultraviolet range, whereas quinoid compounds absorb light from the bands in the visible spectrum and possess color.

The atomic groupings that are associated with color are known as *chromophores*. Chromophoric groups of atoms are usually in a linear sequence that may be simple, branched, or follow a closed ring (quinone). The closed-ring sequence is called a resonance system. The longer the linear sequence, the longer the wavelength at which maximum absorption occurs.

The most important of the chromophoric groups are:
C = C (ethylene group),
C = O (carbonyl group),
C = S (thiazol group),
C = N (cyanic group),
N = N (azo group),
N = O (nitroso group),
NO_2 (nitro group), and
the quinoid group.

The quinoid ring is one of the most important chromophores, and any compound containing the quinoid ring as a constituent will exhibit intense color.

Benzene compounds containing a chromophoric group of atoms possess the property of color and are known as *chromogens*. Although chromogens possess color and can apparently transfer color to a substance placed in them, that color can be quickly and easily removed. The color will not bind to the substance. Chromogens, therefore, are not dyes, since they possess no affinity for cloth fibers or tissue components.

AUXOCHROMES

To convert a chromogen into a dye, a further change must take place in the molecule. The addition of another group of atoms called *auxochromes* will give the compound the power of electrolytic dissociation, or the property of forming salts, and will convert that compound into a dye. The auxochromic groups of atoms also determine whether the dye will be acid or basic.

An acid is a substance that can donate or give up a proton (a hydrogen ion, H^+), while a base is a substance that can accept a proton. When an acid and a base unite they form a salt and water which is at neutral pH. For example:

Acid	+	*Base*	=	*Salt*	+	*Water*
HCl	+	NaOH	=	NaCl	+	H_2O
Hydrochloric acid	+	Sodium hydroxide	=	Sodium chloride	+	Water

Ionic bonding is an electrolytic phenomenon whereby a positively charged molecule will tend to attract a molecule with an equal negative charge and vice versa.

An example of a compound being converted first to a chromogen and then to a dye is as follows:

If three hydrogen atoms from the benzene ring are replaced with three chromophores of the nitro group (NO_2), the resultant compound is trinitrobenzene, a chromogen colored yellow (Fig. 4).

The further replacement of a hydrogen atom with another group of atoms from the hydroxyl group (OH), which is an auxochrome, will convert the trinitrobenzene into picric acid, which is a dye (Fig. 5). Picric acid is capable of forming a salt with a base and is not easily removed from fibers or those tissue constituents for which it has an affinity.

There are several groups of auxochromes, some acidic and some basic. The hydroxyl group (OH^-) and the carboxyl group ($COOH^-$) are both acidic, while the amino group ($NH_2{}^+$) is basic.

Several of the chromophoric groups may be slightly auxochromic in nature, but do not possess sufficient strength to be significant.

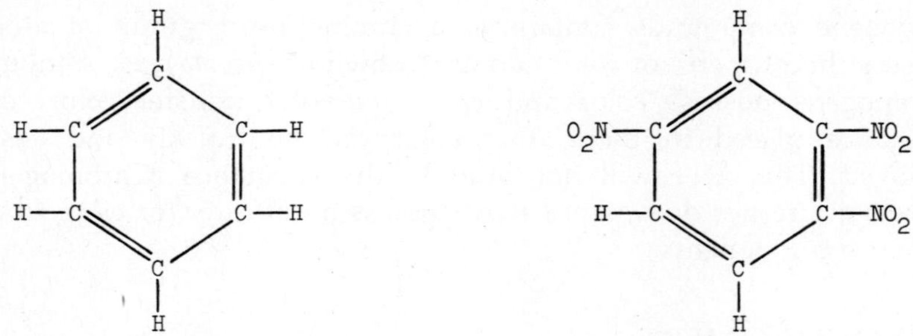

Benzene Trinitrobenzene

Figure 12-4. The conversion of Benzene to Trinitrobenzene.

THE SULFONIC GROUP

The sulfonic (SO_3H) group of atoms is both strongly acidic and salt forming, but it is only feebly auxochromic. However it is extremely important to dye chemistry. This group of atoms has the ability to make an insoluble dye soluble in water, and to convert a basic dye into an acid dye. Basic fuchsin (Rosanilin) is converted to acid fuchsin by the addition of a sulfonic group to the basic fuchsin (Fig. 6).

A compound may contain both a chromophoric group and a sulfonic group, but it is not a dye unless there is a true auxochromic group of atoms present.

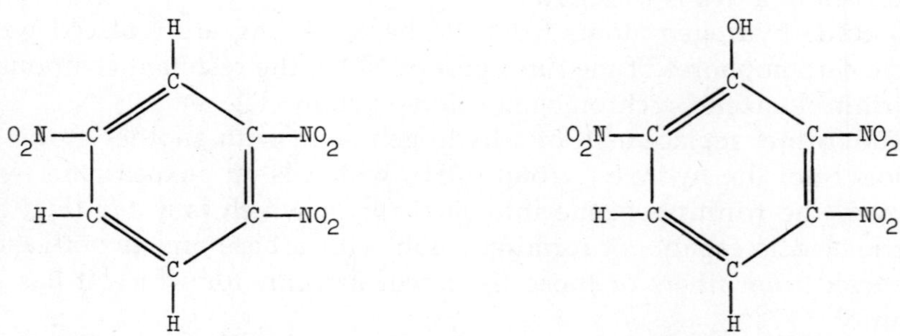

Trinitrobenzene ($C_6H_3N_3O_6$) Picric Acid ($C_6H_3N_3O_7$)

Figure 12-5. The conversion of Benzene to Picric Acid.

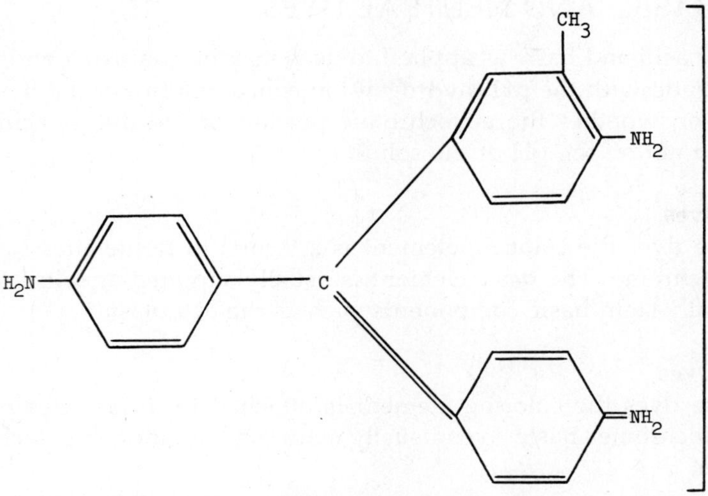

Basic Fuchsin (Rosanilin) $C_{20}H_{20}N_3Cl$

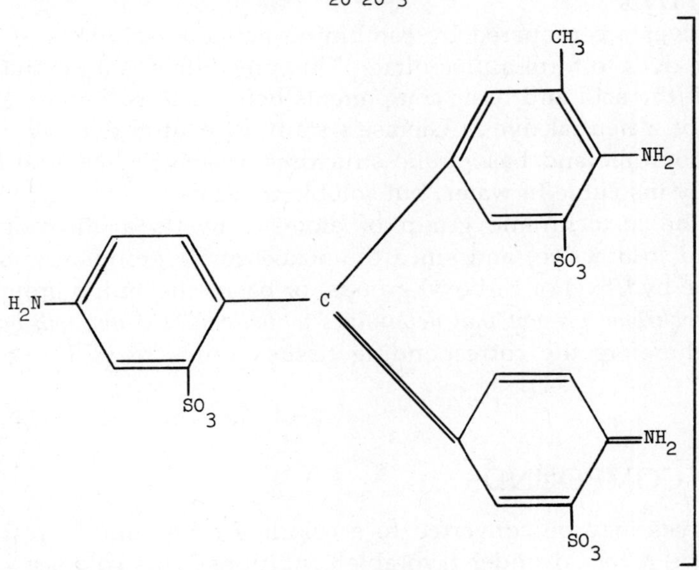

Acid Fuchsin $C_{20}H_{17}N_3O_9S_3Na_2$

Figure 12-6. Comparison of the formulas for Basic Fuchsin and Acid Fuchsin.

Therefore, a dye may be defined as an organic compound consisting of a benzene ring to which has been attached both a chromophoric group(s) of atoms giving the color, and an auxochromic group(s) of atoms giving the dyeing property.

ACID, BASIC, AND NEUTRAL DYES

The terms acid and basic as applied to dyes may be confusing and has nothing to do with the pH (hydrogen ion concentration) of the dye. It depends on whether the auxochromic portion of the dye is acid or basic, and not on the pH of the solution.

Acid Dyes

In these dyes the coloring element is attached to tissue sites by an acid auxochrome. The basic element is usually supplied as salts. Acid dyes usually stain basic components such as the cytoplasm.

Basic Dyes

In these dyes the coloring element is attached to tissue sites by a basic auxochrome. Basic dyes usually stain acid components such as the nuclei.

Neutral Dyes

These dyes are prepared by combining aqueous solutions of acid and basic dyes to form a precipitate. This precipitate is a neutral dye with both the acid and basic components being colored. An excellent example of a neutral dye is Giemsa's stain. A neutral dye will stain both acidophillic and basophillic structures selectively. Neutral dyes are usually insoluble in water, but soluble in alcohol.

Since the auxochromic group of atoms converts a chromogenic compound into a dye, and since the auxochromic groups are either acidic (the hydroxyl or carboxyl groups) or basic (the amino group), *it is the auxochrome present that determines which class the dye will belong to*, and therefore the corresponding tissue groups to which it will bind.

LEUCO-COMPOUNDS

Certain dyes may be converted to a colorless compound, a reaction that can be reversed under favorable conditions. This colorless compound is called a *leuco-compound*.

All chromophoric groups, although differing considerably from one another, possess one property in common. They are all easily reducible. In the language of chemistry, this means that they have an unsatisfied affinity for hydrogen. Combining with hydrogen is the opposite of oxidation and is therefore reduction.

In the quinoid ring, the double bond may break, and hydrogen atoms will attach themselves to the freed valencies; the bond between the nitrogen atoms in the azin group may break and two hydrogen atoms will become attached; or the nitro group (NO_2) may be reduced to an amino group (NH_2). When a chromophore is thus destroyed it loses the property of color, and the prefix *leuco* is applied to the compound.

Under favorable conditions of oxidation this reaction can be reversed. When the chromophore is restored to its original form the compound will regain its color.

Some basic dyes become colorless after losing their acid radical and are termed a *leuco-base*. Similarly, certain acid dyes become colorless when the chromophore is broken during the rearrangement of atoms which occurs on neutralization. These compounds are useful as indicators of hydrogen ion concentration (pH) since this reaction is normally easily reversible.

The breakdown of the basic dyes into leuco-bases occurs mainly in the arylmethane group among the triphenylmethanes. When the molecule is rearranged during neutralization, the result is not a true dye base, but a compound known as a carbinol in which a chromophore does not exist.

Carbinols are important in dye chemistry as intermediates in the preparation of dyes and are often referred to as carbinol bases or color bases of the phenylmethane dyes.

The Classification of Dyes

Although dyes are grouped into natural and synthetic dyes, further classification under the chemical structure of the compound is essential, especially for the synthetic dyes.

Classification is made not, as might be supposed, by the color of the dye, but by the chemical grouping of the chromophore present. Every dye contains at least one group of chromophores, the group of atoms responsible for the color property of the compound.

Only a few of the chromophoric groups require our consideration. They are:

1. The nitro group
2. The quinoid benzene ring
3. The azo group
4. The azin group
5. The indamine group

There are eight major classifications of dyes which are of interest to the biologist. They are:

1. *The Nitroso Group (Quinoneoximes).* These dyes are produced by the action of nitrous acid on phenolic compounds producing nitrosophenol, a compound having the same atoms attached to a benzene ring as does quinoneoxime. The arrangement is different, but the formula is identical. This suggests that the compounds react as quinoneoximes, which accounts for their behavior as dyeing agents, since the quinone benzene ring is a strong chromophore.

2. *The Nitro Group.* The dyes in this group are all acid because the chromophore —NO_2 is so strongly acid in nature.

3. *The Azo Group.* The chromophore in this group is —N=N—, joining either benzene or naphthalene rings. Because the azo group can occur more than once in a molecule, subgroups of disazo, trisazo, or polyazo dyes are formed. The azo chromophore is basic but is not strong enough to make the dyes basic when hydroxyl groups are contained in the compound. Those compounds containing amino groups are strongly basic.

4. *The Thiazole Group.* This is a small group of dyes in which the indamine group —N= is the chromophore.

5. *The Anthraquinone Group.* The dyes in this group include derivatives of anthracene by its oxidation to the chromogen anthraquinone. It is converted into a dye by the addition of hydroxyl groups. It is of interest to note that two of the dyes in this group are natural dyes, occurring in the root of madder.

6. *The Quinone-Imine Group.* The dyes in this group contain two chromophores, the indamine group —N= and the quinoid benzene ring.

7. *The Arylmethane or Phenylmethane Group.* The chromophore for this group is $>$C=NH, joining two benzene rings to form the chromogen. Dyes are formed by the addition of alkylamino groups para to the methane carbon on both benzene rings. Dyes in this group may be either acid or basic, depending on the auxochromic group present in the compound.

8. *The Xanthene Group.* This group of dyes is derived from the compound xanthene and consists of both acid and basic dyes.

Dyes are also identified by name and their color index (C.I.). The color index is a system of identification published by the Society of Dyers and Colourists in England and was revised twenty years ago in a joint effort with the American Association of Textile Chemists and Colorists in an effort to obtain some degree of international standardization. A five-digit system was adopted, with sufficient spacing between groups to allow for the addition of new dyes.

The problem of identifying a dye solely by name is that many dyes have a host of names (synonyms) for the same compound. In the past, manufacturers were only interested in marketing their product and would identify the dye with a name of their own choosing, regardless of what another manufacturer might call it or its preferred nomenclature. The result was confusion. The same dye was frequently used under a different name for different procedures. When identifying a dye by name, the preferred nomenclature should be used (if known) plus the color index.

The Theory of Staining

The reaction between stain and tissue is a very complex subject, and many theories have been put forward to explain this phenomenon. It is not yet fully understood.

Although it is generally accepted that acid dyes stain the basic components of tissue and basic dyes stain the acid components of tissue, this is not always strictly true. Hematoxylin, which is an acid dye, although not used as such, is a strong nuclear (basic) stain when used with a mordant. It does not stain the cytoplasm.

If staining reactions are purely chemical in nature, then in theory the reaction should continue until one or other of the reagents is exhausted. If staining is a purely physical phenomenon, then all staining will take place by either osmosis, capillary attraction, or solubility. The dye would be easily removed from all tissue components, which it is not.

Some staining reactions require the use of either an accentuator, a mordant, or heat, or a combination of these in order to work.

The generally accepted theory is that staining reactions are a combination of both physical and chemical action. The physical theories that have been advanced to explain staining reactions are (1) solubility and (2) adsorption.

The solubility reaction is based on the theory that the dye is more soluble in the substance being stained than it is in the solvent in which it is dissolved. Fat stains are an excellent example of this as they are more soluble in fat than they are in 70 percent alcohol. Solubility is sometimes referred to as absorption.

Adsorption has been called the electrical theory of staining, and is the property by which a large body may attract minute particles to itself, the dye particles penetrating the cell to be deposited on, or form combinations with, various cellular constituents. The reaction may be affected by whether the dye is acid or basic, the pH of the tissue or cellular constituents, or both, and may therefore be selective. It can be seen that when staining with a polychromatic solution, a solution containing more than one dye, eg, Gomori's One-Step Trichrome Solution, the tissue components are stained selectively.

Fixation will also affect the manner in which tissue will react to dyes. Tissue fixed in solutions containing salts of heavy metals, such as mercuric chloride (Zenker's fluid), tend to stain more brilliantly with acid dyes such as eosin, while there appears to be a slight inhibitory effect on the staining of the nuclei by the alum hematoxylins. What has happened is that the isoelectric point (IEP) has shifted.

The isoelectric point is defined as that pH point at which the protein molecule behaves as neither acid nor base, and the positive and negative charges are equalized with the result of a net charge of zero.

Proteins are complex organic nitrogenous compounds consisting essentially of combinations of α-amino acids and their derivatives. They make up approximately one-third of the constituents of cytoplasm, the other two-thirds consisting of lipids and carbohydrates. Proteins are primarily classified into two groups, the simple, naturally occurring proteins consisting of globular proteins, such as albumin and globulin, and fibrous proteins, such as collagen, and the conjugated proteins that consist of simple proteins combined with nonprotein material, for example, nucleoprotein and glycoprotein. Simple proteins yield only α-amino acids and their derivatives on hydrolysis. Upon fixation precipitated protein aggregates are formed.

When the protein molecule is at its IEP with a zero charge, it is said to be amphoteric. This means that it has the capability of shifting to acid (−ve charge) or base (+ve charge) depending upon the pH of the solution in which it is placed. A solution that is more acid than the IEP will shift this towards base and vice versa.

Fixatives containing salts of heavy metals combine with the carboxyl groups leaving the amino groups free. The IEP is shifted to a higher pH (more basic) giving a more positive charge, and the substance is therefore more receptive to acid dyes. It may be said that they have an affinity for acid dyes. Formalin will combine with the basic radicals leaving the carboxyl acid radicals free and shifts the IEP to a lower pH (more acid). Each fixative will tend to give a slightly differing IEP.

Accentuators and Mordants

ACCENTUATORS

Accentuators are substances that cause an increase in the selectivity or in the staining power of a dye, thus making it more intense. They do not form links or lakes between the dye and the tissue, nor do they take any part in the staining reaction, which could occur without the use of the accentuator. Common examples are the phenol in carbol fuchsin and potassium hydroxide used in a methylene blue solution.

Accentuators used in the metallic-salt impregnation methods for the nervous system are often termed accelerators. An example is the veronal used in Cajal's method for axis cylinders.

MORDANTS

A mordant is a substance that causes certain staining reactions to take place by forming a link between the tissue and the stain. This link is often referred to as a "lake." Without the mordant the dye is not capable of binding to and staining the tissue.

Some of the most frequently used mordants in routine staining procedures are the alums incorporated in many of the hematoxylin solutions and Gram's iodine used in the staining of bacteria by Gram's method.

The way in which the accentuators and mordants work is illustrated in Figure 7.

Staining

The purpose of staining is to optically differentiate the cells, cellular constituents, and tissue constituents by variations in color and shades of the same color during microscopic examination.

Tissue and tissue sections may be stained by a variety of methods, many of them allowing selective staining of specific structures or substances. If after treatment with a reagent or a series of reagents or

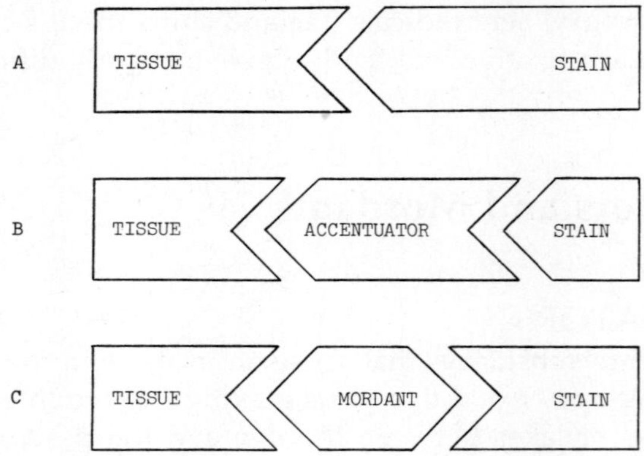

Figure 12-7. Diagramatic illustration of the types of staining reactions: **A.** Direct staining. **B.** Using an accentuator or accelerator. **C.** Using a mordant.

dyes a structure acquires color, it is said to be stained. This coloration is usually homogenous (not particulate) and transparent. Staining techniques fall into the categories described below.

VITAL STAINING

This is the staining of living cellular constituents in the body, *intra vitam* or *in vivo* staining, by injecting a dilute solution of dye into the organ, or by dissociating living (unfixed) tissue in a simple staining solution, *supra vitam* or *in vitro* staining. The method is used to stain cytoplasmic inclusions such as mitochondria and neutral red vacuoles. Some cells, phagocytes, ingest minute particles of dye.

STAINING OF FIXED TISSUE

The majority of the staining techniques employed in the histopathology laboratory fall into this category. They may be subdivided into the following groups:

Direct Staining

The application of a simple dye to stain the tissue in varying shades of a single color.

Indirect Staining

The use of a mordant to facilitate a particular staining method, or the use of an accentuator to improve either the selectivity or the intensity of a stain.

Progressive Staining

The technique whereby stains are applied to the tissue in strict sequence and for specific times. The stain is not washed out or decolorized because there is no overstaining of the tissue constituents. The method is controlled by frequent observation under the microscope.

Regressive Staining

The technique whereby the tissue is overstained, and then the excess stain is removed from all but the structures to be demonstrated. This process is called differentiation, and should always be controlled under the microscope.

IMPREGNATION

Impregnation is not strictly a staining method, but it is one of the techniques employed in demonstrating tissue structures and constituents and should therefore be included. It is the deposition of salts of heavy metals on or around cell and tissue constituents. The results are opaque, and not transparent as when a stain is applied, and particulate rather than homogenous. The obvious example is the silver method for reticulin, and it is applied in many of the neuropathologic methods. The salts of metals most commonly employed are those of gold, lead, osmium, and silver.

HISTOCHEMICAL REACTIONS

A reaction between a colorless solution, frequently a leuco-compound, and a tissue constituent that produces a color reaction to identify that specific substance is a histochemical reaction. An excellent example is the Feulgen reaction for the demonstration of nucleic acid. Also, the reaction between chemical reagents and a substance in the tissue to produce color and thereby identify that substance is considered a histochemical reaction. Perls' prussian blue reaction for the demonstration of hemosiderin, and the Fouchet reaction for bile salts are examples of this.

METACHROMATIC STAINING

Although most cell and tissue constituents stain in varying shades of the color of the dye that is applied, there are certain basic dyes belonging to the aniline group that will differentiate particular tissue components by staining them a different color to that of the original dye. This phenomenon is known as *metachromasy* and the tissue elements reacting in this manner are said to be exhibiting *metachromasia*. These tissue elements are called *chromotropes*.

The generally accepted explanation of this phenomenon is that the change in color is due to polymerization. A high molecular weight appears to be a factor in metachromasia, and sulfated substances are more chromotropic than those containing carboxyl or phosphate groups. Metachromasia can be induced in polysaccharides by treatment with sulfuric acid (sulfation). Mast-cell granules contain heparin which is highly sulfated.

The most important metachromatic dyes are methylene blue, thionin, and toluidine blue. Methyl violet also demonstrates metachromasia, but there is some doubt as to whether this is true metachromasia or a false reaction due to some impurity in the dye.

Amyloid, cartilage, mast-cell granules, and mucin are among the principal tissue components demonstrated by metachromatic staining techniques.

FAT STAINS

The application of a dye that is more soluble in fat than in the solvent in which it is applied.

Differentiation

Differentiation is the process of washing out or removing excess stain until a specific substance or structure is sharply defined and stained differentially from the surrounding tissue.

The reagents commonly employed for differentiating stains are dilute solutions of acids or alkalis in alcohol, solvents such as alcohol or acetone, dilute solutions of mordants, buffer solutions, and even clearing agents such as aniline oil.

Differentiation should be a relatively slow process, and the technician should be able to halt the process at any given point. It should be controlled at all times by observation under the microscope until the desired degree of differentiation is obtained.

BIBLIOGRAPHY

Culling CFA: Handbook of Histopathological and Histochemical Techniques, 3rd ed. Butterworth, London, 1974.

Gurr E: Encyclopedia of Microscopic Stains, Williams & Wilkins, Baltimore, 1960.

Lillie RD: Histopathologic Technic and Practical Histochemistry, 3rd ed. Blakiston Division, McGraw-Hill, New York, 1965.

Lillie RD: H. J. Conn's Biological Stains, 8th ed. Williams & Wilkins, Baltimore, 1969.

THIRTEEN

Basic Staining: The Hematoxylin and Eosin Technique

The hematoxylin and eosin staining technique can well be called the "bread-and-butter" method for the majority of histopathology laboratories. A well-stained and properly differentiated section stained by this technique is possibly the most informative tool of the pathologist. A diagnosis or a request for special stains is made after studying a section stained with hematoxylin and eosin.

Too many technologists and pathologists refer to this technique as the routine staining method in the laboratory. There is nothing routine about this technique and it is a misnomer to refer to it in this manner. It would be more correct to refer to it as the basic staining technique of histopathology. Just because a method is used as the primary technique in the laboratory and is part of the routine in that laboratory, it should not become routine. With this kind of thinking the Warthin Starry technique is routine in a laboratory specializing in the study of spirochetes.

Technically the method is relatively straightforward, but such a wide range of color density is possible with the eosin counterstaining that it is impossible to please everybody. Many pathologists like a vivid, almost fluorescent, eosin; but the requests for density of color varies all the way through the scale from a bright red down to those who express a preference for the more delicate shades of reds and pinks. This latter does allow more cytological detail to be observed. In a busy department with several pathologists, the objective is to produce an end result that is acceptable to each of them. It is impracticable to try and stain each section to suit the taste of every member of the staff.

Alcoholic and acidified solutions of eosin tend to stain much more vividly than do the aqueous solutions, while the addition of phloxin to a solution of eosin will add a variety of shades of red to the tissue constituents. The type of eosin solution employed is a matter of choice.

There are many solutions of hematoxylin, and of these, four are commonly employed as nuclear stains for the hematoxylin and eosin method. Each of them is an alum hematoxylin solution, and whichever one is used is a matter of personal choice. The formula for each is:

Delafield's Hematoxylin[1]

Staining time: 15–20 minutes.

Hematoxylin (C.I. 75290)	4 g
Absolute ethyl alcohol	25 ml
Saturated aqueous solution of aluminum ammonium sulfate (Ammonium alum)	400 ml
Glycerin	100 ml
Absolute ethyl or methyl alcohol	100 ml

Dissolve the hematoxylin in 25 ml of absolute ethyl alcohol with the aid of gentle heat on an electric hotplate. Cool and add the saturated solution of ammonium alum. Allow to stand for four days to one week in an unstoppered flask exposed to sunlight. Shake frequently. Filter and add the glycerin and the remainder of the alcohol. Store in a well-stoppered bottle and allow to ripen for several months.

Ehrlich's Hematoxylin[2]

Staining time: 15–40 minutes.

Hematoxylin (C.I. 75290)	1 g
Absolute ethyl alcohol	100 ml

Dissolve with gentle heat on an electric hotplate.

Aluminum potassium sulfate (Potassium alum)	*to excess*	60 g
Glycerin		100 ml
Distilled water		100 ml

Dissolve with the aid of heat. Mix the two solutions and add:

Glacial acetic acid	10 ml

Ripen by exposure to daylight and warmth for several months in a flask which has been lightly plugged with cotton. Store in a well-stoppered bottle.

Note: Glycerin appears to retard the ripening process and may be added four to six weeks after the date of preparation.

Harris' Hematoxylin[3]
Staining time: 5–20 minutes.

Hematoxylin (C.I. 75290)	1 g
Absolute ethyl alcohol	10 ml

Dissolve with gentle heat on an electric hotplate.

Ammonium or potassium alum	20 g
Distilled water	190 ml

Dissolve in a *large* beaker, not a flask. Add the hematoxylin solution and bring to the boil. When just boiling add:

Mercuric oxide (red)	0.5 g

Plunge immediately into ice cold water. The violent liberation of oxygen will cause the solution to erupt from a narrow mouthed flask—hence the need for a large beaker. When cool add:

Glacial acetic acid	10 ml

Filter and store in a well-stoppered bottle. The hematoxylin is ready for immediate use.

Mayer's Hemalum[4]
Staining time: progressive, 15 minutes; regressive, 40–60 minutes.

Hematoxylin (C.I. 75290)	1 g
Distilled water	1000 ml

Dissolve with gentle heat.

Ammonium or potassium alum	50.0 g
Sodium iodate	0.2 g

Add to the hematoxylin solution and dissolve.

Citric acid	1 g
Chloral hydrate	50 g

Add to the mixture and dissolve.

The solution turns a reddish violet color. The hematoxylin is ready for immediate use. Store in a well-stoppered bottle, and filter before use.

Other alum hematoxylins that are good general nuclear stains and may be considered as alternatives to the more commonly used formulas listed previously are:

1. Bullard's Hematoxylin[5]
2. Lillie's Hematoxylin[6]
3. Mallory's Hematoxylin[7]

Hematoxylin crystals, as obtained from the manufacturer, have no staining properties until they have been "ripened," or *oxidized*, into hematein. Oxidation may be effected by allowing the solution to stand exposed to sunlight and atmospheric oxygen for a period of up to several months, or it may be obtained spontaneously by adding an oxidizing agent. Most laboratories seem to prefer this latter method in preparing their solutions as they are then ready for immediate use. During oxidation the hematoxylin loses two atoms of hydrogen, and its formula changes from $C_{16}H_{14}O_6$ to $C_{16}H_{12}O_6$. Sufficient hematoxylin should be left unoxidized in the solution so that natural oxidation can continue thus prolonging the shelf life and useability of the stain. Completely oxidized hematoxylin becomes colorless.

Commonly used oxidizing agents for hematoxylin solutions are: mercuric oxide (red), sodium iodate, and potassium permanganate.

Hematein in aqueous solution is an amphoteric dye on the alkaline side of its isoelectric point. It functions as an anionic dye, staining cationic tissue components red; but if sufficient acid is added to such a solution the pH will shift to the acid side of its isoelectric point and it will act as a cationic dye, staining anionic tissue components orange. However, hematein is not usually employed for staining in such a solution.

When employed with suitable mordants, hematein forms a dye-lake that functions as a cationic dye and stains anionic tissue components, such as nuclei, blue to blue-black. As can be seen from the preceding formulas, the most frequently employed mordants for alum hematoxylins are ammonium or potassium alum.

Hematein, oxidized hematoxylin, is a dye with an affinity for many tissue components when employed with the appropriate mordant. This mordant may be applied to the tissue immediately prior to the application of the hematein (hematoxylin) as in Heidenhain's iron hematoxylin method (page 252), added to the hematoxylin immediately before the mixture is used as in Weigert's iron hematoxylin method (page 218), or incorporated into the stain when it is made up as in the alum hematoxylin formulas in this chapter.

The various tissue elements demonstrated by hematoxylin (hematein), the appropriate mordant, and some suggested staining methods are listed in Table I.

The hematoxylin stains are, for the most part, used in regressive staining methods; that is, the tissue is overstained and then destained or differentiated until only the desired tissue components retain the stain. They are usually differentiated with either an acid, a mordant, or an oxidizing agent.

A counterstain is employed to impart different colors or shades of a

TABLE I
Hematoxylin Staining Methods

Tissue Element	Mordant (Metal)	Staining Method
Nuclei	Aluminum	Alum hematoxylin & eosin
	Iron	Weigert's iron hematoxylin & Van Gieson
	Tungsten	Phosphotungstic acid hematoxylin (PTAH)
Myelin sheaths	Chromium	Weigert-Pal method
	Iron	Loyez's hematoxylin
Elastic fibers	Iodine and iron	Verhoeff's elastic stain
Myoglia and neuroglia fibrils	Tungsten	Phosphotungstic acid hematoxylin (PTAH)
Mucin	Aluminum	Mayer's mucihematein method
Fibrin	Tungsten	Phosphotungstic acid hematoxylin (PTAH)
Mitochondria	Iron	Heidenhain's iron hematoxylin method
Beta cells	Chromium	Chrome-alum hematoxylin method
Axis cylinders	Lead	Mallory's lead chloride hematoxylin method
Muscle striations	Iron	Heidenhain's iron hematoxylin method
	Tungsten	Phosphotungstic acid hematoxylin (PTAH)
Fibroglia fibrils	Tungsten	Phosphotungstic acid hematoxylin (PTAH)
Collagen	Molybdenum	Mallory's phosphomolybdic acid hematoxylin method[8]

single color to the surrounding tissue components as a contrast to the nuclear staining of the hematoxylin.

The counterstain generally used in conjunction with the alum hematoxylins is eosin, an anionic dye that stains the cationic tissue components. As stated earlier in this chapter, the choice of the depth of color from the eosin counterstain is one of personal preference or a matter of reaching an acceptable compromise with the pathologist.

There are several formulas for eosin solutions, and those in most common use are:

Eosin, Alcoholic Solution

Stock Solution

Eosin Y (C.I. 45380)	1 g
Distilled water	20 ml

Dissolve with gentle heat and allow to cool. Add:

95 percent ethyl alcohol	80 ml

Working Solution

Stock solution	25 ml
80 percent ethyl alcohol	75 ml

Filter before use.

The addition of 0.5 ml glacial acetic acid to each 100 ml of stain will give a deeper shade of red to the tissue.

Eosin, Aqueous Solution

Stock Solutions

Eosin Y (C.I. 45380)	5 g
Water (tap or distilled)	100 ml

It has been stated that the alkalinity of tap water will give superior staining.[9] In either case, a crystal of thymol or a few drops of formalin must be added to the solution to prevent the growth of mold.

Working Solution

Stock solution	1 part
Water	4 parts

Eosin–Phloxine B Solution

Stock Solutions

A Eosin Y (C.I. 45380)	1 g
Distilled water	100 ml
B Phloxine B (C.I. 45410)	1 g
Distilled water	100 ml

Working Solution

Stock eosin solution (A)	100 ml
Stock phloxine solution (B)	10 ml
95 percent ethyl alcohol	780 ml
Glacial acetic acid	4 ml

Make up the working solution as it is needed. This solution should be changed at least once a week and more frequently with heavy use.

Eosin: Precipitated Method

Eosin Y (C.I. 45380)	5 g
Distilled water	1000 ml

Dissolve with the aid of gentle heat and cool.

Add, drop by drop, 8 ml of concentrated hydrochloric acid, shaking gently while the acid is being added. Allow to stand for 24 hours to allow the resultant precipitate to settle and then decant the supernatent fluid.

Wash the precipitate in six changes of distilled water, using at least 500 ml of water for each wash. Dry the washed precipitate at room temperature or at 37 C and dissolve it in 800 ml of 95 percent ethyl alcohol. The solution is now ready for use.

Results with this eosin tend to be brighter than with the standard aqueous solution. Staining time is 30–60 seconds.

THE HARRIS HEMATOXYLIN AND EOSIN STAINING TECHNIQUE

Solutions Required

A. Harris' Hematoxylin.
B. 1 percent Acid Alcohol.
C. Blueing Agent. If the tap water is not alkaline then a blueing agent is required. Either:
   1. 1 percent lithium carbonate (sat. soln.)
   2. 2 percent ammonia (ammonia water)
   3. Scott's tap water substitute:

Sodium bicarbonate	7 g
Magnesium sulfate	40 g
Tap water	2000 ml

   Add 1 percent formalin to prevent the growth of mold.

D. Eosin of choice.

Fixation

Any fixative except for those containing osmium tetroxide.

Method

1. Sections to water. Remove mercuric chloride deposits if present.
2. Harris' hematoxylin for 5 minutes (see first Note).
3. Rinse well in tap water.
4. Differentiate in 1 percent acid alcohol for 5–30 seconds. Control under the microscope until only the nuclei are stained.
5. Rinse quickly in tap water.
6. "Blue" in running tap water for 5 minutes.

   OR

   "Blue" with one of the blueing agents[9] and wash in running tap water for 5 minutes.
7. Eosin for 2–5 minutes (see Notes).

8. Wash in tap water (if an alcoholic eosin is used wash and differentiate in 70 percent alcohol) until the desired shades of red or pink are obtained.
9. Dehydrate, clear, and mount in a resinous medium.

Results

Nuclei	Blue/black
Red blood cells	Orange to pink
Rest of tissue	Shades of red and pink

Notes

1. Following fixation in solutions containing mercuric chloride, and following decalcification, the staining time in hematoxylin should be increased slightly.
2. It is important to remove the ammonia completely from the section if this has been used as a blueing agent. Ammonia has a slight inhibitory effect on eosin.
3. If alcoholic eosin prepared by the precipitation method is used the staining time should be reduced to 15 or 30 seconds. A rinse of 80 percent alcohol should be used immediately before applying this stain.
4. Following fixation in solutions containing mercuric chloride and following decalcification the staining time in eosin should be reduced slightly.

On occasion a request might be submitted for a hematoxylin stain with a more differential counterstain than eosin. The technique given next is useful in such instances.

MAYER'S HEMATOXYLIN-PHLOXINE-SAFFRON TECHNIQUE[10]

Solutions Required

A. Mayer's Hematoxylin.
B. Saturated Aqueous Picric Acid.
C. 1.5 percent Aqueous Phloxine B (C.I. 45410).
D. 2 percent Alcoholic Saffron (C.I. 75100) in Absolute Ethyl Alcohol.

Fixation

Any fixative except those containing osmium tetroxide.

Method

1. Sections to water. Remove mercuric chloride deposits if present.
2. Saturated aqueous picric acid for 5 minutes.
3. Wash in tap water until all of the yellow is removed.
4. Mayer's hematoxylin for 15 minutes.
5. Wash in running tap water for 20 minutes.
6. 1.5 percent aqueous phloxine B for 2 minutes.
7. Wash in running tap water for 5 minutes.
8. Pass through three changes of absolute alcohol.
9. 2 percent alcoholic saffron for 5 minutes.
10. Rinse with two changes of absolute alcohol.
11. Clear and mount in a resinous medium.

Results

Nuclei	Blue
Red blood cells	Pink
Bone	Yellow
Cartilage	Yellowish green
Muscle	Red
Collagen	Yellow

The most common cause of poor quality staining is poor or inadequate fixation of the tissue. Other causes for poor staining in the hematoxylin and eosin technique are:

1. Over or under ripened hematoxylin.
2. Overused or "worked out" hematoxylin.
3. Over or under differentiation of the hematoxylin.
4. Insufficient blueing following differentiation.
5. Failure to wash the blueing agent out of the section (if one is used) before counterstaining with eosin. This is especially important when ammonia is used as a blueing agent.
6. Insufficient differentiation of the eosin during washing or dehydration.
7. Dilution and contamination of the stains and solutions by "carryover" from the preceding reagent.
8. Insufficient dehydration and clearing of the section.

SUBSTITUTE METHODS FOR THE HEMATOXYLIN AND EOSIN TECHNIQUE: LENDRUM'S CELESTIN BLUE—CHROMOTROPE 2R METHOD[11]

Solutions Required

A. Celestin Blue Solution.

Celestin Blue (C.I. 51050)	0.5 g

5 percent iron alum	100.0 ml

Shake the dye and alum solution in a flask. Boil for three minutes and allow to cool. Add:

Sulfuric acid, concentrated	2 ml
Glycerin	14 ml

B. Acid Alcohol.

70 percent alcohol	100 ml
Hydrochloric acid, conc.	2 ml

C. 1 percent Phosphomolybdic Acid.

D. 1 percent Chromotrope 2R (C.I. 16570) in Absolute ethyl alcohol. Eosin may be used as an alternative counterstain.

Fixation

Zenker's fluid or Bouin's fluid are preferred. 10 percent neutral formalin is acceptable.

Method

1. Sections to water. Remove the mercuric chloride deposit or wash out the picric acid, whichever is applicable.
2. Celestin blue solution for 15 minutes. A longer time is necessary following formalin fixation. Control under the microscope.
3. Differentiate in acid alcohol until only the nuclei are stained. Control under the microscope.
4. Wash in running tap water for 1 minute.
5. Mordant in the 1 percent phosphomolybdic acid for 1–2 minutes.
6. Wash well in water.
7. Absolute alcohol for 1 minute, two changes.
8. 1 percent Chromotrope 2R for 2 minutes, or eosin.
9. Dehydrate, clear, and mount.

Results

Nuclei	Bluish purple
Cytoplasm	Pink
Collagenous elements	Bright red

REFERENCES

1. Delafield J: Hämatoxylin. Z Wiss Mikrosk 2:288, 1885
2. Ehrlich P: Hämatoxylinlösung. Z Wiss Mikrosk 3:150, 1886
3. Harris HF: On the rapid conversion of hematoxylin into hematein in staining reactions. J Appl Mikcrosc 3:777–80, 1900

4. Mayer P: Notiz über Hamatein und Hämalaum, Z Wiss Mikrosk 20:409–11, 1904
5. Lillie RD: Histopathologic Technic and Practical Histochemistry, 3rd Ed. New York, McGraw-Hill, 1965, pp 174–75
6. Lillie RD: An improved acid hematoxylin formula, Stain Technol 17:89, 1942
7. Mallory FB: Pathological Technique, Philadelphia, Saunders, 1938, p 70
8. Mallory FB: Pathological Technique, Philadelphia, Saunders, 1938, p 156
9. Drury RAB, Wallington EA: Carleton's Histological Technique, 4th ed. London, Oxford University Press, 1967, p 129
10. Luna LG (Ed): Manual of Histologic Staining Methods of the A.F.I.P., 3rd ed. New York, McGraw-Hill, 1968, p 39
11. Lendrum AC: Celestin blue as a nuclear stain, J Pathol Bacteriol 40:415–16, 1935

BIBLIOGRAPHY

Culling CFA: Handbook of Histopathological and Histochemical Techniques, 3rd ed. London, Butterworth, 1974

Lillie RD: Histopathologic Technic and Practical Histochemistry, 3rd ed. New York, McGraw-Hill, 1965

Thompson SW: Selected Histochemical and Histological Methods, Springfield, Ill, Thomas, 1966

FOURTEEN

Methods for the Demonstration of Connective Tissue and Muscle

Connective Tissue

Connective tissue is, as the name implies, tissue that connects, supports, and binds together all other tissue. All connective tissue is derived from the embryonic mesenchyme cell and is made up of cells, fibers, and matrix, supported in an intercellular amorphous ground substance composed of a mixture of mucopolysaccharides. The cells usually associated with connective tissue are plasma cells, mast cells, and fibroblasts.

There are three types of fiber in connective tissue that we are frequently required to demonstrate. They are collagen (white fibers), which occur as wavy fibrils either singly or in bundles; elastic (yellow fibers), which occur as fine fibers or sheets of fibers as seen around blood vessels; and reticular (argyrophilic fibers), which consist of fine branching fibers supporting the cells and tissues.

Basement membranes which are both argyrophilic and P.A.S.-positive are closely associated with reticular fibers. They are located between the epithelial surfaces and their supporting connective tissue.

Matrix is normally associated with bone and cartilage.

The majority of the methods used to demonstrate connective tissue constituents stain the various structures in contrasting colors, or varying shades of the same color. This permits easy identification of the various components.

Probably the most used counterstain for connective tissue methods is the picro-fuchsin solution of Van Gieson. It is frequently used in conjunction with Weigert's iron hematoxylin (Van Gieson's method) and is the couterstain of choice in the methods for elastic fibers. This solution stains the collagen fibers in varying shades of red; the red blood cells, yellow; and the smooth muscle, yellow.

Methods for the Demonstration of Collagen

VAN GIESON'S METHOD[1]

Fixation

Ten percent neutral buffered formalin is acceptable, but fixatives containing mercuric chloride will give more brilliant results.

Solutions Required

A. Weigert's Iron Hematoxylin:

Solution A

Hematoxylin (C.I.75290)	1 g
Absolute ethyl alcohol	100 ml

Solution B

30 percent ferric chloride	4 ml
Hydrochloric acid (conc.)	1 ml
Distilled water	100 ml

Let both solutions stand for six weeks before use. For use mix:

Solution A	1 part
Solution B	1 part

Once mixed the stain will not keep for more than 24 hours.

B. Van Gieson's Stain:

Solution A

Acid fuchsin (C.I.42685)*	1 g
Distilled water	100 ml

Solution B

Saturated aqueous picric acid

For use with connective tissue mix:

Solution A	10 ml
Solution B	90 ml

* Ponceau S (C.I.27195) may be substituted for acid fuchsin, but does not give as precise results.

This mixture is best ripened for several weeks before use. For immediate use a combination of 50 ml of saturated aqueous picric acid and 7.5 ml of 1 percent acid fuchsin gives precise staining. For use with tissue from the nervous system mix:

Solution A	15 ml
Solution B	15 ml
Distilled water	70 ml

Method

1. Sections to alcohol.
2. Weigert's iron hematoxylin for 15 minutes.
3. Wash in running tap water for 5 minutes.
4. Rinse in distilled water.
5. Van Gieson's stain for 3 minutes.
6. Rinse in distilled water.
7. Rinse in 70 percent alcohol.
8. Dehydrate rapidly, clear, and mount.

Results

Nuclei	Blackish brown to gray
Collagen	Red
Smooth muscle	Yellow
Red blood cells	Yellow

Notes

1. Picric acid, in addition to being a fixative and a stain, will also act as a differentiating agent. If the times given for this method are strictly adherred to, the need to differentiate the hematoxylin in 1 percent acid alcohol is eliminated. Differentiation of the hematoxylin is done by the picric acid in the Van Gieson's stain.
2. Differentiation of the collagen and smooth muscle may be accomplished, if further differentiation is desired, during steps 6 and 7. Van Gieson's stain consists of acid fuchsin which is readily soluble in water and picric acid which is readily soluble in alcohol. It follows that the accentuation of either the collagen or the smooth muscle can be obtained very easily by washing in the appropriate solvent to remove more dye from the other component.
3. It is important that the picric acid solution is a saturated solution.
4. If desired, the sections can be postfixed in mercuric chloride prior to staining. *Remove the precipitate.*

The actual staining mechanism of the polychromatic (containing more than one dye) staining solution of Van Gieson or other connective tissue stains is not fully understood. Theories put forward suggest that the penetrating powers of the dyes vary in relationship to their acidity or basicity, their molecular weights, and in the penetrability of the tissue structures being stained.

Acid fuchsin and picric acid are both acid (anionic) dyes and stain the basic (cationic) tissue components selectively. Picric acid is much more acid than an equal percentage solution of acid fuchsin, and has more penetrating power per unit of time even though acid fuchsin is the more intense dye. In the time allowed for Van Gieson's stain the acid fuchsin is only able to stain the more easily penetrable component (collagen) by either masking or displacing the picric acid. If the acid fuchsin does penetrate the cytoplasm and smooth muscle, it does not do so with sufficient accumulation to mask the picric acid, unless the picric acid used was *not* in saturated solution. In this instance the smooth muscle and cytoplasm will take on an orange tinge.

When two anionic dyes are used in the same solution, or paired together in the same method, the dye with the higher molecular weight has a tendency to stain the more easily penetrated tissue structures, ie., collagen, while the dye with the lower-molecular-weight stains the cytoplasm of the cells and other less easily penetrated structures. Acid fuchsin has a molecular weight of 585 and picric acid has a molecular weight of 229.

Another factor to consider is aggregation. When dyes are dispersed in solution in particles larger than a single anion it is known as aggregation. Those dyes which form large aggregates are used to stain collagen while those dispersed as single ions stain the background.

MASSON'S TRICHROME METHOD (MODIFIED)[2]

Fixation

Ten percent neutral buffered formalin, Zenker's fluid, or Bouin's fluid.

Solutions Required

A. Weigert's Iron Hematoxylin (page 218).

B. 1 percent Acid Alcohol:

Hydrochloric acid, (conc.)	1 ml
70 percent ethyl alcohol	99 ml

C. Masson's Acid Fuchsin:

Acid fuchsin (C.I.42685)	1 g
Glacial acetic acid	1 ml
Distilled water	to 100 ml

OR

Acid Fuchsin/Biebrich Scarlet Solution:

1 percent Biebrich scarlet (C.I.26905), aq. soln.	90 ml
1 percent Acid fuchsin (C.I.42685), aq. soln.	10 ml
Glacial acetic acid	1 ml

D. 1 percent Phosphomolybdic Acid:

Phosphomolybdic acid	1 g
Distilled water	100 ml

OR

Phosphomolybdic Acid–Phosphotungstic Acid Solution:

Phosphomolybdic acid	2.5 g
Phosphotungstic acid	2.5 g
Distilled water	100 ml

E. Aniline Blue Solution:

Aniline blue, wat. sol. (C.I. 42755)	2.5 g
Glacial acetic acid	2.5 ml
Distilled water	97.5 ml

OR

2 percent Light Green Solution:

Light green SF, yellowish (C.I. 42095)	2 g
Glacial acetic acid	1 ml
Distilled water	99 ml

F. 1 percent Acetic Acid:

Glacial acetic acid	1 ml
Distilled water	99 ml

Method

1. Sections to water.
2. *If formalin fixed*, mordant as follows:
   a. Overnight at room temperature in Bouin's fluid.
   b. One hour at 56 C in Bouin's fluid (preheated).
3. Wash until the yellow coloration is removed.
4. Weigert's iron hematoxylin for 15 minutes.
5. Rinse in tap water.
6. Differentiate in 1 percent acid alcohol until only the nuclei are stained. Control under the microscope.
7. "Blue" in running tap water for 5–10 minutes.

8. Rinse in distilled water.
9. Masson's acid fuchsin for 5 minutes.

   OR

   Acid fuchsin/Biebrich scarlet solution for 5 minutes.
10. Rinse in distilled water.
11. Differentiate and mordant with 1 percent phosphomolybdic acid for 5 minutes. Discard the solution after use.
    Note: If the 2 percent light green solution is to be used as the counterstain a rinse in distilled water is necessary after this step.

    OR

    Differentiate in the phosphomolybdic acid–phosphotungstic acid solution for 10–15 minutes. Discard the solution after use.
    Note: If the 2 percent light green solution is to be used as the counterstain differentiation should be done in 5 percent phosphotungstic acid for 15 minutes. Rinse. *Differentiation should be controlled under the microscope*.
12. Aniline blue solution for 5 minutes.

    OR

    2 percent light green solution for 2–3 minutes.
13. Rinse off excess stain in distilled water.
14. Wash well in 1 percent acetic acid for 1–3 minutes. This step is intended to remove any excess or overlying blue or green from the cytoplasmic structures. Control under the microscope.
15. Dehydrate, clear, and mount.

Results

Nuclei	Brownish black
Muscle	Red
Cytoplasm	Red
Keratin	Red
Collagen	Blue or green
Mucin	Blue or green

Aniline blue and acid fuchsin are both impure mixtures of several dye substances and possess anionic as well as cationic groups and are regarded as amphoteric dyes. In acid solution they stain cationic components of tissue. In Masson's method acid fuchsin is applied as a stronger solution and for a longer unit of time than in Van Gieson's method, allowing it to stain the less penetrable tissue components. After removal from the collagen fibers (easily penetrable) and the mordanting of these fibers with the differentiating solution, the acid fuchsin is replaced with a dye of a higher molecular weight. Aniline blue (mol wt 737) and light green (mol wt 792) have a much higher molecular weight than acid fuchsin (mol wt 585), which in turn has a higher molecular weight than picric acid (mol wt 229) (see Van Gieson's method and discussion).

GOMORI'S ONE-STEP TRICHROME METHOD[3]

Fixation

Ten percent neutral buffered formalin.

Solutions Required

A. Weigert's Iron Hematoxylin (see page 218).
B. Gomori's Trichrome Stain:

Chromotrope 2R (C.I. 16570)	0.6 g
Light green SF, yellowish (C.I. 42095)*	0.3 g
Glacial acetic acid	1.0 ml
Phosphotungstic acid	0.8 g
Distilled water	100.0 ml

Method

1. Sections to water.
2. Mordant as follows:
   Overnight at room temperature in Bouin's fluid.
   OR
   1 hour at 56 C in Bouin's fluid (preheated).
3. Wash until the yellow coloration is removed.
4. Weigert's iron hematoxylin for 10 minutes. (Harris' hematoxylin may be substituted with the staining time extended to 20 minutes.)
5. Wash in tap water.
6. Trichrome stain for 20 minutes.
7. Rinse well in 0.5 percent acetic acid.
8. Rinse in distilled water.
9. Dehydrate, clear, and mount.

Results

Nuclei	Brownish black (or blue/black)
Muscle fibers	Red
Collagen	Green

* Aniline blue (C.I. 42755) may be substituted for light green if desired. Collagen will then stain blue.

PICRO-TRICHROME METHOD*

Fixation

Ten percent neutral formalin and Bouin's fluid are satisfactory, but Helly's fluid gives the best results.

Solutions Required

A. Weigert's Iron Hematoxylin (see page 218)
B. Picro-Orange Solution:

Orange G (C.I. 16230)	1 g
Saturated picric acid in 80 percent ethyl alcohol	400 ml

C. Acid Fuchsin-Biebrich Scarlet Solution (see page 221).
D. 5 percent Phosphotungstic Acid:

Phosphotungstic acid	5 g
Distilled water	100 ml

E. 1 percent Acetic Acid.
F. 2 percent Light Green in 1 percent Acetic Acid (see page 221)

Method

1. Sections to water.
2. Weigert's iron hematoxylin for 15 minutes.
3. Wash in running tap water for 5 minutes.
4. Rinse in 70 percent alcohol.
5. Picro-orange solution for 5–8 minutes.
6. Wash in tap water until only the RBCs are stained yellow. Control under the microscope.
7. Acid fuchsin-Biebrich scarlet solution for 5 minutes.
8. Rinse in distilled water.
9. Place into 5 percent phosphotungstic acid for 10 minutes, *two changes of 5 minutes each* appear best.
10. Rinse thoroughly in distilled water.
11. 2 percent light green solution for 2 minutes.
12. Rinse in 1 percent acetic acid to remove the excess stain.
13. Dehydrate, clear, and mount.

Results

Nuclei	Brownish black
Muscle	Red
Collagen	Green
RBCs	Yellow

* Modification by G. Brown.

HEIDENHAIN'S AZAN STAIN[4]

Fixation

Helly's fluid, Zenker's fluid, Bouin's fluid, or Carnoy's fluid.

Solutions Required

A. 1 percent Azocarmine B Solution.

Azocarmine B (C.I. 50090)	1 g
Distilled water	100 ml

Bring to the boil and cool to 56 C. Filter, and cool to room temperature. Add:

Glacial acetic acid	1 ml

B. 0.1 percent Aniline/Alcohol:

Aniline	1 ml
95 percent ethyl alcohol	1000 ml

C. 1 percent Acetic Acid in 95 percent Ethyl Alcohol.
D. 5 percent Phosphotungstic Acid.
E. Aniline Blue–Orange G Solution:

Aniline blue, wat. sol. (C.I. 42755)	0.5 g
Orange G (C.I. 16230)	2.0 g
Glacial acetic acid	8.0 ml
Distilled water	to 100.0 ml

Heat to dissolve the ingredients and filter when cool. Dilute 1:3 with distilled water for use.

Method

1. Sections to water.
2. If formalin fixed, mordant overnight in Zenker's fluid.
3. Remove the mercuric chloride deposit and wash in running water for 5 minutes.
4. Azocarmine stain at 56–60 C for 1 hour. Cool for 20 minutes.
5. Wash in distilled water.
6. Differentiate in 0.1 percent aniline/alcohol until the nuclei stand out clearly and the cytoplasm and connective tissue are a pale pink. Control under the microscope. Takes up to 1 hour.
7. Arrest the differentiation by rinsing thoroughly in 1 percent acetic acid in 95 percent alcohol.
8. Mordant in 5 percent phosphotungstic acid for 1 hour.
9. Aniline blue-orange G solution for 1 hour. Use undiluted for pituitary and pancreas.
10. Wash in distilled water.
11. Dehydrate, clear, and mount.

Results

Nuclei and RBCs	Red
Collagen and reticulin	Deep blue
Mucin	Blue
Muscle	Orange to red
Neuroglia	Pale red
Basophilic granules	Deep blue
Acidophilic granules	Orange to red

Methods for the Demonstration of Elastic Fibers

WEIGERT'S RESORCIN-FUCHSIN METHOD[5]

Fixation

Ten percent neutral formalin, formal sublimate, or alcohol.

Solutions Required

A. Weigert's Resorcin-Fuchsin Stain:

Rosanilin (*basic fuchsin*) (C.I. 42510)	2 g
Resorcin (*resorcinol*)	4 g
Distilled water	to 200 ml

Place in a large porcelain evaporating dish and bring to the boil. Slowly add 25 ml of 29 percent ferric chloride ($FeCl_3$), stir, and boil for a further 2–5 minutes. Cool and filter. Discard the filtrate and place the filter paper containing the precipitate into the original dish to dry. When dry, add 200 ml of 95 percent ethyl alcohol and heat gently on an electric hotplate until the precipitate is dissolved. Remove the filter paper and add 4 ml of concentrated hydrochloric acid. Cool and filter. Make up the volume to 200 ml with 95 percent ethyl alcohol. This solution is stable for several months.

OR

Hart's Modification of Weigert's Elastic Stain.[6] This is simply a dilution of Weigert's stain:

Weigert's elastic stain	10–30 ml
2 percent hydrochloric acid in 70 percent ethyl alcohol	90–70 ml

OR

Sheridan's Modificaton of Weigert's Elastic Stain.[7] In place of Rosanilin (basic fuchsin), substitute as follows:

Crystal violet (C.I. 42555)	2 g
Dextrin	2 g

Make up in exactly the same way as Weigert's stain.

B. Van Gieson's Stain (see page 218).

Method

1. Sections to 70 percent alcohol.
   Note. If Hart's or Sheridan's modifications are used, take sections to water and oxidize as follows:
   a. 0.5 percent potassium permanganate for 5 minutes.
   b. Wash in water.
   c. Bleach in 5 percent oxalic acid for 5 minutes.
   d. Wash in tap water for 3 minutes followed by several rinses in distilled water.
2. Weigert's elastic stain for 3 hours to overnight at room temperature. Hart's modification of Weigert's elastic stain should be left overnight at room temperature and Sheridan's modification may be left for 1 hour at 56 C, or preferably overnight at room temperature.
3. Rinse off the excess stain with 95 percent alcohol and examine under the microscope. If the staining is diffuse, differentiate in 1 percent acid alcohol until the elastic stands out clearly.
4. Wash in tap water.
5. Rinse in distilled water.
6. Counterstain with Van Gieson's stain for 3 minutes.
7. Rinse in distilled water.
8. Dehydrate, clear, and mount.

Results

Elastic fibers	
(Weigert's)	Dark blue-black
(Hart's)	Blue-black
(Sheridan's)	Deep green
Collagen	Red
Muscle	Yellow
RBCs	Yellow

The mechanism of this staining reaction is not really understood, but it is thought that the resorcin–fuchsin–ferric chloride mixture in acid solution forms an iron–resorcin lake. It is known that other cationic dyes such as crystal violet may be used as a substitute for basic fuchsin, and that other phenolic compounds may be substituted for resorcin.

Oxidizing with the potassium permanganate–oxalic acid sequence may improve the staining results, but is not essential to the reaction.

TAENZER-UNNA ORCEIN METHOD[8]

Fixation

Any well-fixed tissue.

Solutions Required

A. Taenzer's Orcein:

Synthetic orcein (certified dye)	1 g
70 percent ethyl alcohol	100 ml
Hydrochloric acid, conc.	1 ml

This solution is stable for many months.

B. Mallory's Borax-Methylene Blue:

Methylene blue (C.I. 52015)	1 g
Sodium borate (borax)	1 g
Distilled water	100 ml

Dilute for use as follows:

Borax-methylene blue solution	1 part
Distilled water	9 parts

C. 0.5 percent Colophonium (Rosin) in 95 percent Ethyl Alcohol

Method

1. Sections to alcohol.
2. Orcein stain for 30 minutes at 37 C or 2 hours to overnight at room temperature.
3. Rinse thoroughly in 70 percent alcohol.
4. Wash in running tap water for 5-10 minutes.
5. Rinse in distilled water.
6. Borax-methylene blue stain for 5 minutes.
7. Rinse in distilled water.
8. Differentiate in 0.5 percent colophonium in 95 percent alcohol for about 2 minutes. Keep the slide in motion and control under the microscope.
9. Dehydrate rapidly in absolute ethyl alcohol, clear, and mount.

Results

Elastic fibers	Dark brown to purple
Nuclei	Blue

This method is specific for elastic fibers, but the mechanism of the staining reaction is not known. However, synthetic orcein does give better and more reliable results than does the natural dye.

HUMBERSTONE'S ELASTIC TISSUE STAIN[9]

Fixation

Ten percent formalin or formal sublimate.

Solutions Required

A. Elastic Tissue Stain:

Victoria blue 4R (C.I. 42563)	1 g
Ethyl violet (C.I. 42600)	1 g

Dissolve in 200 ml of boiling distilled water and add in order:

Resorcin	4.0 g
Dextrin	0.5 g
30 percent ferric chloride, freshly prepared	25 ml

Boil for 3 minutes. Cool rapidly and filter. Discard the filtrate. Wash the precipitate with at least six changes of distilled water and transfer the filter paper containing the precipitate to the original beaker. Add 100 ml of 95 percent ethyl alcohol and boil gently on an electric hotplate (or in a water bath) for 15 minutes to dissolve the precipitate. Cool, filter, and make up to 350 ml with 95 percent ethyl alcohol. Add:

Phenol	10 g
Hydrochloric acid, conc.	4 ml

The stain is stable and appears to improve with age.

B. Van Gieson's Stain (see page 218).

Method

1. Sections to water.
2. 0.25 percent potassium permanganate for 10 minutes.
3. Rinse with distilled water.
4. 5 percent oxalic acid for 3 minutes.
5. Wash thoroughly in distilled water.
6. Rinse with 95 percent alcohol.
7. Elastic stain overnight at room temperature.
8. Rinse in 90 percent ethyl alcohol to remove excess stain.
9. Rinse in distilled water.
10. Van Gieson's stain for 3 minutes.
11. Rinse in distilled water.
12. Dehydrate, clear, and mount.

Results

Elastic fibers	Greenish-blue to blue-black
Collagen	Red
Muscle	Yellow

Note

1. Fixation in formalin which has been buffered with disodium hydrogen orthophosphate and sodium dihydrogen orthophosphate gives poor staining results.
2. Oxidizing with the potassium permanganate-oxalic acid sequence is essential to this method.
3. The mechanism of the staining reaction is not understood, but it is probably similar to that of Weigert's elastic stain.

VERHOEFF'S STAIN FOR ELASTIC TISSUE[10]

Fixation

Ten percent formalin, Helly's fluid, and Zenker's fluid.

Solutions Required

A. Verhoeff's Elastic Stain:

5 percent alcoholic hematoxylin	20 ml
10 percent aqueous ferric chloride	8 ml
Iodine solution	8 ml
Iodine	2 g
Potassium iodide	4 g
Distilled water	100 ml

Bale's modification also works well:

5 percent alcoholic hematoxylin	5 ml
10 percent aqueous ferric chloride	1 ml
Iodine solution	1 ml

B. 2 percent Aqueous Ferric Chloride.

C. Van Gieson's Stain (see page 218).

Method

1. Sections to alcohol.
2. Verhoeff's elastic stain for 15–30 minutes.
3. Rinse in distilled water.
4. Differentiate in 2 percent aqueous ferric chloride, controlling under the microscope, until only nuclei and elastic fibers are stained.

5. Rinse in distilled water.
6. "Blue" in running tap water for 10 minutes.
7. Rinse in distilled water.
8. Van Gieson's stain for 3 minutes.
9. Rinse in distilled water.
10. Dehydrate, clear, and mount.

Results

Nuclei	Black
Elastic fibers	Black
Collagen	Red
Muscle	Yellow
RBCs	Yellow

Note

1. Mercuric chloride pigment need not be removed prior to staining. It is dissolved by the iodine in the staining solution.
2. It is best to underdifferentiate slightly. Fine elastic fibers are easily decolorized.
3. The stain is not stable and must be prepared from the stock solutions each time it is required.

It is thought that the elastic tissue is easily penetrated by the stain in the form of a metallic-dye lake. The iodine possibly acts as both an oxidizing agent, thus accelerating the conversion of hematoxylin to hematein, and as a trapping agent for the cationic dye-lake, thus retarding its extraction during differentiation with the mordant (ferric chloride) in which it is readily soluble.

IRON GALLEIN METHOD FOR ELASTIC[11]

Fixation

Ten percent neutral buffered formalin.

Solutions Required

A. Iron Gallein Staining Solution:

Solution A

Gallein (C.I. 45445)	1 g
Ethylene glycol	20 ml
Dissolve and add:	
Absolute ethyl alcohol	80 ml

Solution B

Ferric chloride, 29 percent aq.	4 ml
Distilled water	95 ml
Hydrochloric acid, conc.	1 ml

For use mix:

Solution A	1 part
Solution B	1 part

B. 2 percent Ferric Chloride
C. Van Gieson's Stain (see page 000)

Method

The staining procedure is exactly the same as for Verhoeff's method. Apply the freshly prepared iron gallein solution for 30 minutes at room temperature.

Results

Nuclei	Black
Elastic fibers	Black
Collagen	Red
Muscle	Yellow
RBCs	Yellow

GOMORI'S ALDEHYDE FUCHSIN METHOD[12]

Fixation

Ten percent formalin and Bouin's fluid are preferred. Avoid fixatives containing chromates.

Solutions Required

A. Aldehyde Fuchsin Solution:

Rosanilin (*basic fuchsin*) (C.I. 42510)	0.5 g
Distilled water	30.0 ml
Absolute ethyl alcohol	70.0 ml

Dissolve and add:

Hydrochloric acid, conc.	1.0 ml
Paraldehyde (USP)	1.0 ml

Allow to stand until the solution becomes a deep violet color, about 24 hours. Store in the refrigerator.

B. Van Gieson's Stain (see page 218).

Method

1. Sections to water.
2. Lugol's iodine for 10 minutes.
3. Rinse in tap water.
4. 5 percent sodium thiosulfate for 5 minutes.
5. Wash well in tap water.
6. Rinse in 70 percent alcohol.
7. Aldehyde fuchsin stain for 5 minutes to 2 hours. The time used depends upon which tissue constituent is to be stained:

Elastic fibers	10–30 min
Mast cell granules	5–10 min
Pancreatic beta cells	15–30 min
Pituitary beta cells	30 min to 2 hr

8. Rinse in 70 percent alcohol, several changes.
9. Rinse in distilled water.
10. Van Gieson's stain for 3 minutes.
11. Rinse in distilled water.
12. Dehydrate, clear, and mount.

Results

Elastic fibers	Deep purple
Mast cell granules	Violet to purple
Pancreatic beta cells	Purple
Pituitary beta cells	Purple
Collagen	Red
Muscle	Yellow
RBCs	Yellow

The staining reaction of this method is not fully understood, but it is known that the paraldehyde and rosanilin form a Schiff-type reagent which shows an inexplicable affinity for elastic fibers, staining them a deep purple.

As can be seen the method has several applications apart from the staining of elastic fibers.

MOVAT'S PENTACHROME METHOD[13]

Fixation

Ten percent neutral buffered formalin, Bouin's fluid, or Zenker's fluid.

Solutions Required

A. 1 percent Alcian Blue Solution:

Alcian blue (C.I. 74240)	1 g
Distilled water	100 ml
Glacial acetic acid	1 ml

B. Alkaline Alcohol Solution:

Ammonium hydroxide	10 ml
95 percent alcohol	90 ml

C. Resorcin–Fuchsin Stain:

Weigert's elastic stain (see page 226)	10 ml
70 percent alcohol	100 ml
Hydrochloric acid, conc.	2 ml

D. Weigert's Iron Hematoxylin (see page 218)

E. Woodstain Scarlet–Acid Fuchsin Solution:

Solution A

Brilliant crocein MOO (*Woodstain scarlet*) (C.I. 27290)	0.1 g
Distilled water	99.5 ml
Glacial acetic acid	0.5 ml

Solution B

Acid fuchsin (C.I. 42685)	0.1 g
Distilled water	99.5 ml
Glacial acetic acid	0.5 ml

For use dilute as follows:

Solution A	8 parts
Solution B	2 parts

F. 0.5 percent Acetic Acid.

G. 5 percent Aqueous Phosphotungstic Acid.

H. Alcoholic Saffron Solution:

Saffron (Safran du Gatinais) (C.I. 75100)	6 g
Absolute ethyl alcohol	100 ml

Store in a tightly stoppered container to prevent hydration. Place in an oven at 58–60 C for 48 hours before use to extract the saffron.

Method

1. Sections to distilled water.
2. Alcian blue solution for 20 minutes.
3. Wash in running tap water for 5 minutes.
4. Alkaline alcohol for 2 hours. This converts the alcian blue into the insoluble pigment monastral fast blue.
5. Wash in running tap water for 10 minutes.
6. Rinse in 70 percent alcohol.
7. Resorcin–fuchsin overnight at room temperature.
8. Wash in running tap water for 10 minutes.
9. Rinse in distilled water.
10. Weigert's iron hematoxylin for 15 minutes.
11. Rinse thoroughly in tap water followed by a rinse in distilled water.
12. Woodstain scarlet–acid fuchsin solution for 5 minutes. The nuclei are differentiated in this solution.
13. Rinse in 0.5 percent acetic acid.
14. Differentiate in 5 percent phosphotungstic acid for 10–20 minutes. Control under the microscope until the collagen is pale pink and the background substance, which has been stained red, is bluish again.
15. Rinse in 0.5 percent acetic acid.
16. Rinse thoroughly in three changes of fresh, absolute ethyl alcohol.
17. Alcoholic saffron solution for 5–15 minutes.
18. Dehydrate in three changes of absolute ethyl alcohol.
19. Clear in three changes of xylene. Examine under the microscope, and if the collagen is not yellow enough repeat steps 16–19.
20. Mount.

Results

Nuclei	Black
Elastic fibers	Dark purple to black
Collagen	Yellow
Reticulin fibers	Yellow
Ground substance	Blue to bluish green
Fibrinoid	Red
Muscle	Red

Methods for the Demonstration of Reticulin Fibers

Reticulin fibers, which are argyrophilic, are best demonstrated by silver impregnation methods. As most of the silver techniques for reticulin are similar, only two reliable methods will be given in this text.

Studies with electron microscopy have suggested that reticulin is young collagen, either as single fibers or small bundles of fibers. It may be demonstrated by the periodic acid Schiff (PAS) reaction in certain situations due to a carbohydrate component, which may also be one of the reasons for its affinity to silver. As stated, the silver reticulin methods are all similar and follow the same sequence: oxidation, mordanting or sensitization, impregnation, reduction, toning, and fixing, a procedure very similar to photographic processing.

Sections that are to be stained by the silver impregnation methods should always be fixed to the slide with an adhesive, or they may be coated with a thin celloidin solution immediately prior to staining (see page 178). This is because alkaline silver solutions have a strong tendency to lift sections right off of the slide.

WILDER'S METHOD FOR RETICULIN FIBERS[14]

Fixation

Ten percent neutral buffered formalin, Helly's fluid, or Zenker's fluid.

Solutions Required

A. 10 percent Phosphomolybdic Acid.
B. 1 percent Aqueous Uranium Nitrate.
C. Ammoniacal Silver Nitrate Solution. To 5 ml of 10.2 percent silver nitrate add 28 percent ammonia, drop by drop, until the resultant precipitate is almost dissolved. Add 5 ml of 3.1 percent sodium hydroxide. Dissolve the resultant precipitate by adding more 28 percent ammonia, drop by drop, until the solution is faintly opalescent. Make up to 50 ml with distilled water. Use immediately.
D. Reducing Solution:

40 percent formaldehyde	0.5 ml
1 percent uranium nitrate, aq.	1.5 ml
Distilled water	50.0 ml

Make up freshly for use.
E. 0.2 percent Gold Chloride.
F. 5 percent Sodium Thiosulfate.
G. A counterstain as desired.

Method

1. Sections to distilled water.
2. Oxidize in 10 percent phosphomolybdic acid for 1 minute.
3. Wash in running water for 2 minutes.
4. Rinse in distilled water.
5. Sensitize in 1 percent uranium nitrate for 2–5 seconds.
6. Wash thoroughly in distilled water.
7. Ammoniacal silver nitrate solution for 1 minute.
8. Dip into 95 percent alcohol.
9. Place into the reducing solution for 1 minute.
10. Rinse thoroughly in distilled water.
11. Tone in 0.2 percent gold chloride for 1 minute. The sections should turn a pale lavender color. Control under the microscope.
12. Rinse in distilled water.
13. 5 percent sodium thiosulfate for 5 minutes.
14. Wash in running tap water for 5 minutes.
15. Counterstain if desired.
16. Dehydrate, clear, and mount.

Results

Reticulin	Black
Collagen	Pale rose

GORDON AND SWEETS' METHOD FOR RETICULIN[15]

Fixation

Any well-fixed tissue.

Solutions Required

A. Acidified Potassium Permanganate Solution:

1 percent potassium permanganate	47.5 ml
3 percent sulfuric acid	2.5 ml

I have found that 0.5 percent potassium permanganate works equally well.
B. 5 percent Oxalic Acid.
C. 2 percent Ferric Ammonium Sulfate.
D. Ammoniacal Silver Nitrate Solution. To 5 ml of 10 percent silver

nitrate add concentrated ammonia (S.G. 0.880), drop by drop, until the resultant precipitate is just dissolved. Add 5 ml of 3 percent sodium hydroxide and dissolve the resultant precipitate by adding more ammonia, drop by drop, until the solution is faintly opalescent. Make up to 50 ml with distilled water.

E. 10 percent Neutral Formalin.
F. 0.2 percent Gold Chloride.
G. 5 percent Sodium Thiosulfate.
H. Counterstain as desired.

Method

1. Sections to water.
2. Oxidize in acidified potassium permanganate for 1–7 minutes.
3. Wash in distilled water.
4. Bleach until white in 5 percent oxalic acid.
5. Wash in running tap water for 2 minutes.
6. Rinse thoroughly in distilled water.
7. Mordant (sensitize) in 2 percent Ferric ammonium sulfate for 10 minutes.
8. Rinse in distilled water.
9. Impregnate in ammoniacal silver nitrate solution for 7–10 seconds.
10. Wash in distilled water.
11. Reduce in 10 percent Neutral formalin for 30 seconds.
12. Wash in distilled water.
13. Tone in 0.2 percent Gold chloride for 1 minute.
14. Wash in distilled water.
15. Fix in 5 percent Sodium thiosulfate for 2–5 minutes.
16. Wash in running tap water for 5 minutes.
17. Counterstain if desired.
18. Dehydrate, clear, and mount.

Results

Reticulin fibers	Black

Note

1. The ammoniacal solution may be used for up to 30 days, although the staining time may have to be increased by several seconds.[16]
2. It has been reported that this solution must be handled with care at all times as it is *explosive*.[17]

Methods to Demonstrate Basement Membranes

JONES' PERIODIC ACID-METHENAMINE SILVER METHOD (P.A.M.), MODIFIED[18,19]

Fixation

Ten percent neutral buffered formalin, Bouin's fluid, or 4 percent buffered paraformaldehyde.

Solutions Required

A. 0.5 percent Periodic Acid.

B. Methenamine* Silver Solution:

A	5 percent sodium borate	5 ml
	Distilled water	25 ml
B	3 percent methenamine solution	25 ml
	5 percent silver nitrate	3 ml

Add solution A to solution B. The mixture will turn cloudy at first, but will clear with gentle agitation. Prepare freshly from the stock solutions and place into a water bath at 60 C.

C. 0.2 percent Gold Chloride.

D. 3 percent Sodium Thiosulfate.

Method

1. Sections to distilled water.
2. 0.5 percent periodic acid for 11 minutes.
3. Rinse in distilled water.
4. Methenamine silver solution for 30–80 minutes at 60 C. Start checking the sections after 30 minutes. Rinse with warm distilled water and control under the microscope until the basement membranes appear black.
5. Rinse in warm distilled water and allow to cool.
6. Tone in 0.2 percent gold chloride for up to 3 minutes. The sections will appear gray.
7. Rinse in distilled water.
8. 3 percent sodium thiosulfate for 5 minutes.
9. Wash very thoroughly in distilled water.
10. Counterstain with the Harris hematoxylin and eosin method.
11. Dehydrate, clear, and mount.

Results

Nuclei	Blue/black
Basement membranes	Black
Background	Shades of pink

* I prefer FISHER (TM) Methenamine.

LILLIE'S ALLOCHROME METHOD[20]

Fixation

Any well-fixed tissue.

Solutions Required

A. 0.5 percent Periodic Acid.
B. Schiff's Reagent (see page 304).
C. 0.5 percent Sodium Metabisulfite.
D. Weigert's Iron Hematoxylin (see page 218).
E. Picric Acid–Methyl Blue Solution:

Picric acid, sat. aq. soln.	250.0 ml
Methyl blue (C.I. 42780)	0.1 g

Method

1. Sections to distilled water.
2. 0.5 percent periodic acid for 10 minutes.
3. Wash in running tap water for 5 minutes.
4. Schiff's reagent for 10–15 minutes.
5. 0.5 percent sodium metabisulfite for 3 changes of 2 minutes each.
6. Wash in running tap water for 10 minutes.
7. Weigert's iron hematoxylin for 2 minutes.
8. Wash in running tap water for 10 minutes.
9. Picric acid–methyl blue solution for 6 minutes.
10. Dehydrate from 95 percent alcohol through absolute alcohol, clear, and mount.

Results

Nuclei	Black, gray, or brown
Cytoplasm and muscle	Gray, green to greenish-yellow
Collagen	Blue
Reticulin	Blue
Basement membranes	Red

Note

Valuable for differentiating between reticulin and basement membranes.

Methods for Connective Tissue Cells

FIBROBLASTS

Fibroblasts give rise to all types of connective tissue and they produce fibroglia fibrils intimately connected with the cytoplasm of the cell.

These fibrils run over the surface of the fibroblast and extend out along its processes. They are very delicate, definitely separated from one another, and seem to pass from cell to cell. Fibroglia fibrils are most evident when the fibroblast is multiplying readily, such as in granulation tissue, organization of fibrin, and in fibrosarcomas. They can only be demonstrated in *absolutely fresh* tissue, that is, placed into fixative immediately on removal from the living tissue. Autopsy specimens are useless.

Phosphotungstic acid hematoxylin stains the fibrils blue, and they may also be demonstrated by the method given below.

MALLORY'S ACID FUCHSIN STAIN[21]

Fixation

Zenker's fluid.

Solutions Required

A. 1 percent Aqueous Acid Fuchsin (C.I. 42685)
B. 0.1 percent Potassium Permanganate.

Method

1. Sections to distilled water.
2. 1 percent aqueous acid fuchsin for 1 hour at 56 C or overnight at room temperature.
3. Drain, and differentiate in 0.1 percent potassium permanganate for 40–60 seconds. Do not exceed this time or the section will be completely decolorized.
4. Dehydrate in 95 percent alcohol followed by absolute alcohol, clear, and mount.

Results

Nuclei	Red
Fibroglia fibrils	Red
Collagen	Pale reddish yellow
Elastic	Lemon yellow
RBCs	Purplish red

MAST CELLS

The function of these cells is not fully known, but it is known that mast cells produce heparin (a sulfated mucopolysaccharide that accounts for their metachromasy) and histamine. Mast cells contain an indented nucleus and coarse basophilic and metachromatic granules in the cytoplasm. These granules are well demonstrated metachromatically with polychrome methylene blue, toluidine blue, or thionin, and may be demonstrated as basophilic structures with the Giemsa stain.

The methods given below are recommended.

TOLUIDINE BLUE METHOD[22]

Fixation

Carnoy's fluid, absolute alcohol, or 10 percent neutral formalin. Frozen sections give the best results.

Solution Required

A. 0.5 percent Aqueous Toluidine Blue (C.I. 52040).

Method

1. Sections to water.
2. 0.5 percent toluidine blue for 3–5 minutes.
3. Rinse in distilled water.
4. Dehydrate rapidly in absolute ethyl alcohol.
5. Clear and mount.

Results

Nuclei	Blue
Mast cell granules	Red to purple

Note

The reaction of the dye is strong with mast cell granules and is relatively resistant to ethanol. Other substances should be dehydrated in butanol or mounted in an aqueous medium.

A MODIFIED THIONIN TECHNIQUE[23]

Fixation

Ten percent neutral formalin.

Solutions Required

A. 1 percent Aqueous Thionin (C.I. 52000). For use dilute as follows:

1 percent thionin solution	0.3 ml
Tap water	50.0 ml

B. 0.2 percent Acetic Acid.
C. Saturated Solution of Tartrazine (C.I. 19140) in Cellosolve (2-Ethoxyethanol).

Method

1. Sections to water.
2. Thionin solution for 20 minutes.
3. Rinse in tap water.
4. Differentiate in 0.2 percent acetic acid until the background is clear and the mast cell granules and nuclei appear red to purple. Control under the microscope.
5. Rinse in tap water.
6. Rinse briefly in absolute ethyl alcohol to destroy the nuclear metachromasia.
7. Tartrazine solution for 20–30 seconds.
8. Rinse quickly in tap water.
9. Dehydrate in absolute ethyl alcohol, clear, and mount.

Results

Nuclei	Blue
Mast cell granules	Red to purple
Background	Yellow

GIEMSA'S STAIN (MODIFIED)[24]

Fixation

Any well-fixed tissue.

Solutions Required

A. Giemsa Stain, Gurr's Improved R.66.* Purchase as a readymade stock solution. Dilute for use:

Giemsa stain	1 part
Tap water	49 parts

B. 0.001 percent (1:1000) Acetic Acid.

Method

1. Sections to distilled water.
2. Dilute Giemsa stain overnight at room temperature.
3. Rinse in distilled water.

* Available from Bio/Medical Specialties, Santa Monica, California.

4. Differentiate in 1:1000 acetic acid, controlling under the microscope.
5. Dehydrate rapidly in two changes of absolute ethyl alcohol, clear, and mount.

Results

Nuclei	Blue
Mast cell granules	Deep blue
Eosinophilic granules	Red
Cytoplasm	Pink
Bacteria	Blue

PLASMA CELLS

Plasma cells have a large oval cytoplasm with the nucleus often located at one pole of the cell. A good hematoxylin and eosin stain is adequate for the identification of these cells, but they may be stained specifically. Unna's method employing methyl green and pyronin was introduced in 1910 and has since been modified by many workers. This stain can be very capricious. Trevan and Sharrock's modification is recommended for tissue fixed in an alcoholic fixative or formalin, while Jordan and Baker's modification is recommended for Zenker-fixed tissue. In both of these modifications the methyl green should be washed with several changes of chloroform in a separating funnel to extract the methyl violet, a product of methyl green, from this dye. This process will take at least eight washings until the chloroform is almost colorless.

METHYL GREEN-PYRONIN METHOD FOR PLASMA CELLS[25,26]

Fixation

Carnoy's fluid, alcoholic formalin, 10 percent formalin, or Zenker's fluid.

Solutions Required

A. Jordan and Baker's Methyl Green–Pyronin Solution:

0.5 percent pyronin Y (C.I. 45005), aq.	37 ml
0.5 percent methyl green (C.I. 42585), aq.	13 ml
Acetate buffer, pH 4.8	50 ml

OR

Trevan and Sharrock's Methyl Green–Pyronin Solution:

5 percent pyronin Y (C.I. 45005), aq.	35 ml
2 percent methyl green (C.I. 42585), aq.	20 ml
Distilled water	500 ml

For use, dilute with an equal volume of acetate buffer, pH 4.8
Note: The methyl green must be washed with chloroform before the aqueous solutions are prepared. The acetate buffer is prepared as follows:

0.1N acetic acid	80 ml
0.1N sodium acetate	120 ml

B. Acetone.
C. Acetone–Xylol (equal parts).

Method

1. Sections to distilled water.
2. Methyl green–pyronin stain for 15-60 minutes. (Jordon and Baker's modification is recommended after Zenker fixation).
3. Rinse quickly in distilled water.
4. Blot almost dry with fluffless filter paper.
5. Rinse the slide rapidly with two changes of acetone. About 1-2 seconds for each rinse.
6. Rinse quickly in acetone–xylol mixture.
7. Clear in fresh xylene and mount.

Results

Nuclei	Green
Cytoplasm	Rosy red
Deoxyribonucleic acid (DNA)	Green
Ribonucleic acid (RNA)	Rosy red

Note

Methyl green is considered specific for deoxyribonucleic acid (DNA), and pyronin will specifically demonstrate ribonucleic acid (RNA) if it is controlled by ribonuclease extraction. Pyronin Y is preferred to Pyronin B as it stains less diffusely.

HITCHCOCK AND EHRLICH'S METHOD FOR PLASMA CELLS[27]

Fixation

Zenker's fluid is preferred although 10 percent formalin will suffice.

Solutions Required

A. Malachite Green Solution:

Malachite green (C.I. 42000)	0.3 g
Distilled water	15.0 ml

B. Acridine Red Solution:

Acridine red (C.I. 45000)	0.9 g
Distilled water	45.0 ml

Mix solutions A and B for use. Filter.

Method

1. Sections to distilled water.
2. Malachite green–acridine red mixture for 30–60 seconds if fixed in Zenker's fluid. Formalin fixed tissue requires 5 minutes.
3. Rinse quickly in distilled water.
4. Dehydrate rapidly in absolute ethyl alcohol, clear, and mount.

Results

Nuclei of plasma cells	Blue-green
Cytoplasm	Crimson

Other cells in lighter shades.

Methods for Bone and Cartilage

Excellent sections can be produced from properly decalcified bone. These are normally stained by the hematoxylin and eosin method (see page 212) or the Van Gieson method (see page 218). The marrow cells are best demonstrated with one of the modifications of the Giemsa stain. Ground sections may sometimes be required for the study of lamallae and canaliculi, although this technique is being replaced with the methods for undecalcified sections of plastic embedded bone.

The technique for ground sections is as follows:

Method

1. Fix the specimen in 10 percent formalin.
2. Cut a very thin slice of the bone and macerate to remove any superfluous tissue.
3. Wash thoroughly and air dry.
4. Grind between two pieces of pumice or on a glass plate that has been smeared with carborundum paste until the specimen is paper thin and almost transparent.
5. Wash thoroughly and dry.

6. Place a small piece of balsam on a slide and another piece on a coverslip. Heat until the balsam just melts.
7. Place the specimen into the balsam on the coverslip and press into the balsam on the slide.

Results

Lacunae and canaliculi	Filled with air
Lamallae	Brown/black lines

Note

If desired, the lacunae and canaliculi can be filled with colored celloidin. After step 3 soak the bone in ether for 1–2 days and then place into celloidin that has been colored with basic fuchsin for 2–3 days. Transfer to 80 percent alcohol for 2–3 days and proceed with step 4. Lacunae and canaliculi show up red.

Plastic embedded sections of undecalcified bone require special preparation and embedding procedures if thin sections are to be obtained for microscopic examination. Such sections, properly stained, show a degree of detail that is impossible to obtain with ground sections or decalcified paraffin sections.

Undecalcified bone sections for plastic embedding may be processed in the following manner[28]:

Method

1. Specimens no larger than 20 × 15 × 8 mm should be fixed and thoroughly dehydrated in acetone for 24–36 hours. At least four changes of acetone are required.
2. Infiltrate under vacuum in catalyzed monomer and leave for 18 hours (overnight) at 5 C.

   The monomer is prepared by mixing methyl and butyl methacrylate in equal parts and filtering through three changes of calcium chloride (8 mesh), using Whatman No. 1 filter paper, to dehydrate the solution. Store at 5 C.

   Note. Should the specimens fail to infiltrate properly and the blocks are not fully polymerized, the monomer should be washed as follows: In a separating funnel mix five parts of monomer to one part of washing solution:

Sodium chloride	20 g
Sodium hydroxide	5 g
Distilled water	100 ml

   and shake vigorously. Allow to separate and drain off the bottom layer of washing solution. Repeat this procedure several times. The solution should now be cleared of inhibitor (hydroquinone).

Pour into a beaker containing a two-inch layer of anhydrous calcium chloride and stir thoroughly. Filter as before.

3. Discard the monomer solution and replace with the partial polymer solution. Place the specimen in an open dish in a desiccator and reduce the pressure to 9 mm of mercury. Leave for five minutes. Repeat this step until all of the air has been extracted from the specimen. Remove the container from the desiccator and cover. Leave overnight at 5 C.

   The partial polymer is prepared by dissolving 5 g of benzoyl peroxide (the catalyst) in 1000 ml of monomer and filtering. Heat in a water bath at 70–80 C under an exhaust hood with constant stirring. After about two hours the solution will become slightly syrupy and refraction waves will appear. When the solution attains the consistency of glycerine prepolymerization is complete. Remove from the heat and cool rapidly to room temperature, cover, and store at 5 C.
4. Embed in metal molds, silicon rubber molds, or glass slide molds. Orientate the specimen and add sufficient partial polymer to cover the specimen. Subject to alternating vacuum and pressure until all air is removed. Fill the mold with polymer and place in an oven at 48 C. As the block shrinks during curing, more polymer is added periodically until the desired height is obtained. This usually takes about 24–36 hours.
5. Sections are cut on a motor-driven Jung Model K microtome equipped with tungsten carbide-tipped knives. During sectioning both the knife edge and the block are kept flooded with 70 percent alcohol and the sections are guided up the blade of the knife as they are cut.
6. The cut sections are laid on gelatinized slides and gently teased until the wrinkles have been removed. The slide is then exposed to warm xylene fumes in a covered pan for approximately two hours to further spread and flatten the section.
7. Most staining methods are applicable to these sections. Sections are hydrated in the same manner as paraffin sections as methacrylate is soluble in xylene.

As stated earlier the hematologic elements in the bone marrow may be demonstrated by one of the modifications of the Giemsa stain. Two modifications are given, the second method being used at the University of Texas Medical Branch for bone marrow biopsies.

WOLBACH'S GIEMSA METHOD[29]

Fixation

Zenker's fluid is preferred but any well-fixed tissue is acceptable.

Solutions Required

A. Giemsa Solution:

Giemsa stock (Wolbach's Modification)*	1.25 ml
Methyl alcohol	1.50 ml
Distilled water	50.00 ml

B. Rosin-alcohol solution:

10 percent colophonium (rosin) in absolute ethyl alcohol	5 ml
95 percent ethyl alcohol	40 ml

Method

1. Sections to distilled water.
2. Dilute Giemsa solution overnight.
3. Differentiate in the rosin-alcohol solution until the sections appear pinkish. Control under the microscope.
4. Dehydrate in absolute alcohol and clear in two changes of xylene. Mount.

Results

Nuclei	Blue
Other tissue elements	Shades of pink
Rickettsia	Purple
Bacteria	Blue

MODIFIED GIEMSA FOR BONE MARROW BIOPSIES[30]

Fixation

Any well-fixed tissue. Undecalcified formalin fixed soft tissue should be mordanted in Bouin's fluid for one hour at 60 C or overnight at room temperature.

Solutions Required

A. Giemsa Solution:

Giemsa stock (Wolbach's Modification)*	2.5 ml
Distilled water	47.5 ml

B. 0.05 percent Acetic Acid.

Method

1. Sections to distilled water.
2. 5 percent Giemsa solution for 45-60 minutes.

* This is best purchased ready made.

3. Rinse in distilled water.
4. Wash well and differentiate in 0.05 percent acetic acid. The section will shed a blue haze and appear pinkish. Control under the microscope.
5. In a coplin jar, dehydrate through 95 percent alcohol to which 2 drops of glacial acetic acid have been added for 5–10 seconds.
6. In a coplin jar, dehydrate through absolute ethyl alcohol to which 2 drops of glacial acetic acid have been added for 5–10 seconds.
7. Dehydrate through neutral absolute ethyl alcohol for 5–10 seconds.
8. Clear in two changes of xylene and mount.

Note. The section should be examined under the microscope after step 4, and again after step 8. If it appears too blue, steps 6 through 8 should be repeated.

Results

Nuclei	Blue
Cytoplasm	Pink
Eosinophilic granules	Bright pink to red
Other tissue elements	Shades of pink

CARTILAGE

Cartilage may be demonstrated by the hematoxylin and eosin method. Ehrlich's hematoxylin is particularly useful in demonstrating the cement lines of bone and the mucopolysaccharide content of cartilage, but the strong staining of the basophilic material may obscure the nuclear detail. The use of Weigert's iron hematoxylin may give more precise nuclear staining.

Methods for the Demonstration of Muscle

Muscle fibers and connective tissue fibers differ from each other in both structure and function. While connective tissue fibers are intercellular, noncontractile, and bind tissues, the muscle fibers are contractile and the fibers are cells. The purpose of muscle is to move parts of the body by its contractions, whether voluntary or involuntary.

Three types of muscle are distinguishable. They are:

1. Smooth muscle
2. Skeletal muscle
3. Cardiac muscle

SMOOTH MUSCLE

Smooth muscle is nonstriated, involuntary muscle, with sustained rhythmic contractions that do not require impulses from the central nervous system for contraction. It is located in the alimentary, respiratory, and urogenital tracts, around glandular organs, and the ciliary muscle of the eye, and in blood vessels.

Smooth muscle is easily demonstrated by the hematoxylin and eosin method, and the connective tissue stains described earlier in the chapter.

SKELETAL MUSCLE

Skeletal muscle is striated, voluntary muscle, which only moves on receiving impulses from the central nervous system. It is the locomotory muscle that moves the parts of the body, and, as its name implies, is attached to the bones by tendons. It is distributed all over the body, including the abdominal wall and the diaphragm. Muscle with the same morphologic appearance as skeletal muscle can be found in various places such as the tongue. As it is not attached to bone, this is more accurately termed voluntary muscle.

Skeletal muscle is demonstrated by the hematoxylin and eosin method and the connective tissue stains. The cross-striations may be demonstrated by Heidenhain's iron hematoxylin or the phosphotungstic acid hematoxylin (PTAH) method.

CARDIAC MUSCLE

Cardiac muscle is striated, involuntary muscle, although the rate of contraction is regulated by impulses from the central nervous system. The contractions are not sustained as there is a pause between each contraction. This muscle is only found in the heart.

Cardiac muscle is demonstrated by the same methods as skeletal muscle.

HEIDENHAIN'S IRON HEMATOXYLIN METHOD[31]

Fixation

Ten percent neutral formalin for cross-striations in muscle, Flemming's fluid minus acetic acid for mitochondria.

Solutions Required

A. 5 percent Ferric Ammonium Sulfate (iron alum).
B. Heidenhain's Hematoxylin:

Hematoxylin (C.I. 75290)	1 g
Absolute ethyl alcohol	20 ml
Distilled water	180 ml

Dissolve with gentle heat on an electric hotplate and ripen for 3–4 weeks. Filter before use.

C. 1 percent Ferric Ammonium Sulfate.
D. Counterstain of choice.

Method

1. Sections to water.
2. Mordant in 5 percent ferric ammonium sulfate for 3 hours to overnight.
3. Rinse in distilled water.
4. Heidenhain's hematoxylin for 1–6 hours.
   Note. Staining for 45 minutes at 45 C also gives good results.
5. Wash in running tap water for 2–5 minutes.
6. Rinse in distilled water.
7. Differentiate in 1 percent ferric ammonium sulfate. Control under the microscope.
8. Wash in running tap water for 10–20 minutes.
9. Counterstain if desired. Rinse in distilled water.
10. Dehydrate, clear, and mount.

Results

Nuclei	Black
Mitochondria	Black
Mitotic figures	Black
Muscle striations	Black
RBCs	Black

MALLORY'S PHOSPHOTUNGSTIC ACID HEMATOXYLIN (PTAH)[32]

Fixation

Zenker's fluid is preferred, but 10 percent neutral formalin will suffice. *Note*: After Zenker fixation the mercuric chloride deposit must be dissolved with Lugol's iodine, *but under no circumstances* should the iodine be removed with sodium thiosulfate as this will ruin the stain. The iodine should be removed by washing in alcohol.

Solutions Required

A. 0.5 percent Potassium Permanganate.
B. 5 percent Oxalic Acid.
C. Mallory's Phosphotungstic Acid Hematoxylin.

Hematoxylin (C.I. 75290)	1 g
Phosphotungstic acid	20 g
Distilled water	1000 ml

Dissolve the solids in separate portions of distilled water, mix together, and stand in the light for several weeks to ripen. Spontaneous ripening can be obtained by adding 0.177 g potassium permanganate. This solution is ready for immediate use.

Method

1. Sections to water.
2. Remove the mercuric chloride deposits if Zenker fixed.
3. Wash in distilled water.
4. 0.5 percent potassium permanganate for 5 minutes.
5. Wash well in distilled water.
6. 5 percent oxalic acid until bleached white. This takes up to 5 minutes.
7. Wash well in two changes of distilled water.
8. Phosphotungstic acid hematoxylin overnight at room temperature.
9. Rinse well in 95 percent alcohol.
10. Dehydrate in absolute alcohol, clear and mount.

Results

Nuclei	Deep blue
Fibrin	Blue
Cross-striations	Blue
Collagen	Reddish
Elastic fibers	Bluish

METHOD FOR DEMONSTRATING MYOCARDIAL ISCHEMIA[33]

Fixation

Ten percent neutral formalin.

Solutions Required

A. Harris' Hematoxylin. (see page 208).
B. 0.1 percent Aqueous Basic Fuchsin (*Rosanilin* C.I. 42510).
C. Acetone.
D. 0.1 percent Picric Acid in Acetone.

Method

1. Sections to water.
2. Harris' hematoxylin for 30 seconds.
3. Wash in tap water.
4. Rinse in distilled water.
5. 0.1 percent basic fuchsin for 3 minutes.
6. Rinse in distilled water.
7. Rinse in acetone.
8. Differentiate in 0.1 percent picric acid in acetone for 15 seconds. Increase the time by one second for each succeeding section and discard the solution after five sections have been differentiated.
9. Rinse in acetone.
10. Clear in xylene and mount.

Results

Nuclei	Blue
Normal muscle	Yellow
Ischemic muscle	Red
RBCs	Red

REFERENCES

1. Van Gieson I: Laboratory notes of technical methods for the nervous system. NY Med J 50:57–60, 1889
2. Masson PJ: Some histological methods. Trichrome stainings and their preliminary technique. J Technol Method 12:75–90, 1929
3. Gomori G: A rapid one-step trichrome stain. Am J Clin Pathol 20:661–64, 1950
4. Heidenhain M: Über die Mallorysche Bindegewebsfärbung mit Karmin und Azokarmin als Vorfarben. Z Wiss Mikrosk 32:361–72, 1915
5. Weigert C: Ueber eine Methode zur Färbung elastischer Fasern. Zentralbl Allg Pathol 9:289–92, 1898
6. Hart K: Die Färbung der elastischen Farsen mit dem von Weigert angengebenen Farbstoff. Zentralbl Allg Pathol 19:1–3, 1908
7. Sheridan WF: Weigert's elastic tissue stain prepared with crystal violet. J Technol Method 12:123, 1929
8. Mallory FB: Pathological Technique. Philadelphia, Saunders, 1938, p 171
9. Humberstone GCW, Humberstone FD: An elastic tissue stain. J Med Lab Technol 26:99–101, 1969

10. Verhoeff FH: Some new staining methods of wide applicability; including a rapid differential stain for elastic tissue. JAMA 50:876-77, 1908
11. Churukian CJ, Schenk EA: Iron gallein elastic method-a substitute for Verhoeff's elastic tissue stain. Stain Technol 51:213-17, 1976
12. Gomori G: Aldehyde-Fuchsin: a new stain for elastic tissue. Am J Clin Pathol 20:665-66, 1950
13. Movat HZ: Demonstration of all connective tissue elements in a single section. Arch Pathol 60:289-95, 1955
14. Wilder HC: An improved technique for silver impregnation of reticulum fibers. Am J Pathol 11:817-19, 1935
15. Gordon HB, Sweets HH: A simple method for the silver impregnation of reticulum. Am J Clin Pathol 12:545, 1936
16. Brown GG: Ammoniacal silver hydroxide solution: a one-month test period on its usability for impregnating connective tissue fibers. Stain Technol 44:247-49, 1969
17. Wallington EA: The explosive properties of ammoniacal-silver solutions. J Med Lab Technol 22:220-23, 1965
18. Jones DB: Inflammation and repair of glomerulus. Am J Pathol 27:991-1009, 1951
19. Jones DB: Nephrotic glomerulonephritis. Am J Pathol 33:313-29, 1957
20. Lillie RD: The allochrome procedure. A differential method segregating the connective tissues, collagen, reticulum and basement membranes into two groups. Am J Clin Pathol 21:484-88, 1951
21. Mallory FB: Pathologic Technique. Philadelphia, Saunders, 1938, p 151
22. Kramer H, Windrum GM: The metachromatic staining reaction. J Histochem Cytochem 3:227-37, 1955
23. Cook HC: A modified thionin technique for mast cells in tissue sections. J Med Lab Technol 18:188-89, 1961
24. Gurr GT: Biological Staining Methods, 7th ed. London, George T. Gurr, 1963, p 31
25. Jordan BM, Baker JR: A simple pyronine/methyl green technique. Q J Microsc Sci 96:177-179, 1955
26. Trevan DJ, Sharrock A: A methyl green-pyronin-orange G stain for formalin-fixed tissues. J Pathol Bacteriol 63:326-29, 1951
27. Hitchcock CH, Ehrlich W: A new method for differential staining of plasma cells and of other basophilic cells. Arch Pathol 9:625-630, 1930
28. Urban KH: Processing and cutting of undecalcified bone specimens. Histotechnology Topics, ASCP Educational Center Program, August 1973

29. Wolbach SB: Studies on Rocky Mountain Spotted Fever. J Med Res 41:1-197, 1919
30. Brown GG: A Modified Giemsa Stain for Bone Marrow Biopsies. Galveston, University of Texas Medical Branch, 1976
31. Heidenhain M: Noch einmal über die Darstellung der Centralkörper durch Eisenhämatoxylin nebst einigen allgemeinen Bemerkungen über die Hämatoxylinfarben. Z Wiss Mikrosk 13:186-99, 1896
32. Mallory FB: A contribution to staining methods. J Exp Med 5:15-20, 1900
33. Lie JT, Holley KE, Kampa WR, Titus JL: New histochemical method for morphologic diagnosis of early stages of myocardial ischemia. Mayo Clin Proc 46:319-37, 1971

BIBLIOGRAPHY

Clayden EC: Practical Section Cutting and Staining, 4th ed. London, Churchill, 1962

Culling CFA: Handbook of Histopathological and Histochemical Techniques, 3rd ed. London, Butterworth, 1974

Drury RAB, Wallington EA: Carleton's Histological Technique, 4th ed. London, Oxford University Press, 1967

Freeman WH, Bracegirdle B: An Atlas of Histology, London, Heinemann, 1966

Hoskins MM, Bevelander G: Outline of Histology, 3rd ed. St. Louis, Mosby, 1955

Mallory FB: Pathological Technique. Philadelphia, Saunders, 1938

Thompson SW: Selected Histochemical and Histological Methods, Springfield, Ill, Thomas, 1966

FIFTEEN

Cell Products, Special Cells, and Cytoplasmic Inclusions

Keratin

Skin is composed of two layers, the *epidermis*, or outer layer, and the *dermis*. The epidermis has an outer covering of *keratin* that is a fibrous protein derived from dead flattened cells. This may be hard, as in nails and hair, very tough as on the feet (particularly on the great toe and heel) and calluses, or soft as on the majority of the skin. Hard and tough keratin may be softened by immersing it in Perenyi's fluid (page 43) or four percent phenol either prior to or following processing.

Keratin stains strongly with picric acid as in the Van Gieson stain, is generally P.A.S. positive, and is Gram positive.

A METHOD FOR KERATIN AND MUCIN-LIKE SUBSTANCES (MODIFIED BY G. BROWN)[1]

Fixation

10 percent neutral formalin.

Solutions Required

A. Harris' Hematoxylin (page 208).
B. 1 percent Acid Alcohol.
C. Eosin–Phloxin Solution (page 211).
D. Alcian Green in Acetic Acid:

Alcian green 2GX* (*No color index*)	1.0 g
Distilled water	99.5 ml
Glacial acetic acid	0.5 ml
Thymol crystals	0.02 g

Filter before use.

E. Ethanolic Saffron:

Saffron* (C.I. 75100)	0.25 g
Absolute ethyl alcohol	100.00 ml

Place in a flask, preferrably fitted with a reflux condenser and boil in a water bath to dissolve as much of the powder as possible. Make up to 100 ml with fresh absolute alcohol and filter. Keep in a well-stoppered bottle.

Method

1. Sections to water.
2. Stain as for the hematoxylin and eosin method, but extend the staining time in eosin-phloxin to 3 minutes.
3. Rinse in distilled water.
4. Alcian green solution for 5 minutes.
5. Rinse thoroughly in distilled water. The section should have a pink color to the naked eye.
6. Rinse in 95 percent ethyl alcohol.
7. Ethanolic saffron for 5 minutes.
8. Dehydrate in two changes of absolute ethyl alcohol, clear in xylol, and mount.

Results

Nuclei	Blue/black
Acid mucopolysaccharides	Green
Connective tissue	Yellow to Orange
Keratin	Red
Other tissue elements	Shades of pink and red

* Obtainable from Roboz Surgical Instrument Co., Washington, D.C.

DANE'S METHOD FOR PREKERATIN, KERATIN, AND MUCIN[2]

Fixation

10 percent neutral formalin.

Solutions Required

A. Mayer's Hemalum (page 208).
B. Phloxine (C.I. 45405), 1 percent aq. soln.
C. Alcian Blue (C.I. 74240), 0.5 percent solution in 0.5 percent Acetic Acid.
D. Orange G Solution:

Orange G (C.I. 16230)	0.5 g
Phosphotungstic acid	2.0 g
Distilled water	100.0 ml

Method

1. Sections to distilled water.
2. Mayer's hemalum for 10 minutes.
3. Blue in running tap water for 10 minutes.
4. Rinse in distilled water.
5. Phloxine solution for 3 minutes.
6. Rinse thoroughly in distilled water to remove excess phloxine.
7. Alcian blue solution for 5 minutes.
8. Wash in running tap water for 2 minutes.
9. Rinse in distilled water.
10. Orange G solution for 13 minutes.
11. Dehydrate through two changes of 95 percent alcohol, five dips in each.
12. Dehydrate through two changes of absolute ethyl alcohol, fifteen dips in each.
13. Clear in xylene and mount.

Results

Nuclei	Orange to brown
Acid mucopolysaccharides	Pale blue
Keratin and prekeratin	Orange to red-orange

Fibrin

Fibrin is a product of the fibrinogen of blood plasma. In its early stages of development it is seen as delicate fibrils or a network of fine threads, developing into coarser threads and amorphous masses. While young fibrin can be demonstrated fairly specifically, older masses of fibrin stain as collagen.

A similar substance found in rheumatic lesions and in blood vessels has been termed *fibrinoid*. This is because its staining reactions are similar to those of fibrin. It has been postulated that this is in fact fibrin in a later stage of development.[3]

Fibrin stains strongly with eosin, is yellow with Van Gieson's stain, is moderately P.A.S. positive, and may be demonstrated by Mallory's PTAH method (page 252), although older fibrin will stain red as does collagen. Weigert modified Gram's stain by utilizing aniline oil with xylene as the differentiating agent. Fibrin will stain Gram positive and dense collagen may also stain Gram positive as it is difficult to remove the Gram's stain from it without overdifferentiating the fibrin.

WEIGERT'S METHOD FOR FIBRIN (MODIFIED)[4]

Fixation

Ten percent neutral formalin, formol alcohol, Carnoy's fluid, or absolute alcohol.

Solutions Required

A. 5 percent Aqueous Solution of Eosin (C.I. 45380).

B. Aniline Gentian Violet Solution:

Solution A

Methyl violet (C.I. 42535)	5 g
Absolute ethyl alcohol	10 ml

Grind the dye in a mortar and gradually add the alcohol.

Solution B

Aniline oil	2 ml
Distilled water	88 ml

Mix solutions A and B, stand for 24 hours, and filter.

C. Gram's Iodine:

Iodine	1 g
Potassium iodide	2 g
Distilled water	300 ml

Dissolve the potassium iodide in a little of the distilled water, add the iodine and dissolve. Add the remainder of the distilled water.

D. Aniline–Xylene:

Aniline oil	50 ml
Xylene	50 ml

Method

1. Sections to water.
2. 5 percent aqueous eosin for 5 minutes.
3. Rinse in tap water.
4. Aniline gentian violet solution for 5 minutes.
5. Gram's iodine for 5 minutes.
6. Rinse in tap water.
7. Blot *nearly* dry with fluffless filter paper.
8. Differentiate with aniline-xylene until no more color comes away. Agitate the slide by rocking throughout this step. The section should appear pinkish.
9. Clear in fresh xylene, two changes, and mount.

Results

Fibrin	Blue/black
Gram positive organisms	Blue/black
Rest of tissue	Shades of pink

Note

The nuclei may be stained with lithium carmine instead of using eosin as a general counterstain.

MARTIUS-SCARLET-BLUE (MSB) METHOD FOR FIBRIN[3]

Fixation

Fixatives containing mercuric chloride are preferred, but postmordanting will give acceptable results.

Solutions Required

A. Celestine Blue Solution:

Celestine blue (C.I. 51050)	0.5 g
5 percent iron alum	100.0 ml

Boil for three minutes, cool, filter, and add:

Glycerin	14.0 ml

This stain is stable for six months.

Note. The difference between this solution and that used as a substitute for hematoxylin (page 214) is that the sulfuric acid is omitted.

B. Mayer's Hemalum (page 208).

C. Weigert's Iron Hematoxylin (page 218). This may be used as a substitute for solutions A and B.

D. 1 percent Hydrochloric acid in 70 percent alcohol.

E. Martius Yellow Solution:

Martius yellow (C.I. 10315)	0.5 g
Phosphotungstic acid	2.0 g
Distilled water	5.0 ml
Absolute ethyl alcohol	95.0 ml

F. Crystal Ponceau Solution:

Crystal ponceau 6R (C.I. 16250)	1.0 g
Glacial acetic acid	2.5 ml
Distilled water	97.5 ml

G. 1 percent aq. Phosphotungstic Acid.

H. Aniline Blue Solution:

Aniline blue WS (C.I. 42755)	0.5 g
Glacial acetic acid	1.0 ml
Distilled water	99.0 ml

Method

1. Sections to water.
2. Remove the mercuric chloride deposits.
3. Wash in running tap water for 5 minutes.
4. Weigert's iron hematoxylin for 15 minutes,

   OR

   a. Celestine blue solution for 5 minutes.
   b. Rinse in distilled water.
   c. Mayer's hemalum for 5 minutes.
5. Wash well in running water.
6. Differentiate in 1 percent acid alcohol for 5–10 seconds.
7. Blue in running tap water for 5 minutes.
8. Rinse in 95 percent alcohol.
9. Martius yellow solution for 2 minutes.
10. Rinse in distilled water.
11. Crystal ponceau solution for 10 minutes.
12. Rinse in distilled water.
13. 1 percent phosphotungstic acid for 5 minutes.
14. Rinse well with distilled water.
15. Aniline blue solution for 10 minutes.

16. Rinse in distilled water.
17. Dehydrate, clear, and mount.

Results

Nuclei	
Weigert's hematoxylin	Gray
Mayer's hemalum/celestine blue	Blue/black
Fibrin	Bright red
Muscle	Red
Connective tissue	Blue
RBCs	Yellow

Calcium

Calcium salts are normally present in bone and teeth, but in some pathologic conditions deposits of calcium and areas of calcification are formed in tissues normally devoid of these salts. It is often desirable to positively identify these deposits as calcium, and although calcium will stain an intense blue with the alum hematoxylins, more specific methods should be employed for their definite identification. The calcium salts normally found in animal tissues are calcium carbonate, calcium oxalate, and calcium phosphate.

The specific methods for the identification of calcium salts fall into two groups: metal substitution, as in the Von Kossa method, and a dye–lake reaction, as in the alizarin red and purpurin methods. In these later methods the pH of the staining solution is critical for the accurate and positive identification of calcium salts in tissue sections. The staining procedures for both alizarin red and purpurin are similar, but alizarin red is easier to control and gives better permanent mounts than does purpurin. It is the preferred method when employing dyes to demonstrate calcium salts. However, it should be noted that alizarin red does not stain calcium oxalate salts, which are demonstrated by the Von Kossa method. The Von Kossa method substitutes silver for calcium when silver nitrate is reduced by light. Calcium carbonate can be demonstrated by the Von Kossa method but requires prolonged exposure.

THE VON KOSSA METHOD FOR CALCIUM SALTS (MODIFIED)[5]

Fixation

Ten percent neutral formalin or absolute alcohol.

Solutions Required

A. 1.5 percent Aqueous Silver Nitrate.
B. 5 percent Sodium Thiosulfate.
C. 1 percent Aqueous Neutral Red (C.I. 50040).

Method

1. Sections to distilled water.
2. 1.5 percent silver nitrate. Expose to direct sunlight or a desk lamp for 30 minutes.
3. Rinse in distilled water.
4. 5 percent sodium thiosulfate for 3–5 minutes.
5. Rinse in distilled water.
6. 1 percent Neutral red for 5 minutes.
7. Rinse in distilled water.
8. Dehydrate, clear, and mount.

Results

Nuclei	Red
Calcium salts	Black
Background	Pale pink

ALIZARIN RED S STAIN FOR CALCIUM[6]

Fixation

Ten percent neutral formalin or absolute alcohol.

Solutions Required

A. Alizarin Red Stain:

Alizarin red S (C.I. 58005)	2 g
Distilled water	100 ml

Adjust the pH of the solution to between 4.1 and 4.3 by adding concentrated ammonia, drop by drop, stirring constantly and with the electrodes remaining in the solution. The stain will turn a deep iodine color and is stable for 12 months.

B. Acetone.
C. Acetone–Xylene Mixture:

Acetone	20 ml
Xylene	20 ml

Method

1. Sections to distilled water.
2. Alizarin red S solution for 30 seconds to 5 minutes. The section should be examined at 30 second intervals under the microscope until the calcium deposits are stained orange-red. The end point is when the desired intensity of staining is reached.
3. Drain off the excess stain.
4. Blot dry with fluffless filter paper.
5. Flood the slide with acetone for 20 seconds.
6. Flood the slide with acetone–xylene mixture for 20 seconds.
7. Clear the slide in fresh xylene and mount.

Results

Sites of calcium deposits	Covered by a birefringent orange-red precipitate

Urates: Uric Acid Crystals

Uric acid crystals occur in the tissues, particularly the joints, as acid sodium urate. The crystals are seen in lesions associated with gout.

Urates are soluble in aqueous solutions, slightly soluble in weak alcoholic solutions, but insoluble in absolute alcohol and concentrated ammonia. They are also birefringent.

Because of their solubility in aqueous solutions, the tissue must be fixed in either 95 percent or absolute alcohol.

DeGALANTHA'S METHOD FOR URATES[7]

Fixation

95 percent or absolute ethyl alcohol.

Solutions Required

A. 20 percent Silver Nitrate.
B. Developing Solution:

3 percent gelatin (warmed until melted)	10 ml
20 percent silver nitrate	3 ml
2 percent hydroquinone	2 ml

Method

1. Sections at 8μ to absolute alcohol.
2. 20 percent silver nitrate for 1–4 hours in bright sunlight or exposed to a strong (100 w) electric light until the urates turn a bright rose color.
3. Flood the slide with the developing solution until the urates turn black and the connective tissue becomes yellowish/brown.
4. Wash in warm water to remove all traces of the gelatin.
5. Dehydrate, clear, and mount.

Results

Uric acid crystals	Black
Background	Yellowish/brown

METHENAMINE SILVER METHOD FOR URATES[8]

Fixation

95 percent or absolute ethyl alcohol.

Solutions Required

A. Methenamine Silver Solution:

Solution A

3 percent methenamine solution	100 ml
5 percent silver nitrate	5 ml

Shake well until the white precipitate disappears. Store in the refrigerator.

Solution B

Boric acid	1.6 g
Sodium borate (Borax)	1.3 g
Distilled water	200.0 ml

Store in the refrigerator.

Solution C

Working Solution:

Solution A	25 ml
Solution B	5 ml
Distilled water	20 ml

Prepare fresh for each use.

B. 2 percent Sodium Thiosulfate.

C. Counterstain of Choice.

Method

1. Sections to alcohol.
2. Working solution of buffered silver at 45 C in the dark for 1–2 hours.
3. Rinse in distilled water.
4. 2 percent sodium thiosulfate for 2 minutes.
5. Wash in running tap water for 5 minutes.
6. Counterstain if desired.
7. Dehydrate, clear, and mount.

Results

Urates	Black

The Pancreatic Cells

The function of the pancreas is to secrete digestive enzymes and to produce insulin. Because autolysis is extremely rapid in this gland, prompt fixation is essential, especially if specific cells are to be demonstrated. These cells are the *alpha* (α) cells, *beta* (β) cells, and D cells of the islets of Langerhans and the *zymogen granules* found in the acinar cells. These granules are strongly acidophillic and stain P.A.S. positive. They may be fixed with 10 percent neutral formalin, Helly's fluid, and formal sublimate, but solutions containing acetic acid must be avoided. The hematoxylin and eosin method will adequately demonstrate the pancreatic tissue, but it will not differentiate specific islet cells. These require special methods.

Alpha cells, beta cells, and D cells are found in the *islets of Langerhans*, the beta cells being involved in the production of insulin. The exact function of alpha and D cells is not fully understood, but it is possible that the alpha cells are concerned with the production of hormonal substances. Beta cells are P.A.S. negative, stain a deep purple with Gomori's aldehyde fuchsin (page 232), and are orange-brown in the trichrome methods (page 220). The alpha-cell granules stain red with the trichrome methods and the D-cell cytoplasm has an affinity for aniline blue and light green.

GOMORI'S CHROME ALUM HEMATOXYLIN–PHLOXINE METHOD FOR ALPHA AND BETA CELLS[9]

Fixation

Bouin's fluid or Helly's fluid are preferred. Ten percent neutral formalin will suffice with secondary treatment in either of these solutions.

Solutions Required

A. Bouin's Fluid.

B. Acidified Potassium Permanganate Solution:

Potassium permanganate	0.3 g
Distilled water	100.0 ml
Sulfuric acid, conc.	0.3 ml

C. 5 percent Sodium Bisulfite.

D. Chrome Alum Hematoxylin:

Hematoxylin (C.I. 75290), 1 percent aq. sol.	50.0 ml
Chromium potassium sulfate 3 percent aq. soln.	50.0 ml

Add:

Potassium iodate	0.1 g

Boil until a deep blue. The stain is ready for immediate use, and can be used as long as a metallic film forms on the surface of the stain in a coplin jar. Filter before each use.

E. 1 percent Hydrochloric Acid in 70 percent Alcohol.

F. 0.5 percent Aqueous Phloxine B (C.I. 45410).

G. 5 percent Phosphotungstic Acid.

Method

1. Sections to water.
2. Mordant overnight in Bouin's fluid.
3. Wash in running tap water to remove the picric acid.
4. Acidified potassium permanganate solution for 1 minute.
5. Bleach until white in 5 percent sodium bisulfite.
6. Wash well in running water.
7. Chrome alum hematoxylin for 10–15 minutes.
8. Examine under the microscope. Beta cells should stand out a deep blue.
9. Rinse in distilled water.
10. 1 percent acid alcohol for 1 minute.
11. Wash in running tap water until the section appears a clear blue.
12. 0.5 percent Phloxine B for 5 minutes.
13. Rinse in distilled water.
14. 5 percent phosphotungstic acid for 1 minute.
15. Wash in running tap water for 5 minutes. The section should appear red.
16. Differentiate in 95 percent alcohol. Control under the micro-

scope. If the section is too red and the alpha cells are not clearly defined, rinse in 80 percent alcohol for 15–20 seconds.
17. Dehydrate with absolute alcohol, clear, and mount.

Results

Beta cells	Deep blue
Alpha cells	Red
D cells	Pink to red

ALDEHYDE–NEW FUCHSIN–LIGHT GREEN–ORANGE G STAIN FOR ALPHA AND BETA CELLS IN THE PANCREAS[10]

Fixation

Ten percent neutral formalin or Bouin's fluid. Avoid the use of alcoholic fixatives. Beta-cell granules are soluble in alcohol.

Solutions Required

A. Aldehyde–New Fuchsin Solution:

Solution A

New fuchsin (C.I. 42520)	1 g
70 percent ethyl alcohol	100 ml

Solution B

Paraldehyde USP*	2 ml
Hydrochloric acid, conc.	2 ml

Mix solution A and solution B and allow to stand at room temperature for 24 hours or until a deep purple color has formed. Store in the refrigerator. This solution is stable for 1 week to 10 days.

B. Chromic Chloride–Acetic Acid Solution:

Chromic chloride ($CrCl_3 \cdot 6H_2O$)	5 g
2 percent acetic acid	100 ml

The solution turns a pale purple upon standing, but is stable at room temperature for 6 months.

C. Light Green–Orange G Solution:

Light green S.F., yellowish (C.I. 42095)	0.2 g
Orange G (C.I. 16230)	1.0 g

* Must be absolutely fresh.

Phosphotungstic acid	0.5 g
Glacial acetic acid	1.0 ml
Distilled water	99.0 ml

This solution keeps indefinitely.

Method

1. Sections to distilled water.
2. Chromic chloride-acetic acid solution for 72 hours.
3. Rinse thoroughly in three changes of distilled water.
4. Rinse in 70 percent ethyl alcohol.
5. Aldehyde-new fuchsin solution for 6 hours.
6. Rinse thoroughly in 70 percent ethyl alcohol to remove the excess stain.
7. Wash thoroughly in running tap water for 5-10 minutes.
8. Rinse in distilled water.
9. Light Green-Orange G solution for 45 seconds.
10. 95 percent ethyl alcohol for 30 seconds.
11. Dehydrate through two changes of absolute ethyl alcohol, 15 seconds in each.
12. Clear in xylene and mount.

Results

Alpha-cell granules	Orange
Beta-cell granules	Deep blue to purple
Cytoplasm	Unstained to grayish-green

The Pituitary (Hypophysis)

The pituitary or *hypophysis* is located at the base of the brain. It is divided into two lobes in the human: the *pars nervosa*, which is composed of nervous tissue, and the *pars anterior*. The cells of the pars nervosa may be demonstrated by the appropriate neurologic methods, but it is the cells of the pars anterior, the anterior lobe, that the histotechnologist is usually required to demonstrate.

The cells of the pars anterior may be divided into two types by the staining reaction of their cytoplasmic granules. They are (1) the *chromophobe cells*, which contain no stainable granules, and (2) the *chromophil cells*, which do contain stainable granules in their cytoplasm. The chromophil cells are further divided into two groups, the *alpha cells* and the *beta cells*. Distribution of these cells is approximately: chromophobe cells, 53 percent; alpha cells, 34 percent; and beta cells, 13 percent.

The alpha cells produce hormonal substances related to growth and also assist in sugar metabolism. The beta cells also produce hormonal substances, but these are related to the gonads. They also appear to be related to fat metabolism. The exact function of the chromophobe cells is not known, but it is suspected that they play an important role in fetal development in addition to the production of chromophil cells.

The hematoxylin and eosin method on thin sections will give fairly reasonable differentiation of these cells, the alpha cells staining a bright red, the beta cells purplish, and the chromophobes pale pink. Alpha cells are stained red in the trichrome methods and are P.A.S. negative. Beta cells stain blue or green with the trichrome methods, depending upon the counterstain employed, and are P.A.S. and Gram positive following fixation in formalin or Zenker's fluid. It is important that fixation be commenced promptly and completed within 12 hours. Extended fixation tends to show some granular depletion.

Special stains give a better differential picture than the trichrome methods or the hematoxylin and eosin method. These methods will stain the cytoplasmic granules specifically.

P.A.S.-ORANGE G METHOD FOR PITUITARY (MODIFIED)[11]

Fixation

Ten percent neutral formalin, Bouin's fluid, or Helly's fluid.

Solutions Required

A. 1 percent Periodic Acid.
B. Schiff's Reagent (page 304).
C. Sulfurous Acid Rinse (page 304).
D. Harris' Hematoxylin (page 208).
E. 2 percent Orange G* (C.I. 16230) in 5 percent Phosphotungstic Acid.

Method

1. Sections to distilled water.
2. 1 percent periodic acid for 5 minutes.
3. Rinse in distilled water.
4. Schiff's reagent for 15 minutes.

* Orange II (C.I. 15510) may be substituted and gives a deeper color.[12]

5. Place into three changes of sulfurous acid rinse, 2 minutes in each. *A thorough washing in running tap water for 30 minutes may be substituted for this step and step 6.*
6. Wash in running tap water for 10 minutes.
7. Harris' hematoxylin for 30–60 seconds.
8. Rinse in tap water.
9. Rinse in distilled water.
10. Orange G solution for 10 seconds.
11. Dehydrate, clear, and mount.

Results

Nuclei	Blue
Alpha-cell granules	Orange
Beta-cell granules	Deep rose to magenta

Note

A modification of this method which stains *gamma granules* in addition to the alpha- and beta-granules is as follows[13]:

1. Proceed through steps 1–6 of the P.A.S.–Orange G method.
2. 1 percent aqueous orange G for 30 seconds.
3. 5 percent phosphotungstic acid for 30 seconds.
4. Rinse in running tap water for 30 seconds.
5. 1 percent aqueous methyl blue (C.I. 42780) for 1 minute.
6. 1 percent acetic acid. Rinse briefly until no more blue flows from the section.
7. Dehydrate, clear, and mount.

The results of this method are:

Alpha-cell granules	Orange
Beta-cell granules	Deep rose to magenta
Gamma granules	Purple
RBCs	Yellow/orange

A ONE-STEP MSB TECHNIQUE FOR THE ANTERIOR PITUITARY[14]

Fixation

Ten percent neutral formalin.

Solutions Required

A. Celestine Blue Solution (page 261).
B. Mayer's Hemalum (page 208).

C. 1 percent Hydrochloric Acid in 70 percent Alcohol.
D. Martius-Scarlet-Blue Solution:

Solution A

Martius yellow (C.I. 10315)	0.1 g
Phosphotungstic acid	2.0 g
95 percent ethyl alcohol	100.0 ml

Filter before use.

Solution B

Crystal ponceau 6R (C.I. 16250)	1.0 g
Glacial acetic acid	2.5 ml
Distilled water	97.5 ml

Filter before use.

Solution C

Aniline blue WS (C.I. 42755)	0.5 g
Glacial acetic acid	1.0 ml
Distilled water	99.0 ml

Filter before use.

Working Solution:

Solution A	15 ml
Solution B	10 ml
Solution C	15 ml

Allow to stand for 3 days at room temperature before use. This solution is stable for 3 months.

Method

1. Sections to distilled water.
2. Celestine blue solution for 5 minutes.
3. Rinse in distilled water.
4. Mayer's hemalum for 5 minutes.
5. Wash well in running tap water.
6. Differentiate in 1 percent acid alcohol for 5–10 seconds. Control under the microscope.
7. Blue in running tap water for 5 minutes.
8. Rinse in distilled water.
9. MSB solution in a coplin jar for 8 minutes.
10. Rinse rapidly in distilled water.
11. Blot dry.
12. Dehydrate through absolute ethyl alcohol, clear, and mount.

Results

Alpha granules	Cherry red
Beta granules	Blue
Collagen	Pale blue
Colloid	Orange/red
Nuclei	Blue/black
RBCs	Yellow

Juxtaglomerular Cell Granules in the Kidney

These granules are not readily seen with the hematoxylin and eosin method or other routine staining methods.

The juxtaglomerular cells are located at the base of the glomerular tuft or stem and may be seen only in favorable sections. The granules within these cells must be demonstrated with special stains. They are concerned with the production of hormonal substances which function in the control of blood pressure.

BOWIE'S STAIN FOR JG (JUXTAGLOMERULAR) GRANULES[15]

Fixation

Helly's fluid or Smith's fluid; 10 percent formalin, 100 ml; potassium dichromate, 5 g; and glacial acetic acid, 2.5 ml.[16]

Solutions Required

A. 2.5 percent Potassium Dichromate.
B. Bowie's Stock Solution:

Solution A

Biebrich scarlet (C.I. 26905)	1 g
Distilled water	250 ml

Filter into a beaker.

Solution B

Ethyl violet (C.I. 42600)	2 g
Distilled water	500 ml

Filter a small amount of solution B at a time into solution A with frequent stirring. The neutralization end point is reached when the color changes abruptly from red to violet and when a drop placed on filter paper does not show any color other than the precipitate itself. Filter this mixture and dry the precipitate.* Dissolve the precipitate in 95 percent ethyl alcohol to make a 1 percent solution.

C. Xylene–Clove Oil Mixture:

Xylene	25 ml
Clove oil	25 ml

Method

1. Sections to water and remove any mercuric chloride deposits.
2. Wash in running tap water for 5 minutes.
3. Mordant in 2.5 percent potassium dichromate overnight at 40 C.
4. Rinse with distilled water.
5. Immerse in 20 percent ethyl alcohol to which has been added 15 drops (0.5 ml) of Bowie's stock solution per 100 ml of alcohol. Leave overnight.
6. Blot dry with fluffless filter paper.
7. Dip quickly in 2 changes of acetone to remove any excess stain.
8. Differentiate in the xylene–clove oil mixture until the section appears red to reddish purple. Microscopically the renal parenchyma should be red to magenta and the elastic fibers in the vessels should be blue-purple. Juxtaglomerular granules will be the same color as the elastic.
9. Clear in 2 changes of fresh xylene and mount.

Results

JG granules	Deep purple
Elastic	Deep purple
Background	Light red to reddish-brown
RBCs	Amber

Note

The elastic fibers provide a useful criterion for the completion of differentiation as JG granules are not always easily found. RBCs are amber due to the dichromate mordanting.

Paneth Cell Granules

Paneth cells are located at the base of the *crypts of Lieberkuhn* in the small intestine. The cytoplasm of these cells contain coarse, strongly acidophilic granules which can be easily seen with the hematoxylin

* Available commercially from Roboz Surgical Instrument Co., Washington, D.C.

and eosin method, Lendrum's Phloxine-tartrazine method (page 000), and the MSB method (page 000).

Acid fixatives such as Zenker's fluid and Bouin's fluid should be avoided as primary fixatives because the granules are dissolved by these solutions. However, prompt fixation in 10 percent neutral formalin renders the granules resistant to the solvent action of these solutions and they may be employed as secondary fixatives if desired.

Argentaffin or Enterochromaffin Cells

Argentaffin, or enterochromaffin cells, also known as *Kultschitzky* cells, may be found throughout the normal alimentary tract from the esophagus to the anus. They are most easily found in the pyloric glands of the stomach, at the base of the intestinal glands (crypts of Lieberkuhn), and in the mucosa of the appendix. The granules acquired their name because they are argyrophilic, having an affinity for silver (argentaffin), and an affinity for chromium salts (chromaffin).

Argentaffin cell granules have the capability of reducing an ammoniacal silver nitrate solution to produce a visible black deposit of silver on the granules. This capability differentiates them from the argyrophil cells that cannot reduce ammoniacal silver solutions directly, but require the use of a reducing agent such as hydroquinone or formalin. The argyrophil cells are possibly precursors of the argentaffin cells.

Fixation in alcohol, or solutions containing alcohol, *must* be avoided because argentaffin granules are soluble in alcohol. The tissue *must* be fixed in formalin or solutions containing formalin if argentaffin granules are to be demonstrated. This requirement for formalin fixation differentiates the enterochromaffin cells from the true chromaffin cells, which can be demonstrated after fixation in potassium dichromate without treatment in formalin.

Argentaffin granules fixed in formalin will exhibit autofluorescence. Paraffin sections are brought to distilled water and mounted in Apathy's mounting medium. On examination under the fluorescence microscope using a Scott UG-2 exciter filter with a colorless ultraviolet barrier filter, the argentaffin granules will fluoresce a bright golden yellow.

The histochemical reaction is dependent on the presence of 5-hydroxytryptamine (5-HT), which is converted to the tetrahydro-4-carboline derivative by formalin as reported by Holcenberg and Benditt.[17]

Argentaffin granules appear as yellowish-brown granules in certain carcinoid tumors as well as the alimentary tract. They may be demonstrated by the Fontana-Masson method, the Diazo technique, and by Schmorl's method.

MASSON-FONTANA METHOD FOR ARGENTAFFIN GRANULES AND MELANIN[18]

Fixation

Ten percent neutral formalin.

Solutions Required

A. Ammoniacal Silver Nitrate Solution:
To approximately 50 ml of 10 percent silver nitrate add, drop by drop, concentrated ammonia until the resultant precipitate is just dissolved. Add a few drops of silver nitrate until the solution remains slightly cloudy. Stand overnight in the refrigerator and filter before use. *For use* dilute 1 part with 3 parts of distilled water.
B. 0.2 percent Gold Chloride.
C. 5 percent Sodium Thiosulfate.
D. Counterstain if desired.

Method

1. Sections to distilled water.
2. Ammoniacal silver nitrate solution overnight in the dark at room temperature or for 1 hour at 60 C. Sections should turn a light brown.
3. Rinse thoroughly in distilled water.
4. Tone in 0.2 percent gold chloride for 10 minutes.
5. Rinse in distilled water.
6. 5 percent sodium thiosulfate for 5 minutes.
7. Wash in running tap water for 5 minutes.
8. Counterstain if desired.
9. Dehydrate, clear, and mount.

Results

Argentaffin granules	Black
Melanin	Black

Note

Although used widely as an aid to the identification of melanin, this method should not be considered specific. Other procedures should be employed to confirm the findings.

THE DIAZO METHOD FOR ARGENTAFFIN GRANULES[19]

Fixation

Ten percent neutral formalin.

Solutions Required

A. Diazo Reagent:
Prepare fresh for each use.

Fast red B (C.I. 37125)	0.25 g
Distilled water	25.00 ml
Sat. aq. lithium carbonate	10.00 ml

Place in the refrigerator at 4 to 5 C for 10 minutes before use.

B. Harris' Hematoxylin (page 208).

Method

1. Sections to distilled water.
2. Diazo reagent at 4 to 5 C in the refrigerator for 2 minutes.
3. Rinse in distilled water.
4. Wash in running tap water for 2–3 minutes.
5. Harris' hematoxylin for 20–30 seconds.
6. Wash in running tap water for 2 minutes.
7. Dehydrate, clear, and mount.

Results

Nucei	Blue
Argentaffin granules	Orange-red

Note

Alternative diazo salts are:

Fast garnet GBC (C.I. 37210)
Fast red GG (C.I. 37035)

SCHMORL'S METHOD FOR ARGENTAFFIN, CHROMAFFIN, LIPOFUSCIN, AND MELANIN[20]

Fixation

Ten percent neutral formalin for argentaffin. Fixatives containing chromates for chromaffin.

Solutions Required

A. Schmorl's Reagent, freshly prepared:

3 percent ferric chloride	25 ml
1 percent potassium ferricyanide	25 ml

B. 1 percent Aqueous Neutral Red (C.I. 50040)

Method

1. Sections to distilled water.
2. Schmorl's reagent for 15–30 minutes.
3. Wash in running water for 2 minutes.
4. 1 percent aqueous neutral red for 1 minute.
5. Rinse in distilled water.
6. Dehydrate rapidly, clear, and mount.

Results

Nuclei	Red
Argentaffin granules	Blue
Lipofuscin pigment	Blue
Chromaffin (after dichromate)	Greenish-blue
Melanin	Blue

Methods for Argyrophil Cells

GRIMELIUS METHOD FOR ARGYROPHILIA[21]

Fixation: **Bouin's fluid is the preferred fixative. Formalin fixed tissue must be post-fixed in Bouin's fluid overnight before staining.**

Solutions Required

A. 0.1 M Acetate Buffer pH 5.8.

Solution A.

Sodium acetate ($NaC_2H_3O_2$)	1.64 g
Distilled water	to 100.00 ml

OR

Sodium acetate ($NaC_2H_3O_2 \cdot 3H_2O$)	2.72 g
Distilled Water	to 100.00 ml

Solution B.

Glacial Acetic acid	1.2 ml
Distilled water	to 100.0 ml

Working Solution.

Solution A	95.0 ml
Solution B	5.0 ml
Distilled water	100.0 ml

B. 0.05 percent Silver Nitrate Solution.

Silver nitrate	0.05 g
0.1 M Sodium acetate buffer	100.00 ml

C. Bodian's Reducing Solution.

Sodium sulfite, anhydrous	5.0 g
Hydroquinone	1.0 g
Distilled water	100.0 ml

D. 2 percent Sodium Thiosulfate.

Method

1. Sections to distilled water.
2. 0.05 percent Silver nitrate solution for 3 hours at 60C.
3. Transfer directly to Bodian's reducing solution at 60C. for 5 minutes. Examine microscopically. If a black color does not appear, wash in distilled water, fix in 2 percent Sodium thiosulfate for 30 seconds and return to the silver solution for another 30 minutes. Repeat the reducing treatment.
4. Wash in distilled water.
5. Fix in 2 percent sodium thiosulfate for 30 seconds.
6. Rinse in distilled water.
7. Dehydrate, clear, and mount.

Results:

Argyrophil cells of the Gastrointestinal mucosa	Black
α_2 Cells in the Pancreatic islets	Black

PASCUAL'S METHOD FOR ARGYROPHIL CELLS[21]

Fixation

Ten percent neutral formalin or Bouin's fluid.

Solutions Required

A. 0.5 percent Silver Nitrate
   Prepare fresh for use.

B. Bodian's Reducing Solution:

Sodium sulfite, anhydrous	5 g
Hydroquinone	1 g
Distilled water	100 ml

C. Counterstain of choice.

Method

1. Sections to distilled water.
2. 0.5 percent silver nitrate at 60 C for 2 hours, or overnight at room temperature.
3. Rinse in distilled water.
4. Bodian's reducing solution for 5 minutes at 60 C. The solution should be preheated.
5. Rinse in distilled water.
6. Wash in running tap water for 3 minutes.
7. Rinse in distilled water.
8. 0.5 percent silver nitrate for 10 minutes at 60 C. The solution should be preheated if it has previously been used at room temperature.
9. Rinse in distilled water.
10. Repeat step 4.
11. Rinse in distilled water.
12. Counterstain if desired by method of choice.
13. Rinse in distilled water.
14. Dehydrate, clear, and mount.

Results

Argyrophil cells of the gastrointestinal mucosa	Black
Insular A and D cells of the pancreas	Black
Nuclei	As stained

Chromaffin

The adrenal glands are located at the upper pole of each kidney. Upon slicing, the cut surface reveals a yellowish cortex surrounding the reddish medulla. The medulla will turn brown after treatment with chrome salts due to the reduction of these salts by the adrenaline present in the cells.

Chromaffin is a dark brown granular material found normally in the medulla and it may occur in some tumors. It is suspected to contain adrenalin and/or noradrenalin. Because the adrenal is the most susceptible of the tissues to autolysis, it must be fixed promptly upon death or removal from the body. Fixation *must* be commenced within two hours of removal or death.

Chromaffin, like argentaffin, is soluble in alcohol, and fixatives containing alcohol must be avoided as should solutions containing mercuric chloride and acetic acid. Unlike argentaffin, it is not well fixed by formalin, and formalin fixation followed by secondary fixation in dichromate will rarely give satisfactory results. The fixatives of choice are Champy's fluid, Müller's fluid, or Régaud's fluid.

Frozen sections are preferred, although paraffin sections will suffice. Chromaffin is slightly soluble in hot paraffin wax.

After correct fixation, chromaffin granules may be demonstrated by the Giemsa stain, Schmorl's method, the P.A.S. technique, and Weisel's method.

WEISEL'S METHOD FOR CHROMAFFIN GRANULES[22]

Fixation

Müller's fluid, Champy's fluid, or Régaud's fluid. Frozen sections are preferred, but paraffin sections will suffice.

Solutions Required

A. 1 percent Aqueous Toluidine Blue (C.I. 52040).
B. 1 percent Aqueous Safranin O (C.I. 50240).

Method

1. Sections to distilled water.
2. 1 percent aqueous toluidine blue for 20 minutes.
3. Wash in running tap water for 5 minutes.
4. 1 percent aqueous Safranin O for 20 minutes.
5. Rinse in water.
6. Differentiate in 95 percent ethyl alcohol until the section appears blue.
7. Clear and mount.

Results

Nuclei	Red
Chromaffin granules	Greenish
Other cells	Blue

Spermatozoa

Berg's method for spermatozoa incorporates Putt's modification of the carbol-fuchsin solution used in the Ziehl-Neelson method for A.F.B. This gives more intense staining of the spermatozoa when used with a weak differentiating agent such as acetic acid.

Although spermatozoa can be seen when stained by the hematoxylin and eosin method, Berg's method stains them differentially from the surrounding tissue structures.

BERG'S METHOD FOR SPERMATOZOA[23]

Fixation

Ten percent neutral formalin.

Solutions Required

A. Putt's Carbol-Fuchsin Solution:

New fuchsin (C.I. 42520)	1 g
Phenol	5 g
Absolute ethyl alcohol	10 ml
Distilled water	84 ml

Filter before use.

B. Saturated Aqueous Lithium Carbonate Solution (approximately 1 percent).

C. 5 percent Glacial Acetic Acid-Alcohol Solution:

Glacial acetic acid	5 ml
Absolute ethyl alcohol	95 ml

D. 0.5 percent Methylene Blue Solution.

Methylene blue (C.I. 52015)	1 g
Absolute ethyl alcohol	200 ml

Method

1. Sections to distilled water.
2. Putt's carbol-fuchsin solution for 3 minutes.
3. Place directly into saturated lithium carbonate for 3 minutes.
4. Differentiate in alcoholic acetic acid for 5 minutes.
5. Rinse in two changes of absolute ethyl alcohol, 1 minute in each rinse.
6. Methylene blue solution for 30-60 seconds.
7. Rinse rapidly in two changes of absolute ethyl alcohol.
8. Clear in xylene and mount.

Results

Spermatozoa	Brilliant red
RBCs	Pale pink
Other structures	Blue to purple

Sex Chromatin

The sex chromatin or Barr body is present in the nuclei of human females and rarely visible in cells from males. Cells are obtained by gently scraping the inside of the mouth and smearing these cells onto a clean slide which is immediately placed into equal parts of 95 percent ethyl alcohol and ether for 15 minutes to fix. Do not allow the smear to dry.

GUARD'S METHOD FOR SEX CHROMATIN[24]

Fixation

Fresh wet smears are placed into equal parts of 95 percent ethyl alcohol and ether for at least 15 minutes.

Solutions Required

A. Biebrich Scarlet Solution:

Biebrich scarlet (C.I. 26905)	1.0 g
Phosphotungstic acid	0.3 g
Glacial acetic acid	5.0 ml
50 percent ethyl alcohol	95.0 ml

B. Harris' Hematoxylin (page 208).

C. 50 percent Ethyl Alcohol.

D. Fast Green Solution:

Fast green FCF (C.I. 42053)	0.5 g
Phosphomolybdic acid	0.3 g
Phosphotungstic acid	0.3 g
Glacial acetic acid	5.0 ml
50 percent ethyl alcohol	95.0 ml

Method

1. Smears from fixative to 70 percent alcohol for 2 minutes.
2. Harris' hematoxylin for 15 seconds.
3. Biebrich scarlet solution for 2 minutes.

4. 50 percent alcohol for 5 minutes.
5. Fast green solution for 24 hours.
6. Dehydrate, clear, and mount.

Results

Sex chromatin (Barr bodies)	Red
Nuclear chromatin	Blue
Cytoplasm	Green

MOORE'S CRESYL ECHT VIOLET METHOD FOR SEX CHROMATIN[25]

Fixation

Fresh wet smears into equal parts of 95 percent ethyl alcohol and ether.

Solutions Required

A. 1 percent Aqueous Cresyl Echt Violet (C.I. None).

Method

1. Smears from fixative to distilled water.
2. Immerse in cresyl echt violet solution for 5–8 minutes.
3. Differentiate in 95 percent alcohol, 5–8 dips.
4. Continue differentiation in absolute ethyl alcohol for about 1 minute. Control under the microscope until details of the cell structure are clearly defined.
5. Clear in two changes of xylene and mount.

Results

Sex chromatin (Barr bodies)	A deeply stained dot in the nucleus, usually lying against the nuclear membrane

Mitochondria

Mitochondria are rodlike, filamentous, or granular bodies that have a smooth outline and are found in the cytoplasm of the cell. They are lipoprotein in nature and are among the first structures to be affected by autolysis. To ensure their presence for demonstration, early fixation is essential in the appropriate fluids, Helly's fluid or Régaud's fluid.

After proper and prompt fixation they may be demonstrated by a well-differentiated Heidenhain's iron hematoxylin (page 251), the phosphotungstic acid hematoxylin method (page 288,) and by Altmann's aniline acid fuchsin method.

ALTMANN'S ANILINE ACID FUCHSIN METHOD FOR MITOCHONDRIA (MODIFIED)[26]

Fixation

Helly's fluid or Regaud's fluid for 24–48 hours followed by 3 percent potassium dichromate for 4–7 days. Change this solution daily. Wash overnight in running tap water.

Solutions Required

A. Altmann's Aniline Acid Fuchsin Solution:

Aniline	1 ml
Distilled water	20 ml
Acid fuchsin (C.I. 42685)	4 g

Shake the aniline and distilled water thoroughly and allow to stand for a few minutes. Repeat this process over 24 hours and filter. Add the acid fuchsin and shake at intervals over several hours. This solution must be used the day it is prepared.

B. Picric Acid Differentiating Solution A:

Saturated alcoholic picric acid	10 ml
20 percent ethyl alcohol	40 ml

C. Picric Acid Differentiating Solution B:

Saturated alcoholic picric acid	10 ml
20 percent ethyl alcohol	70 ml

Method

1. Sections to absolute alcohol. Dry the bottom of the slide and around the section. Do not allow the section to dry.
2. Place the slide on a staining rack and cover with Altmann's stain. Heat gently with a small flame passed under the slide until steam rises from the stain.
3. Remove the flame and allow the slide to cool for 5–8 minutes.
4. Rinse in distilled water.
5. Picric acid differentiating solution A for 1 minute.

6. Transfer directly to picric acid differentiating solution B for 1 minute.
7. Dehydrate rapidly in two changes of absolute alcohol.
8. Clear in xylene and mount.

Results

Nuclei	Yellow
Nucleoli	Red
Mitochondria	Red
Cytoplasm	Yellow
RBCs	Red

Note

If the section is overdifferentiated it cannot be restained. Take a fresh section and reduce the time in the differentiating solutions.

CAIN'S METHOD FOR MITOCHONDRIA[27]

Fixation

As for Altmann's method (page 286).

Solutions Required

A. Altmann's Aniline Acid Fuchsin Solution (page 286).
B. 0.1 percent Aqueous Sodium Carbonate.
C. 1 percent Aqueous Hydrochloric Acid.
D. 0.5 percent Methyl Blue (C.I. 42780).

Method

1. Sections to distilled water.
2. Place sections into hot (steaming) Altmann's stain for 5–10 minutes.
3. Differentiate in sodium carbonate until the cytoplasm is a pale pink.
4. Dip rapidly into the hydrochloric acid to stop the differentiation and heighten the color.
5. Rinse thoroughly in distilled water.
6. Methyl blue solution for a few (5–10) seconds.
7. Rinse in distilled water.
8. Dip quickly in the hydrochloric acid solution.
9. Rinse thoroughly in distilled water.
10. Dehydrate, clear, and mount.

Results

Nuclei	Blue to green
Mitochondria	Red

PHOSPHOTUNGSTIC ACID HEMATOXYLIN METHOD FOR MITOCHONDRIA

Fixation

Ten percent neutral formalin.

Method

1. Transfer the tissue to 5 percent ferric chloride for 2–5 days. Change to fresh solution daily.
2. Wash in water, and place into several changes of 80 percent ethyl alcohol for 24–48 hours. The alcohol should be changed as it becomes yellow.
3. Process the tissue and cut paraffin sections. Stain with the PTAH method (page 252).

Result

Mitochondria	Deep blue

REFERENCES

1. Kreyberg L, Jareg E: Combined staining method for keratin and mucin-like substances. Histological Definition and Classification of Lung Tumours, 1.W.H.O. International Reference Centre, Geneva, 1967, pp 27–28
2. Dane ET, Herman DL: Hematoxylin-phloxine-alcian blue-orange G differential staining of prekeratin, keratin, and mucin, Stain Technol 38: 97–101, 1963
3. Lendrum AC, Fraser DS, Slidders W, Henderson R: Studies on the character and staining of fibrin, J Clin Path 15: 401–413, 1962
4. Weigert K: Über eine neue Methode zur Färbung von Fibrin und von Microorganismen, Fortschr Med 5: 228–232, 1887
5. von Kossa J: Ueber die im Organismus künstlich entzeugbaren Verkalkungen, Beitr Path Anat 29: 163–202, 1901
6. McGee-Russell SM: Histochemical methods for calcium, J Histochem Cytochem 6: 22–42, 1958

7. DeGalantha E: Technic for preservation and microscopic demonstration of nodules in gout, Am J Clin Pathol 5:165, 1935.
8. Gomori G: Microscopic Histochemistry, University of Chicago Press, Chicago, 1952
9. Gomori G: Observations with differential stains on human islets of Langerhans, Am J Pathol 17:395–406, 1941
10. Sieracki JC, Michael JE, Clark DA: The demonstration of beta cells in pancreatic islets and their tumors, Stain Technol 34:67–69, 1960
11. Pearse AGE: The cytochemical demonstration of gonadotropic hormone in the human anterior hypophysis. J Pathol Bacteriol 61:195–202, 1949
12. Lillie RD: Histopathologic Technic and Practical Histochemistry, 3rd ed. Blakiston Division, McGraw-Hill, New York, 1965, p 303
13. Wilson WD, Ezrin C: Three types of chromophil cells of the adenohypophysis, demonstrated by a modification of the periodic acid-Schiff technique, Am J Pathol 30:891–899, 1954
14. Dawes RE, Hillier MH: A one-stage technique for differentiating the alpha- and beta-cells of the anterior pituitary, J Med Lab Technol 21:62, 1964
15. Pitcock JA, Hartcroft PM: The juxtaglomerular cells in man and their relationship to the level of plasma sodium and to the zona glomerulosa of the adrenal cortex, Am J Pathol 34:863–873, 1958
16. Smith CI: Rapid demonstration of juxtaglomerular granules in mammals and birds, Stain Technol 41:291–294, 1966
17. Holcenberg J, Benditt EP: A new color reaction for tryptamine derivatives. Histochemical application to enterochromaffin cells, Lab Invest 10:144–158, 1961
18. Masson P: Carcinoids (argentaffin-cell tumors) and nerve hyperplasia of the appendicular mucosa, Am J Pathol 4:181–211, 1928
19. Gomori G: Histochemistry of the enterochromaffin substance, J Histochem Cytochem 2:50–53, 1954
20. Schmorl G: Die pathologisch-histologischen untersuchungs methoden, 11th ed. Vogel, Berlin, 1934, p 199
21. Grimelius L: A silver nitrate stain for α_2-cells in human pancreatic islets, Acta Soc Med Upsal 73:243–70, 1968
22. Pascual JSF: A new method for easy demonstration of argyrophil cells, Stain Technol 51:231–235, 1976
23. Weisel J: Beiträge zur Anatomie und Entwicklung der menschlichen Nebenniere, Anat Hefte Abt I 19:481–522, 1902
24. Berg JW: Differential staining of spermatozoa in sections of testis, Am J Clin Pathol 23:513–515, 1953
25. Guard HR: A new technic for differential staining of the sex

chromatin, and the determination of its incidence in exfoliated vaginal epithelial cells, Am J Clin Pathol 32:145–151, 1959
26. Moore KL: *The Sex Chromatin: Its Discovery and Variations in the Animal Kingdom*. Acta Cytol 6:1–12, 1962
27. Altmann R: Die elementarorganismen, Viet, Leipzig, 1890
28. Cain AJ: An easily controlled method for staining mitochondria, Q J Microsc Sci 89:229–231, 1948

BIBLIOGRAPHY

Culling CFA: Handbook of Histopathological and Histochemical Techniques, 3rd ed. Butterworth, London, 1974

Drury RAB, Wallington EA: Carleton's Histological Technique, 4th ed. Oxford University Press, London, 1967

Lillie RD: Histopathologic Technic and Practical Histochemistry, 3rd ed. Blakiston Division, McGraw-Hill, New York, 1965

Mallory FB: Pathological Technique. Saunders, Philadelphia, 1938

McManus JFA, Mowry RW: Staining Methods Histologic and Histochemical. Hoeber, Medical Division, Harper & Row, New York, 1960

Pearse AGE: Histochemistry, Theoretical and Applied, 3rd ed. Little, Brown, Boston, 1968

Thompson SW: Selected Histochemical and Histological Methods. Thomas, Springfield, Ill, 1966

SIXTEEN

Nucleic Acids

Nucleic acids are normally conjugated with basic protein to form nucleoprotein. In order that the nucleic acid may be demonstrated specifically, the proteins must be decomposed by acid hydrolysis, leaving the protein residue and the nucleic acid (DNA).

Nucleic acids consist of three components: phosphoric acid, which is believed to be the mechanism by which nuclei stain with basic dyes (ie, hematoxylin stains chromatin intensely); a sugar; and an organic or nitrogenous base. This phosphoric acid–sugar–organic base linkage is termed a polynucleotide chain and is either a deoxyribose or a ribose polynucleotide depending on which sugar is present. There are only two sugars, D-2-deoxyribose and D-ribose, giving deoxyribonucleic acid (DNA) and ribonucleic acid (RNA), respectively. The organic base consists of two purines, adenine and guanine, and two pyrimidines, thymine, cytosine, or uracil. Ribonucleic acid contains uracil instead of thymine, which is found in deoxyribonucleic acid. Cytosine and the two purines, adenine and guanine, are common to both DNA and RNA.

The DNA molecule is self-replicating, carrying the hereditary characteristics from cell to cell during mitosis through the genes in the chromosomes. Besides being self-replicating, DNA can also form RNA, having the same genetic information, which passes from the nucleus to the cytoplasm.

DNA is found largely in the nucleus, while RNA is found in fairly extensive amounts in the cytoplasm and nucleolus, and is present in small amounts in the chromosomes.

In order to demonstrate nucleic acids specifically a control section must be run in parallel with the test section. The nucleic acid is extracted from the control section which should give a negative result.

Extraction of Nucleic Acids

DNA EXTRACTION

Deoxyribonuclease, although available commercially, is not widely used in histologic technique because it is very expensive. Other methods utilizing reagents already available in the laboratory will give reliable results.

Perchloric Acid. Immersion in a 5 percent solution of perchloric acid at 70 C for 20 minutes will extract both DNA and RNA. Neutralize the acid with 1 percent sodium carbonate for 5 minutes and wash in running tap water for 5 minutes before staining.

Trichloracetic Acid. Immersion in a 5 percent solution of trichloracetic acid at 90 C for 15 minutes will extract both DNA and RNA. The section should be washed thoroughly in running tap water for at least 5 minutes before staining.

RNA EXTRACTION

Ribonuclease. Ribonuclease is available commercially in crystalline form. Immersion in an 0.01 percent solution in glass-distilled water at 37 C for 1 hour will extract RNA. A parallel section must be treated in glass-distilled water under the same conditions and both of these sections stained with the test section. The distilled water should not affect the RNA and this section should give a positive result. DNA is unaffected by ribonuclease.

Crude ribonuclease can be extracted from saliva. Collect a sufficient quantity of human saliva in a suitable container and place it in a cold water bath. Raise the temperature to 80 C and maintain at this temperature for 10 minutes. Cool, centrifuge, and use the supernatent fluid.

Perchloric Acid. Immersion in a 5 percent solution of perchloric acid in the refrigerator at 4 C for 4–18 hours will extract RNA. The Feulgen reaction for DNA will be positive, but it may stain red with the methyl green-pyronin method. Neutralize the perchloric acid with 1 percent sodium carbonate for 5 minutes, followed by washing in running tap water for 5 minutes before staining.

Methods for Demonstrating DNA and RNA

The methyl green–pyronin method is considered specific for RNA when used with the extraction methods given above (page 244). Hitchcock and Ehrlich's method may be used to advantage after Zenker fixation (page 245).

FEULGEN'S METHOD FOR DNA[1]

Fixation

Ten percent neutral formalin, Carnoy's fluid, Newcomer's fluid, or Zenker's fluid. *Not* Bouin's fluid.

Solutions Required

A. N Hydrochloric Acid:

Hydrochloric acid, conc. (sp gr 1.19)	83.5 ml
Distilled water	to 1000.0 ml

Make up in a volumetric flask.

OR

Hydrochloric acid, conc. (sp gr 1.18)	85.0 ml
Distilled water	to 1000.0 ml

B. Schiff's Reagent (page 304).
C. Sulfurous Acid (page 304).
D. 0.5 percent Aqueous Light Green SF (C.I. 42095).

Method

1. Sections to distilled water. Wash control sections in distilled water and run in parallel.
2. Rinse in N hydrochloric acid.
3. Hydrolyze in preheated N hydrochloric acid at 60 C for the optimal time depending on the fixative*:

* *Note*. A further control section should be added at step 3. Place this section in preheated distilled water at 60 C for the same amount of time as the test section being hydrolyzed in N hydrochloric acid. This section should be negative after treatment with Schiff's reagent. Any positive reaction indicates the presence of free aldehydes before acid hydrolysis.

Carnoy's fluid	6–8 minutes
Formalin	8 minutes
Newcomer's fluid	6–8 minutes
Zenker's fluid	5 minutes

4. Wash in distilled water.
5. Schiff's reagent for 30–90 minutes.
6. Sulfurous acid rinse for 1 minute.
7. Rinse in two more changes of sulfurous acid, 2 minutes in each.
8. Rinse well in distilled water.
9. 0.5 percent Light green for 30–60 seconds.
10. Dehydrate, clear, and mount.

Results

DNA	Red to magenta
Other constituents	Green

The theory of this method is that fixed tissues are exposed to acid hydrolysis with N hydrochloric acid at 60 C for an optimum time. This releases aldehyde groups from the deoxyribose of DNA, which after washing in water reacts with Schiff's reagent to produce a stable red to magenta coloration in the nuclear chromatin. It is not understood why RNA does not also become reactive.

REFERENCE

1. Feulgen R, Rossenback H: Mikroskopischchemischer Nachweis einer Nucleinsäure von Typus der Thymonucleinsäure und die darauf beruhende elektive Färbung von Zellkernen in mikroskopischen Präparaten, Z Phys Chem 135:203–248, 1924

BIBLIOGRAPHY

Culling CFA: Handbook of Histopathological and Histochemical Techniques, 3rd ed. Butterworth, London, 1974

Drury RAB, Wallington EA: Carleton's Histological Technique, 4th ed. Oxford University Press, London, 1967

Pearse AGE: Histochemistry, Theoretical and Applied, 3rd ed. Little, Brown, Boston, 1968

Thompson SW: Selected Histochemical and Histological Methods, Thomas, Springfield, Ill, 1966

SEVENTEEN

Carbohydrates

The term *carbohydrates* is used to designate polyhydroxy aldehydes and polyhydroxy ketones, and includes those substances from which these compounds may be obtained by hydrolysis. The original terminology was applied to a group of organic substances composed of carbon, hydrogen, and oxygen, with the hydrogen and oxygen in the proportions to form water, ie, CH_2O. Some of the substances now classified as carbohydrates do not fit this definition, not having hydrogen and oxygen in the ratio of 2:1, but they do have chemical structures and properties similar to carbohydrates, while other compounds which fit the definition structurally do not have the chemical properties of carbohydrates, ie, acetic acid, ($C_2H_4O_2$), and are therefore not included in the classification as carbohydrates.

Carbohydrates are widely distributed throughout both plant and animal tissues, and are classified systematically as mono-, di-, tri-, tetra-, and polysaccharides. This classification is based upon the number of carbohydrates in the compound. A monosaccharide will not yield any additional carbohydrates upon acid hydrolysis, whereas a di-, tri-, tetra-, or polysaccharide will yield two, three, four, or more monosaccharides on acid hydrolysis. A monosaccharide is a sugar (carbohydrate).

The carbohydrates of interest to the histotechnologist are the polysaccharides and the mucoid carbohydrates, which may be subdivided into three groups: mucopolysaccharides, which are polysaccharide-protein complexes that are predominately carbohydrate; mucoproteins, that are polysaccharide-protein complexes which are predominately protein; and mucolipids that are polysaccharide-fat compounds.

Polysaccharides

The only carbohydrate from this group that can be demonstrated by histologic methods is *glycogen*. It is present in the liver, cardiac muscle, skeletal muscle, and many organs in the newborn. Contrary to long-standing belief, glycogen is adequately fixed by the standard formalin solutions and does not require fixation in solutions containing picric acid or alcoholic fixatives, although these may be preferred.

Glycogen may be stained with iodine, Best's carmine method is strongly P.A.S. positive and is labile to diastase.

Mucopolysaccharides

Mucopolysaccharides can be divided into two groups:

1. Neutral mucopolysaccharides. These are P.A.S. positive and react similarly to mucoproteins.
2. Acid mucopolysaccharides. These can be further divided into simple—or nonsulfated acid mucopolysaccharides (carboxylated)—and complex—or sulfated acid mucopolysaccharides.

NONSULFATED (CARBOXYLATED) ACID MUCOPOLYSACCHARIDES

These may be classified by site into epithelial and connective tissue subgroups and by content, based on whether the acid radical is sialic acid or a hexuronic acid.

Epithelial Nonsulfated Acid Mucopolysaccharides

In epithelial nonsulfated acid mucopolysaccharides—often called sialomucins—the acid radical is sialic acid, which is in combination with the reactive carboxyl groups. Most of the sialomucins are labile to sialidase (neuramidase) and those which are resistant may be blocked by hydrolysis with weak hydrochloric acid. Sialic acid is resistant to digestion by hyaluronidase.

Epithelial sialomucins are mostly P.A.S. positive, react with alcian blue at pH 2.5, stain with the colloidal iron method, and metachromatically with toluidine blue.

Connective Tissue Nonsulfated Acid Mucopolysaccharides

Connective tissue nonsulfated acid mucopolysaccharides are rich in hexuronic acid and may contain sialic acid. Hexuronic acid-rich substances contain large quantities of hyaluronic acid, which is labile to hyaluronidase.

Connective tissue nonsulfated acid mucopolysaccharides are P.A.S. negative, react with alcian blue at pH 2.5, stain with the colloidal iron method, and metachromatically with toluidine blue.

SULFATED ACID MUCOPOLYSACCHARIDES

Sulfated acid mucopolysaccharides may also be divided by site into two subgroups: epithelial (epithelial sulfo-mucins) and connective tissue sulfated acid mucopolysaccharides.

Epithelial Sulfated Acid Mucopolysaccharides

Epithelial sulfated acid mucopolysaccharides (epithelial sulfo-mucins) contain sulfate esters, but in a different combination to those in the connective tissue sulfated acid mucopolysaccharides. They are weakly sulfated mucopolysaccharides resistant to digestion by hyaluronidase, and are located in the submandibular salivary glands, and in the duodenal and colonic goblet cells.

This group of acid mucopolysaccharides is generally P.A.S. negative, reacts with alcian blue at pH 1.0, stains with aldehyde fuchsin, colloidal iron, and is metachromatic with toluidine blue.

Connective Tissue Sulfated Acid Mucopolysaccharides

These acid mucopolysaccharides contain either sulfated glucuronic acids, such as chondroitin sulfate and heparin sulfate, or keratin sulfate. Those containing chondroitin sulfate are labile to hyaluronidase, while the connective tissue mucopolysaccharides that do not contain chondroitin sulfate are resistant to digestion by this enzyme.

Connective tissue sulfated acid mucopolysaccharides are both strongly acidic and strongly sulfated, and are located in cartilage, heart valves, the aorta, and skin. They are P.A.S. negative, react with alcian blue at pH 0.5, stain with colloidal iron, aldehyde fuchsin, and are metachromatic with toluidine blue.

Sulfated acid mucopolysaccharides may be differentiated from nonsulfated acid mucopolysaccharides by *methylation* and *saponification*.

Methylation will block both groups of acid mucopolysaccharides by desulfation and esterification of carboxyl groups with the loss of staining by alcian blue. Saponification will de-esterify carboxyl groups and restore staining with alcian blue to the nonsulfated acid mucopolysaccharides, while the sulfated acid mucopolysaccharides will remain unstained.

Mucoprotein

Mucoproteins are polysaccharide–protein complexes that are predominently protein in nature. These substances are similar to *glycoproteins*, the difference between the two substances being that the carbohydrate (hexosamine) content of mucoprotein is more than four percent of its total weight, while the carbohydrate content of glycoprotein is less than four percent of its total weight. It has been demonstrated that the carbohydrates present in these substances are galactose, mannose, fucose, and glucose, with rhamnose also present in mucoproteins. Mucoprotein and glycoprotein cannot be differentiated from each other by histologic methods.

Mucoproteins and glycoproteins may be found in beta cells of the pituitary, basement membranes, reticulin, and collagen. They are P.A.S. positive, but do not react metachromatically when stained with toluidine blue.

Mucolipids

Mucolipids are a mixture of polysaccharides and fatty acid complexes. Normally found in tissues as cerebrosides and gangliosides, they are usually P.A.S. positive and may be demonstrated in frozen sections by the lipid stains.

Blocking Techniques

As can be seen from the preceding discussion, the staining methods employed for the identification of carbohydrates are not very specific. This may be improved by the use of blocking methods and enzyme digestion of certain specific substances in control sections so that they do not react with the stains employed. By comparing these control sections with test sections stained in parallel, the specificity of the staining reactions are improved. The precision and completeness of blocking is open to discussion, and as can be seen in the suggested methods times of exposure vary considerably.

Known positive and negative control sections should *always* be stained in parallel to the test and blocked sections.

ALDEHYDE BLOCKING TECHNIQUE[1]

Sections are taken to water and exposed to periodic acid in the normal manner for the P.A.S. technique. Wash, and place the control section in the following solution:

Aniline	10 ml
Glacial acetic acid	90 ml

Leave in this solution for 30 minutes at room temperature and wash thoroughly in distilled water. Continue with the P.A.S. technique. Only nonaldehyde P.A.S.-positive material will be stained.

ACETYLATION: BLOCKING TECHNIQUE FOR 1:2 GLYCOL GROUP[2]

A 1:2 glycol group (carbohydrate) is a P.A.S.-positive substance that will give a P.A.S.-negative reaction after acetylation. The procedure is reversible by saponification (treatment with potassium hydroxide).

The following method is recommended:

1. Label three sections A, B, and C. Bring down to water.
2. Place sections A and B in the following solution:

Acetic anhydride	13 ml
Pyridine	20 ml

   Leave for 1–24 hours at room temperature. One hour is usually sufficient, but a longer period may be required.
3. Wash sections A and B in water.
4. Place section B into 0.1 N potassium hydroxide for 45 minutes at room temperature (saponification).
5. Wash section B in water.
6. Stain all three sections by the P.A.S. technique.

Results

Section A	P.A.S. negative
Section B	P.A.S. positive
Section C	P.A.S. positive

This indicates that the reaction is due to 1:2 glycol grouping and not to preformed aldehydes.

METHYLATION AND SAPONIFICATION

Methylation blocks the staining of both nonsulfated acid mucopolysaccharides and sulfated acid mucopolysaccharides. The staining of the nonsulfated mucopolysaccharides is restored by saponification.

Method

1. Sections to alcohol.
2. Place into 1 percent hydrochloric acid in methyl alcohol for 4–12 hours (methylation).
3. Rinse in alcohol.
4. Place into 0.1 N potassium hydroxide for 45–60 minutes at room temperature, (saponification). Sections have a tendency to float off of the slides during saponification and it may be advisable to celloidinize them before this step.
5. Wash in water.
6. Stain by the appropriate method (Alcian blue).

Results

Nonsulfated acid mucopolysaccharides	Blue
Sulfated acid mucopolysaccharides	Unstained

ACID HYDROLYSIS TO REMOVE SIALIC ACID[3]

Method

1. Bring two sections to water, labeled A and B.
2. Place section A in sodium acetate-hydrochloric acid buffer at pH 2.5 for 2 hours at 75 C. Place section B in M/1 sodium acetate for 2 hours at 75 C.
3. Wash in distilled water.
4. Stain with Alcian blue at pH 2.5.

Results

Loss of staining by Alcian blue in section A indicates that sialic acid groups were present.

SIALIDASE DIGESTION FOR THE REMOVAL OF SIALIC ACID[4]

Method

1. Bring two sections to water. Label A and B.
2. Place section A into the following solution:

Sialidase (Neuramidase: *V. cholera* 500 units/ml)*	1 ml
M/10 phosphate buffer, pH 6.0	4 ml

Place section B into M/10 phosphate buffer, pH 6.0. Incubate both sections at 37 C for 5–10 hours.

3. Wash in distilled water.
4. Stain with Alcian blue, pH 2.5.

Results

Section A	
Sialidase labile sialomucins	Unstained
Other acid mucopolysaccharides	Blue
Section B	
Acid mucopolysaccharides	Blue

HYALURONIDASE DIGESTION:

This enzyme will digest hyaluronic acid and chondroitin sulfates A and C.

Method

1. Bring two sections to water. Label A and B.
2. Place section A into the following solution:

Hyaluronidase* (bovine testes 300 units/mg)	20 mg
M/10 phosphate buffer, pH 6.6	10 ml

Place section B into M/10 Phosphate buffer, pH 6.6. Incubate both sections at 37 C for 3 hours.

3. Wash well in distilled water.
4. Stain with Alcian blue at pH 2.5.

Results

Section A	
Hyaluronic acid and chondroitin sulfates a and C	Unstained
Other acid mucopolysaccharides	Blue
Section B	
Acid mucopolysaccharides	Blue

* Available from Calbiochem, La Jolla, California.

DIASTASE DIGESTION FOR THE REMOVAL OF GLYCOGEN[5]

Diastase is readily available in the form of saliva. However it is sometimes difficult to collect enough to digest several sections. Chewing on a few pellets of paraffin wax will stimulate the production of saliva and up to 35 ml can be collected in this manner. Diastase is also available commercially.

1. Section to water.
2. Place the section into:
   a. Saliva,
   b. 0.1 percent diastase of malt in distilled water, or
   c. 0.1 percent diastase of malt in M/10 phosphate buffer at pH 6.0.

   Incubate at 37 C for 30 minutes.
3. Wash in tap water for 5 minutes.
4. Celloidinize if desired.
5. Stain by Best's carmine method or the P.A.S. technique.

Results

Diastase digested section	Glycogen removed
Undigested section	Glycogen red

BEST'S CARMINE METHOD FOR GLYCOGEN[6]

Fixation

Ten percent neutral formalin, Bouin's fluid, Gendre's fluid, and Carnoy's fluid.

Solutions Required

A. Weigert's Iron Hematoxylin (page 218).

B. Best's Carmine:

Stock solution

Carmine (C.I. 75470)	2 g
Potassium carbonate	1 g
Potassium chloride	5 g
Distilled water	60 ml

Grind the carmine in a mortar, and add, together with the other salts, to the water. Boil gently in a large flask (to avoid frothing) for 5 minutes. Cool and add:

Ammonia, conc.	20 ml

Store in a dark bottle in the refrigerator. The stain will keep for approximately three months.

Working solution:

Best's carmine stock solution	2 parts
Ammonia, conc.	2 parts
Absolute methyl alcohol	3 parts

C. Best's Differentiator:

Absolute ethyl alcohol	80 ml
Absolute methyl alcohol	40 ml
Distilled water	100 ml

D. 1 percent Hydrochloric Acid in 70 percent Alcohol.

Method

1. Sections to alcohol.
2. Celloidinize if desired (page **178**).
3. Weigert's iron hematoxylin for 15 minutes.
4. Wash in tap water.
5. Differentiate in acid alcohol until only the nuclei are stained. Control under the microscope.
6. Blue in running water for 5 minutes.
7. Best's carmine for 10 minutes.
8. Differentiate in Best's differentiator until no more color comes away.
9. Rinse in 80 percent alcohol.
10. Remove celloidin if used.
11. Dehydrate, clear, and mount.

Results

Nuclei	Blue/gray
Glycogen	Red

Note

A known positive control should be stained in parallel with the unknown, plus an unknown which has been digested with diastase.

THE PERIODIC ACID SCHIFF REACTION (P.A.S.)[7]

The periodic acid Schiff reaction (P.A.S.) is based on the fact that periodic acid will oxidize certain tissue elements (ie, 1:2 glycol groups, CHOH-CHOH) to produce aldehydes (CHO) by cleavage of the carbon-carbon bonds where these carbon atoms have adjacent hydroxyl ($-OH$) groups or adjacent hydroxyl and amino ($-NH_2$) groups. These aldehydes react with the colorless Schiff reagent and are colored a deep red to magenta.

This method may be used to demonstrate glycogen as well as many other substances; but because it is not specific for glycogen, control sections must be processed in parallel with the test. Two controls are used, one being a known positive for glycogen and the other being a duplicate of the test section. This duplicate section is subjected to digestion with diastase prior to staining to remove any traces of glycogen. Any coloration in the test section which is not seen in the digested control section is assumed to be glycogen.

The P.A.S. method may be used to demonstrate mucins, fungi, amyloid, hyaline, and basement membranes.

Fixation

Ten percent neutral formalin, Carnoy's fluid, Bouin's fluid, or Gendre's fluid.

Solutions Required

A. 0.5 percent Periodic Acid.

B. Schiff's Reagent:

Rosanilin *basic fuchsin* (C.I. 42510)	1 g
Distilled water	200 ml

Boil the distilled water and add the rosanilin. Stir until dissolved. Cool to 50 C, filter, and add:

N Hydrochloric acid	20 ml

Cool to 25 C and add:

Sodium metabisulfite (anhydrous)	1 g

Allow to stand for 24 hours (the solution should turn a pale straw color) and filter through activated charcoal. The filtrate should be colorless (water white). Store in the refrigerator.

C. Sulfurous Acid Rinse:

10 percent sodium metabisulfite	6 ml
N Hydrochloric acid	5 ml
Distilled water	100 ml

D. Harris' Hematoxylin (page 208).

Method

1. Sections to distilled water.
2. 0.5 percent periodic acid for 5 minutes.
3. Wash in distilled water.

4. Schiff's reagent for 15 minutes.
5. Rinse in three changes of sulfurous acid rinse, 2 minutes in each rinse.
6. Wash in running tap water for 5 minutes.
7. Harris' hematoxylin for 30–60 seconds.
8. Wash in running tap water for 5 minutes.
9. Dehydrate, clear, and mount.

Results

Nuclei	Blue
P.A.S.-positive material	Deep red to magneta

Note

A control section may be processed to test the Schiff's reagent. Place this section in 0.5 percent potassium iodate for 5 minutes and wash thoroughly in water. After treatment with the Schiff's reagent it should remain colorless.

BAUER-FEULGEN METHOD FOR GLYCOGEN[8]

The oxidizing agent used in this method is 4 percent chromic acid (chromium trioxide). Chromic acid has a tendency to continue oxidizing the newly formed aldehyde groups to carboxylic acids and other breakdown products except for glycogen. Other carbohydrate substances are over-oxidized and are either not stained or have the intensity of the staining greatly reduced. Oxidize for 30 minutes.

After oxidizing with chromic acid continue from step 3 of the P.A.S. method.

Results

Nuclei	Blue
Glycogen	Deep red to magenta

SOUTHGATE'S MUCICARMINE METHOD FOR EPITHELIAL MUCIN[9]

Fixation

Ten percent neutral formalin.

Solutions Required

A. Harris' Hematoxylin.
B. 1 percent Hydrochloric Acid in 70 percent Alcohol.

C. Southgate's Mucicarmine:

Carmine (C.I. 75470)	2 g
Aluminum hydroxide	2 g
50 percent ethyl alcohol	200 ml

Dissolve the carmine and aluminum hydroxide in the 50 alcohol and add:

Aluminum chloride, anhydrous	1 g

This may cause violent frothing, and a wide-mouthed flask or beaker should be used. Bring to the boil and boil for exactly $2\frac{1}{2}$ minutes. Cool and filter. For use dilute as follows:

Mucicarmine solution	1 part
Distilled water	4 parts

Note. It is sometimes difficult to obtain a good batch of this stain. When a good batch of carmine is obtained it should be kept exclusively for this solution. Carmine alum lake may be tried as a substitute for carmine.

Method

1. Sections to water.
2. Harris' hematoxylin for 5 minutes.
3. Rinse in tap water.
4. Differentiate in 1 percent acid alcohol until only the nuclei are stained. Control under the microscope.
5. Wash and blue in running tap water for 5 minutes.
6. Southgate's mucicarmine for 30–60 minutes.
7. Rinse in tap water.
8. Dehydrate, clear, and mount.

Results

Nuclei	Blue
Epithelial mucin	Red
Gastric mucin	Red
Capsule of cryptococcus	Red

Note

This may be the best method for cryptococci.

MAYER'S MUCIHEMATEIN METHOD FOR MUCINS (MODIFIED)[10]

Fixation

Absolute ethyl alcohol preferred.

Solution Required

Mayer's Mucihematein.

Hematoxylin (C.I. 75290)	1.0 g
70 percent ethyl alcohol	100.0 ml

Dissolve and add:

Aluminum chloride	0.5 g
1 percent sodium iodate, aq.	5.0 ml

This ripens the solution immediately. Make up to 500 ml. with 70 percent ethyl alcohol. The solution is stable for 4–6 months.

Method

1. Sections to distilled water.
2. Mucihematein for 15 minutes.
3. Wash well in distilled water. At least 5 minutes.
4. Dehydrate, clear, and mount.

Results

Epithelial mucin	Deep blue-violet
Connective tissue mucin	Lighter violet
Cartilage matrix	Lighter violet

ALCIAN BLUE METHODS FOR ACID MUCOPOLYSACCHARIDES[11]

Fixation

Ten percent neutral formalin.

Solution Required

Alcian Blue (pH 2.5):

Alcian blue (C.I. 74240)	1 g
3 percent acetic acid	100 ml

OR

Alcian Blue (pH 1.0):

Alcian blue (C.I. 74240)	1 g
0.1 N Hydrochloric acid	100 ml

OR

Alcian Blue (pH 0.5):

Alcian blue (C.I. 74240)	1 g
0.5 N Hydrochloric acid	100 ml

Filter before use. These solutions are stable for approximately 2 weeks.

Method

1. Sections to distilled water.
2. Desired Alcian blue solution for 30 minutes.
3. *IF Alcian blue (pH 2.5) was used*, wash in distilled water. *IF Alcian blue (pH 1.0 or 0.5) was used*, BLOT DRY with filter paper.
4. Dehydrate rapidly, clear, and mount.

Results

Alcian blue (pH 2.5)

Most acid mucopolysaccharides	Blue

Alcian blue (pH 1.0)

Sulfated acid mucopolysaccharides	Blue

Alcian blue (pH 0.5)

Strongly sulfated acid mucopolysaccharides	Blue

Alcian blue is a water-soluble copper phthalocyanin dye compound which, when used in an acid solution, has a strong affinity for acid mucopolysaccharides. It may be made selective by lowering the pH. It is believed to stain by salt linkage to acidic groups. (Readers should see Refs. 12 and 13 for discussions on Alcian blue.)

P.A.S. ALCIAN BLUE METHOD[14]

Fixation

Ten percent neutral formalin.

Solutions Required

A. Alcian blue (pH 2.5) (page 307).
B. 0.5 percent Periodic Acid.
C. Schiff's Reagent (page 304).
D. Sulfurous Acid Rinse (page 304).

Method

1. Stain with the Alcian blue method (page 307).
2. Stain with the P.A.S. method (page 304).

Results

Acid mucopolysaccharides	Blue
P.A.S.-positive substances	Deep red to magenta

TOLUIDINE BLUE METHOD FOR ACID MUCOPOLYSACCHARIDES[15]

Fixation

Ten percent neutral formalin or formol alcohol.

Solutions Required

A. 0.25 percent Toluidine Blue in Michaelis' Veronal Buffer (pH 4.5):

Toluidine blue (C.I. 52040)	0.25 g
Veronal buffer (pH 4.5)	100.0 ml

B. Michaelis' Veronal Buffer (pH 4.5):

Sodium acetate	19.43 g
Sodium barbiturate	29.43 g
Distilled water	to 1000.0 ml

For use at pH 4.5 mix:

Veronal acetate solution	5.0 ml
M/10 Hydrochloric acid	11.0 ml
Distilled water	9.0 ml

Method

1. Sections to distilled water.
2. Buffered toluidine blue solution for 10 seconds.
3. Rinse in distilled water.
4. Blot completely dry with fluffless filter paper.
5. Clear in xylene and mount.

If the section fails to clear, repeat steps 4 and 5.

Results

Acid mucopolysaccharides	Pink to purple
Other metachromatic substances	Pink to purple
Nuclei	Blue

ALDEHYDE FUCHSIN–ALCIAN BLUE METHOD FOR SULFATED AND CARBOXYLATED ACID MUCOPOLYSACCHARIDES[16]

Fixation

Ten percent neutral formalin.

Solutions Required

A. Aldehyde Fuchsin Solution (page 232).
B. Alcian Blue pH 2.5 (page 307).

Method

1. Sections to water.
2. Rinse in 70 percent alcohol.
3. Aldehyde fuchsin solution for 20–30 minutes.
4. Rinse thoroughly in 70 percent alcohol.
5. Rinse thoroughly in distilled water.
6. Alcian blue solution, pH 2.5, for 30 minutes.
7. Rinse thoroughly in distilled water.
8. Dehydrate, clear, and mount.

Results

Strongly sulfated acid mucopolysaccharides	Deep purple
Weakly sulfated acid mucopolysaccharides	Light purple
Carboxylated acid mucopolysaccharides	Blue

Note

Aldehyde fuchsin is not specific for sulfated acid mucopolysaccharides. A control section should be subjected to methylation and saponification prior to staining. Sites that remain aldehyde fuchsin negative in the control and are positive in the test section may be assumed to be sulfated acid mucopolysaccharides.

MOWRY'S MODIFICATION OF THE COLLOIDAL IRON STAIN FOR ACID MUCOPOLYSACCHARIDES[17]

Fixation

Ten percent neutral formalin. *Avoid* bichromate fixatives.

Solutions Required

A. 12 percent Acetic Acid.
B. Colloidal Iron Solution:

Stock Solution

29 percent ferric chloride solution	4.4 ml
Distilled water	250.0 ml

Boil the distilled water. Into the boiling water pour the ferric chloride solution and stir. When the solution turns red remove from the heat and allow to cool. This solution is stable for several months.

Working Solution

Glacial acetic acid	5 ml
Distilled water	15 ml
Stock colloidal iron	20 ml

C. Hydrochloric Acid–Potassium Ferrocyanide Solution:

2 percent hydrochloric acid	20 ml
2 percent potassium ferrocyanide	20 ml

D. 1 percent Aqueous Neutral Red. (C.L. 50040)

Method

1. Sections to water.
2. Rinse in 12 percent acetic acid.
3. Colloidal iron solution, freshly prepared, for 60 minutes.
4. Rinse in four changes of 12 percent acetic acid for 3 minutes in each rinse.
5. Hydrochloric acid–potassium ferrocyanide solution for 20 minutes.
6. Wash in running tap water for 5 minutes.
7. 1 percent Neutral red for 1 minute.
8. Rinse in distilled water.
9. Dehydrate, clear, and mount.

Results

Acid mucopolysaccharides	Blue
Nuclei	Red

Note

The counterstain is a matter of choice and some workers prefer either a P.A.S. or the Feulgen reaction.

REFERENCES

1. Lillie RD, Glenner GG: Histochemical blockade by aniline in glacial acetic acid, J Histochem Cytochem 5:167–169, 1957
2. McManus JFA, Cason JE: Carbohydrate histochemistry studied by acetylation techniques. I. Periodic acid method, J Exp Med 91:651–654, 1950
3. Quintarelli G, Tsuiki S, Hashimoto, Y, Pigman W: Studies of sialic acid-containing mucins in bovine submaxillary and rat sublingual glands, J Histochem Cytochem 9:176–183, 1961

4. Spicer SS, Warren L: The histochemistry of sialic acid containing mucoproteins, J Histochem Cytochem 8:135–137, 1960
5. Lillie RD: On the destruction of cytoplasmic basophilia (ribonucleic acid) and of the metachromatic basophilia of cartilage by the glycogen splitting enzyme malt diastase. A histochemical study, Anat Rec 103:611–633, 1949
6. Best F: Über Karminfärbung des Glykogen und der Kerne, Z Wiss Mikrosk 23:319–322, 1906
7. McManus JFA: Histological and histochemical uses of periodic acid, Stain Technol 23:99, 1948
8. Bauer H: Mikroskopisch-Chemischer Nachweiss von Glykogen und Einigen Anderen Polysacchariden, Z Mikrosk Anat Forsch 33:143–159, 1933
9. Southgate HW: Note on preparing mucicarmine, J Pathol Bacteriol 30:729, 1927
10. Laskey AM: A Modification of Mayer's mucihematein technic, Stain Technol 25:33–34, 1950
11. Lev R, Spicer SS: Specific staining of sulfate groups with alcian blue at low pH, J Histochem Cytochem 12:309, 1964
12. Scott JE: Histochemistry of Alcian Blue. 2. Structure of Alcian Blue 8GX, Histochemie 30:215, 1972
13. Scott JE: Alcian dyes–ICI Cease manufacture and release details of composition, Histochemie 37:379, 1973 pp. 379–80
14. Mowry RW: Alcian blue technics for the histochemical study of acidic carbohydrates, J Histochem Cytochem 4:407, 1956
15. Vassar PS, Culling CFA: Fibrosis of the breast, Arch Pathol 67:128–133, 1959
16. Spicer SS, Meyer DB: Histochemical differentiation of acid mucopolysaccharides by means of combined aldehyde fuchsin–alcian blue staining, Am J Clin Pathol 33:453, 1960
17. Mowry RW: Improved procedure for the staining of acidic polysaccharides by Müller's colloidal-(hydrous)-ferric oxide and its combination with the Feulgen and periodic acid Schiff reactions, Lab Invest 7:566–576, 1958

BIBLIOGRAPHY

Bancroft JD: Histochemical Techniques, 2nd ed. Butterworths, London, 1975.

Barka T, Anderson PJ: Histochemistry: Theory, Practice, and Bibliography, Hoeber Medical Division, Harper & Row, New York, 1963

Culling CFA: Handbook of Histopathological and Histochemical Techniques, 3rd ed. Butterworth, London, 1974

Drury RAB, Wallington EA: Carleton's Histological Technique, 4th ed. Oxford University Press, London, 1967

Lillie RD: Histopathologic Technic and Practical Histochemistry, 3rd ed. Blakiston Division, McGraw-Hill, New York, 1965.

McManus JFA, Mowry RW: Staining Methods: Histologic and Histochemical, Hoeber Medical Division, Harper & Row, New York, 1960

Pearse AGE: Histochemistry, Theoretical & Applied, 3rd ed., Little, Brown, Boston, 1968

Thompson SW: Selected Histochemical and Histological Methods, Thomas, Springfield, Ill, 1966

EIGHTEEN

Amyloid

Amyloid is an abnormal, intra- and intercellular substance, chemically related to cartilage, that is insoluble in water, alcohol, ether, and weak acids. When stained by the hematoxylin and eosin method, amyloid is seen as a pink-staining homogenous substance, and as such cannot be distinguished with any degree of certainty from other forms of hyaline degeneration. Special stains are absolutely essential for the positive identification of amyloid.

In its fresh state, amyloid is a firm translucent substance that is deposited between parenchymatous cells in connective tissue and closely resembles hyaline in its general appearance. When observed in the spleen it has a characteristic appearance that has been described as "sago spleen." It may also be known as "waxy degeneration." Common sites of amyloid deposits are the liver, skin, lymph nodes, kidneys, and the pancreas. It was a frequent sequel to chronic suppurative and inflammatory conditions, and its appearance in the skin is often an indication of amyloidosis elsewhere. When associated with chronic suppurative or inflammatory conditions, it is called secondary or typical amyloidosis. When amyloidosis occurs as a primary disease and is not associated with any known predisposing disorder, it is known as primary or atypical amyloidosis, or paraamyloid, and as such is often seen in cardiac muscle.

Virchow, in 1854, proposed the term amyloid from the Latin *amylum* meaning starch and the Greek *eidos* meaning form, because of its affinity for iodine, a characteristic of starch, and also because of its gross appearance in tissue. It is this affinity for iodine that differentiates amyloid from hyaline in its fresh state.

Iodine in solution with potassium iodide (Gram's or Lugol's solutions are excellent) will stain fresh amyloid a deep mahogany. This color is changed to a violet-blue after treatment with three percent sulfuric acid, although several minutes may be necessary for the color change to occur. This affinity for iodine should not be taken as an indication that amyloid is starch. For example, iodine has been used extensively for the microscopic demonstration of glycogen since 1826.

What is amyloid? In 1926 amyloid was described as "an abnormal intercellular substance chemically related to the ground substance of cartillage with definite physical and chemical properties," and 40 years later we read that amyloid is "a hyaline-like, structureless translucent substance, possibly chondroitin sulfuric acid." The exact chemical composition of amyloid is as yet unknown. It is believed to be a mixture of protein, glycoprotein, other polysaccharides, and occasionally lipids. Giles and Calkins (1955)[1] studied deposits of almost pure amyloid and their investigations have shown that it is chiefly protein in content. They also discovered that amyloid contains approximately four percent carbohydrates, of which 1.5 percent are amino-sugars. Other investigators have given support to their theory that chondroitin sulfates are possibly not a significant carbohydrate content, but the fact that the mucopolysaccharide component is sulfated was established by Kennedy in 1962[2] using labeled sulfate in radioautographic techniques. It has also been theorized that amyloid may be the product of normal or abnormal plasma cells producing pathologic protein, and that a precipitate of protein and mucopolysaccharides may form amyloid. Another suggestion is that amyloid is the result of an immunologic disturbance and may therefore be the product of a local antigen–antibody reaction.

Amyloidosis is easily induced in experimental animals by several substances, the most common of these being casein-rich substances, which may be administered by either feeding or injection. These techniques cause abnormal stimulation of the protein synthesizing function of the reticulo-endothelial system.

Examination of amyloid by electron microscopy and its birefringence when stained with cotton dyes such as Congo red or Sirius red suggest a peculiar crystalline type of structure. Fibers with the tinctorial properties of collagen suggest an incomplete form of protein fiber formation, or because of its affinity for cotton dyes it may possibly bear some relationship to cellulose fibers.

From this discussion we emerge with a few facts about amyloid that are in general acceptance. Amyloid is possibly a complex of protein, glycoprotein, and sulfated mucopolysaccharides, having some form or structure. It is insoluble in water, alcohol, ether, and dilute acids, and is not digested by either pepsin or hydrochloric acid.

The oldest known method for demonstrating amyloid is with iodine, not only in its fresh state but also in sections. Iodine is still used today for staining museum preparations of whole organs. This method was followed by the use of either methyl violet or crystal violet as a metachromatic reaction, and was originated by Mayer in 1896.[3] Neither of these dyes are pure and the method is therefore not a true metachromatic reaction, even though it retains this terminology. To obtain a true metachromatic reaction with amyloid, it should be stained with a weak solution of thionin or toluidine blue following peptic digestion. It has been suggested that the peptic digestion removes a glycoprotein block from the acid mucopolysaccharides.

The use of cotton dyes in the form of Congo red was introduced by Benhold in 1922.[4] This method has been modified many times since then. Unfortunately, Congo red has a tendency to stain collagen in addition to amyloid, but amyloid stained with Congo red has a green birefringence under polarized light and this should always be used to confirm the staining reaction when this method is used.

In 1948 King[5] introduced a silver technique applicable to frozen sections.

Fluorescent staining using Thioflavin T or S was introduced by Vassar and Culling (1959).[6] Amyloid gives a blue-green fluorescence. The authors have no explanation for the affinity of this dye and amyloid.

Sweat and Puchtler[7] employed Sirius red, another cotton dye, in 1965. This stains amyloid with more specificity than does Congo red without the secondary staining of collagen or other structures. It is also birefringent under polarized light, and this should be used to confirm the staining results.

Methods for the Demonstration of Amyloid

LANGHANS' IODINE METHOD (MODIFIED)[8]

Fixation

Ten percent neutral formalin or absolute alcohol.

Solutions Required

A. 1 percent Acetic Acid.
B. Iodine Solution:

Gram's iodine	3 ml
Distilled water	97 ml

Method

1. Sections to water.
2. 1 percent acetic acid for 1–2 minutes.
3. Iodine solution for 10–15 minutes.
4. Wash in distilled water and mount in an aqueous medium.

Results

Amyloid	Mahogany brown

LIEB'S CRYSTAL VIOLET STAIN FOR AMYLOID[9]

Fixation

Ten percent neutral formalin or absolute alcohol.

Solution Required

Crystal Violet Solution:

Stock Solution, Saturated

Crystal violet (C.I. 42555)	14 g
95 percent ethyl alcohol	100 ml

Working Solution

Stock solution	10 ml
Distilled water	300 ml
Hydrochloric acid	1 ml

Method

1. Sections to water.
2. Working Crystal violet solution for 1–2 minutes. Control under the microscope.
3. Wash well in tap water.
4. Either:

   Mount in Highman's medium

   OR

   Allow to air dry. Clear in xylene and mount.

Results

Amyloid	Purplish
Other elements	Blue

HIGHMAN'S METHYL VIOLET METHOD[10]

Fixation

Ten percent neutral formalin or absolute alcohol.

Solutions Required

Highman's Methyl Violet Solution:

Methyl violet (C.I. 42535)	0.1 g
Distilled water	97.5 ml
Glacial acetic acid	2.5 ml

Method

1. Sections to water.
2. Highman's methyl violet solution for 15–30 minutes. Control under the microscope.
3. Wash well in tap water.
4. Either:

   Mount in Highman's medium

   OR

   Allow to air dry, clear in xylene and mount.

Result

Amyloid	Red to purple

PUCHTLER'S ALKALINE CONGO RED METHOD, MODIFIED[11]

Fixation

Ten percent neutral formalin, absolute alcohol, or Carnoy's fluid.

Solutions Required

A. Harris' Hematoxylin (page 208).
B. Congo Red Solution:

Stock Solution

Congo red (C.I. 22120)	1 g
1 percent sodium chloride in 80 percent alcohol	200 ml

Stir thoroughly until solution is reasonably complete. Filter. This solution is stable for many months. (Puchtler *et al* used saturated sodium chloride and advised that the solution should stand for 24 hours before use).

Working Solution

Stock Congo red solution	100 ml
1 percent sodium hydroxide	1 ml

Method

1. Sections to water.
2. Harris' hematoxylin for 2 minutes.
3. Wash thoroughly in running tap water.
4. Rinse in 80 percent alcohol.
5. Alkaline Congo red solution for 20 minutes.
6. Dehydrate through 3 changes of absolute ethyl alcohol, clear, and mount.

Results

Nuclei	Blue
Amyloid	Orange/Red
Elastic fibers	Paler Orange/Red

MODIFICATION OF PUCHTLER'S ALKALINE CONGO RED METHOD FOR AMYLOID[12]

Fixation

Ten percent neutral formalin, absolute alcohol, or Carnoy's fluid.

Solutions Required

A. Harris' Hematoxylin (page 208).

B. Congo Red in Buffered Ethanol:

Buffer Solution

M/10 Glycine, NH_2CH_2COOH (mol wt 75.07) (7.507 g in distilled water to 1000 ml)	30 ml
M/10 Sodium chloride, NaCl (mol wt 58.5) (5.85 g in distilled water to 1000 ml)	30 ml
M/10 Sodium hydroxide, NaOH (mol wt 40.0) (4.0 g in distilled water to 1000 ml)	40 ml

Working Solution

Congo red (C.I. 22120)	1 g
Buffer solution (pH 10)	100 ml
Absolute ethyl alcohol	100 ml

C. 70 percent Alcohol.

Method

1. Sections to water.
2. Harris' hematoxylin for 2 minutes.
3. Wash thoroughly in running tap water.

4. 0.5 percent Congo red in buffered ethanol for 10–20 minutes.
5. Rinse and differentiate in 70 percent alcohol for a few seconds.
6. Dehydrate, clear, and mount.

Results

Nuclei	Blue
Amyloid	Bright pink to red

SIRIUS RED METHOD FOR AMYLOID[7]

Fixation

Ten percent neutral formalin, absolute alcohol, or Carnoy's fluid.

Solutions Required

A. Alkaline Alcohol:

80 percent ethyl alcohol	100 ml
1 percent sodium hydroxide	1 ml

B. Sirius Red Solution:

Sirius red F3B (C.I. 35780)	2 g
Sodium chloride	1 g
Distilled water	200 ml

C. Buffer Solution, pH 9.0:

1.24 percent boric acid	8 ml
1.9 percent sodium borate	32 ml

D. Harris' Hematoxylin (page 208).

Method

1. Sections to 80 percent alcohol.
2. Alkaline alcohol solution* for 1–1½ hours.
3. Rinse in distilled water.
4. Sirius red solution at 60 C for 1–1½ hours.
5. Rinse in buffer solution, pH 9.0.
6. Wash in running tap water for 5 minutes.
7. Harris' hematoxylin for 2 minutes.
8. Wash in running tap water for 5 minutes.
9. Dehydrate, clear, and mount.

* Sections tend to float free in this solution.

Results

Nuclei	Blue
Amyloid	Pink to red
Background	Unstained

THIOFLAVIN T METHOD FOR AMYLOID[6]

Fixation

Ten percent neutral formalin.

Solutions Required

A. Harris' Hematoxylin (page 208).
B. 1 percent Aqueous Thioflavin T (C.I. 49005).
C. 1 percent Acetic Acid.

Method

1. Sections to water.
2. Harris' hematoxylin for 2 minutes. This quenches nuclear fluorescence.
3. Wash in running tap water for 3 minutes.
4. Rinse in distilled water.
5. 1 percent aqueous thioflavin T for 3 minutes.
6. Rinse in distilled water.
7. Differentiate in two changes of 1 percent acetic acid, for 10 minutes in each.
8. Rinse in distilled water.
9. Either

A. Mount in Apathy's medium,

OR

B. Dehydrate, clear, and mount in a nonfluorescent medium, eg, UVinert.

10. Examine by UV microscopy using either:

A. BG-12 exciter filter with an OG-4 and/or OG-5 barrier filters.

OR

B. UG-1 or a UG-2 exciter filter with a colorless UV filter.

Results

Amyloid	Bright yellow on a black background
Amyloid	A brighter yellow on a blue background

REFERENCES

1. Giles RB, Calkins E: Studies of the composition of secondary amyloid, J Clin Invest 34:1476–1482, 1955
2. Kennedy JS: Sulphur-35 in experimental amyloidosis, J Pathol Bacteriol 83:165–181, 1962
3. Mayer P: Über Schleimfärbung, Mitt Zool Stat Neapel 12:303–330, 1896
4. Benhold H: Eine spezifische Amyloidfärbung mit Kongorot, Munchen Med Wchnschr 2:1537–1538, 1922
5. King LS: Atypical amyloid disease with observations on a new silver stain for amyloid, Am J Pathol 24:1095–1116, 1948
6. Vassar PS, Culling CFA: Fluorescent stains, with special reference to amyloid and connective tissues, Arch Pathol 68:487–498, 1959
7. Sweat F, Puchtler H: Demonstration of amyloid with direct cotton dyes, Arch Pathol 80:613–620, 1965
8. Langhans T: Ueber glykogen in pathologischen neubildungen und den menschlichen eihäuten, Virchous Arch [Pathol Anat] 120:28–67, 1890
9. Lieb E: Permanent stain for amyloid, Am J Clin Pathol 17:413–414, 1947
10. Highman B: Improved methods for demonstrating amyloid in paraffin sections, Arch Pathol 41:559–562, 1946
11. Puchtler H, Sweat F, Levine M: On the binding of Congo red by amyloid, J Histochem Cytochem 10:355–363, 1962
12. Eastwood H, Cole KR: Staining of amyloid by buffered Congo red in 50% ethanol, Stain Technol 46:208–209, 1971

BIBLIOGRAPHY

Bancroft JD: Histochemical Techniques, 2nd ed. Butterworths, London, 1975

Culling CFA: Handbook of Histopathological and Histochemical Techniques, 3rd ed. Butterworth, London, 1974

Thompson SW: Selected Histochemical and Histological Methods, Thomas, Springfield, Ill, 1966

NINETEEN

Lipids

The term lipid is difficult to define. A lipid is generally considered to be an organic substance that is insoluble in water, is soluble or partially soluble in acetone, alcohol, chloroform, ether, or other fat solvents, and which has a greasy feel. Because of this solubility in organic solvents most methods for demonstrating lipids are restricted to frozen section techniques.

Lipids occur normally as a component of all tissues and are usually in the form of stored lipids or as lipid structures such as myelin. They may be bound to protein (lipoproteins) or carbohydrates (glycolipids) or exist as droplets in the storage cells and consist solely of lipid. In general, lipids are defined as being compounds of long-chain fatty acids with an alcohol, and although any classification is hypothetical, it is generally accepted that they may be classified as (1) simple lipids, (2) compound lipids, and (3) derived lipids.

Simple lipids are saturated and unsaturated long-chain fatty acids with alcohols. A fatty acid with one or more double bonds is unsaturated and a fatty acid with no double bonds is saturated. Saturated fats are solid at ordinary temperatures, while unsaturated fats are liquid and therefore oils. They are divided into two groups: *neutral lipids*, comprising fats and oils in which the alcohol is glycerol (triglycerides), and *waxes*, which are esters of fatty acids and higher alcohols. Simple lipids may be demonstrated by the Sudan dyes or the Oil Red O method.

Compound lipids are lipids that contain a nonlipid substance in addition to the long-chain fatty acids and alcohol. They may be divided into two groups, *phospholipids* and *glycolipids*.

Phospholipids (*phosphatides*) are lipids containing a phosphoric acid-nitrogenous base with a fatty acid and alcohol. They can be divided into:

Lecithins
Kephalins
Plasmals
Sphingomyelin

Glycolipids are lipids containing sphingosin (a complex alcohol), a molecule of sugar (usually galactose but sometimes glucose), and a single fatty acid chain. These can be differentiated from phospholipids by the P.A.S. reaction following acetylation to block the aldehydes. Phospholipids are P.A.S. negative.

Glycolipids may be divided into two groups which cannot be differentiated from each other by histochemical methods. They are

Cerebrosides
Gangliosides

As can be seen from their name, these substances are located in the nervous system.

Derived lipids are derivatives of simple lipids and compound lipids. They contain fatty acids that are produced by hydrolysis of these lipids. The fatty acids may be saturated, such as palmitic or stearic acids, or unsaturated, such as oleic acid. Sterols, monohydroxy alcohols of high molecular weight, are usually included in the classification of derived lipids. The most important of these being cholesterol.

The Identification of Lipids

Lipids can be differentiated from other substances using a number of techniques, both physical and histochemical. The histologic identification of lipids utilizes the following methods:

Solubility. Lipids are mostly soluble in organic solvents. Fresh tissue is extracted with a solvent for up to 48 hours, fixed with formalin for 24 hours, washed thoroughly, then frozen sections are cut and stained for comparison with unextracted sections. Some of the extraction methods may be considered specific.

1. Hot chloroform-methanol (2:1) will extract the majority of lipids.
2. Cold acetone will extract triglycerides, cholesterol, and cholesterol esters.

3. Hot acetone will extract cerebrosides.
4. Hot ether will extract the majority of phospholipids.

The temperature of the solvent is usually 60 C, but in some instances may be the boiling point of the solvent.

Examination with Polarized Light. This is not very specific, but cholesterol esters give a characteristic Maltese-cross birefringence.

Reduction of Osmium Tetroxide. The reduction of osmium tetroxide (OsO_4) from a colorless solution to black osmium dioxide (OsO_2) is of limited value except when the structures being studied are known to contain lipid.

Staining with Fat-Soluble Dyes. These are the Sudan dyes and Oil Red O. The methods are based on the fact that the dye is more soluble in the lipid than it is in the solvent employed.

Histochemical and Other Methods. Examples are the P.A.S. method for glycolipids and the chemical demonstration of cholesterol.

SUDAN IV (SCHARLACH R) METHOD FOR NEUTRAL LIPIDS[1]

Fixation

Ten percent neutral formalin. Frozen sections at 10μ.

Solutions Required

A. 70 percent Ethyl Alcohol.
B. Herxheimer's Fat Stain:

Sudan IV (C.I. 26105)	1 g
70 percent ethyl alcohol	50 ml
Acetone	50 ml

Mix and store in a tightly stoppered bottle. Filter before use.

C. Harris' Hematoxylin (page 208).

Method

1. Collect frozen sections into distilled water.
2. Rinse briefly in 70 percent ethyl alcohol.
3. Sudan IV solution for 5 minutes. Keep covered.
4. Rinse in 70 percent ethyl alcohol until no more stain comes away. Up to 1 minute.
5. Wash in distilled water. Hold the section beneath the surface until it sinks.

6. Harris' hematoxylin for 30 seconds.
7. Wash in tap water.
8. Rinse in distilled water.
9. Mount onto a clean slide from distilled water. Drain off the excess water and mount in glycerin jelly.

Results

Nuclei	Blue
Neutral fat	Red

A MODIFIED OIL RED O STAIN FOR NEUTRAL FATS[2]

Fixation

Ten percent neutral formalin. Frozen sections at 10μ.

Solutions Required

A. Oil Red O Solution:

Oil Red O (C.I. 26125)	0.16 g
80 percent acetic acid	100.00 ml

B. 70 percent Acetic Acid.
C. Harris' Hematoxylin (page 208).

Method

1. Collect frozen sections into distilled water.
2. Filtered Oil Red O solution for 5–10 minutes.
3. Rinse in distilled water.
4. Examine under the microscope. If understained return to the Oil red O solution. If overstained rinse in 70 percent acetic acid. Wash in tap water.
5. Harris' hematoxylin for 30 seconds.
6. Wash in tap water.
7. Rinse in distilled water.
8. Mount onto a clean slide from distilled water.
9. Drain off the excess water and mount in glycerin jelly.

Results

Nuclei	Blue
Lipids	Orange/Red

LILLIE AND ASHBURN'S OIL RED O METHOD FOR LIPID MATERIAL[3]

Fixation

Ten percent neutral formalin. Frozen sections at 10μ.

Solutions Required

A. 60 percent Isopropyl Alcohol.
B. Oil Red O Solution:

Stock Solution

Saturated solution of Oil red O (C.I. 26125) in Absolute isopropyl alcohol*

Working Solution

Stock solution	6 ml
Distilled water	4 ml

Allow to stand for 10 minutes. Filter before use.

C. Harris' Hematoxylin (page 208).

Method

1. Collect frozen sections into distilled water.
2. Rinse in 60 percent isopropyl alcohol.
3. Working solution of Oil red O for 10 minutes.
4. Wash in 60 percent isopropyl alcohol.
5. Rinse in distilled water.
6. Harris' hematoxylin for 30 seconds.
7. Wash in tap water.
8. Rinse in distilled water.
9. Mount sections onto clean slides from distilled water.
10. Drain off the excess water and mount in glycerin jelly.

Results

Nuclei	Blue
Lipid material	Orange/Red

Note

Oil red O will often stain fine droplets of lipid material far better than the Sudan methods.

* *Note*. Instead of using isopropyl alcohol as the solvent for this dye, *propylene glycol* may be used as a substitute. The procedure for making up the solution and the method are the same as for the Sudan black method (page 328).

SUDAN BLACK METHOD FOR LIPID MATERIAL[4]

Fixation

Ten percent neutral formalin. Frozen sections at 10μ.

Solutions Required

A. Sudan Black Solution:

Sudan black B (C.I. 26150)	0.5 g
Propylene glycol (U.S.P.)	100.0 ml

Add a small amount of propylene glycol to the dye and mix. Add the remaining propylene glycol slowly and gradually heat to 95 C, stirring constantly. Filter through two thicknesses of Whatman's No. 2 filter paper while still hot and allow to cool. This solution keeps indefinitely. Always filter before use.

B. 100 percent Propylene Glycol.
C. 85 percent Propylene Glycol in Distilled Water.
D. 1 percent Aqueous Neutral Red (C.I. 50040).

Method

1. Collect frozen sections into distilled water. Take paraffin sections to distilled water.
2. 100 percent propylene glycol for 3 minutes.
3. Sudan black solution: frozen sections for 5 minutes; paraffin sections for 8–16 hours.
4. 85 percent propylene glycol for 2 minutes.
5. Wash in distilled water.
6. 1 percent aqueous neutral red for 30–60 seconds.
7. Wash in distilled water.
8. Mount frozen sections onto a clean slide.
9. Drain off excess water and mount in glycerin jelly.

Results

Nuclei	Red
Lipids	Blue/black to black
Myelin	Black

NILE BLUE SULFATE METHOD FOR FATTY ACIDS[5]

Fixation

Fix blocks of tissue in formol-calcium for 48 hours. Transfer to 5 percent potassium dichromate to which has been added 1 percent calcium chloride, leave for 18 hours. Wash in running tap water for 1-2 hours and take frozen sections at 10μ.

Solutions Required

A. 1 percent Aqueous Nile Blue A (C.I. 51180).
B. 0.2 percent Aqueous Nile Blue A (C.I. 51180).
C. 1 percent Acetic Acid.

Method

1. Collect three frozen sections into distilled water.
2. *Section 1*
   Stain with Oil red O (page 327).
   Section 2
   1 percent aqueous Nile blue A for 5 minutes at 60 C.
   Section 3
   0.2 percent aqueous Nile blue A for 5 minutes at 60 C.
3. Rinse sections 2 and 3 in distilled water at 60 C.
4. Rinse sections 2 and 3 in 1 percent acetic acid at 60 C for 30 seconds.
5. Rinse in distilled water at room temperature.
6. Mount sections onto clean slides.
7. Drain off excess water and mount in glycerin jelly.
8. Examine all three sections and compare. If sections 2 and 3 are identical, only section 3 need be examined. Any blue stained areas in sections 2 and 3 that are stained red in section 1 may be assumed to be fatty acids.

Results

Neutral fat	Pink to red
Fatty acids	Blue
Section 1	
All lipids	Red to orange

FISCHLER'S METHOD FOR FATTY ACIDS[6]

Fixation

Ten percent neutral formalin. Frozen sections at 10μ.

Solutions Required

A. Saturated Aqueous Solution of Copper Acetate.
B. Weigert's Lithium Hematoxylin:

Solution A

Hematoxylin (C.I. 75290)	10 g
Absolute ethyl alcohol	100 ml

Solution B

Sat. aq. lithium carbonate	10 ml
Distilled water	90 ml

Working Solution

Solution A	1 part
Solution B	1 part

C. Weigert's Differentiator:

Sodium borate (Borax)	4 g
Potassium ferricyanide	5 g
Distilled water	200 ml

This solution is stable.

Method

1. Collect frozen sections into distilled water.
2. Copper acetate solution for 24 hours at 37 C.
3. Wash thoroughly in distilled water.
4. Weigert's lithium hematoxylin for 20 minutes.
5. Differentiate in Weigert's differentiating solution until the red blood cells just lose their color.
6. Wash thoroughly in distilled water. Mount onto clean slides.
7. Mount in glycerin jelly.

Results

Fatty acids and soaps	Dark blue

Note. Hemosiderin and calcium deposits are also stained blue.

BENDA'S METHOD FOR FAT NECROSIS (MODIFIED)[7]

Fixation

Ten percent neutral formalin. Frozen sections at 10μ.

Solutions Required

A. Weigert's Copper Mordant:

Copper acetate	10 g
Fluorchrome*	5 g

* Chromium fluoride.

Distilled water	200 ml
Glacial acetic acid	10 ml

Dissolve the fluorochrome in boiling water, withdraw the flame, and add the acetic acid. Add the copper acetate and stir until dissolved.

B. Harris' Hematoxylin (page 208).
C. Herxheimer's Fat Stain (page 325).
D. 70 percent Alcohol.

Method

1. Collect frozen sections into distilled water.
2. Weigert's copper mordant for 30 minutes.
3. Wash in several changes of distilled water.
4. Harris' hematoxylin for 1 minute.
5. Wash well in tap water.
6. Rinse in 70 percent alcohol.
7. Fat stain for 5 minutes.
8. Rinse in 70 percent alcohol until no more color comes away.
9. Wash in distilled water. Mount sections onto clean slides.
10. Mount in glycerin jelly.

Results

Nuclei	Blue
Fat necrosis	Green shades
Neutral fat	Orange/Red

ACID HEMATEIN METHOD FOR PHOSPHOLIPIDS[8]

Fixation

Fix blocks of tissue in 10 percent formalin containing 1 percent anhydrous calcium chloride. Transfer to the postchroming solution, 5 percent potassium dichromate containing 1 percent calcium chloride for 18 hours. Transfer to fresh postchroming solution for 24 hours at 60 C. Wash in running tap water for 6 hours and cut frozen sections at 10μ.

Solutions Required

A. Postchroming Solution:

Potassium dichromate	5 g
Calcium chloride, anhyd.	1 g
Distilled water	100 ml

B. Acid Hematein Solution:

Hematein (C.I. 75290)	50 mg
1 percent sodium iodate	1 ml
Distilled water	49 ml

Heat until boiling. Cool and add:

Glacial acetic acid	1 ml

C. Differentiating Solution:

Sodium borate (Borax)	0.25 g
Potassium ferricyanide	0.25 g
Distilled water	100.0 ml

Method

1. Collect frozen sections into distilled water.
2. Postchroming solution for 1 hour at 37 C.
3. Wash well in distilled water, 5 minutes.
4. Acid hematein solution for 5 hours at 60 C.
5. Rinse well in distilled water.
6. Differentiating solution for 18 hours at 37 C.
7. Wash in tap water for 10 minutes.
8. Rinse in distilled water. Drain off the excess water and mount in glycerin jelly.

Results

Phospholipids	Dark blue

Note. Other material may stain blue. This method is only specific when a control is submitted after pyridine extraction.

PYRIDINE EXTRACTION

Fixation

Fix in dilute Bouin's fluid:

Saturated aq. picric acid	50 ml
Formaldehyde	10 ml
Glacial acetic acid	5 ml
Distilled water	35 ml

Method

1. Wash tissue block in 70 percent alcohol for 1 hour.
2. Wash tissue block in 50 percent alcohol for 30 minutes.

3. Wash in running tap water for 30 minutes.
4. Place into Pyridine for 1 hour at room temperature.
5. Transfer to fresh Pyridine for 1 hour at room temperature.
6. Transfer to fresh Pyridine for 24 hours at 60 C.
7. Washing in running tap water for 2 hours.
8. Cut frozen sections and stain by the Acid hematein method.

Note. These sections should be negative after staining. Any blue staining is not due to phospholipids.

PEARSE'S METHOD FOR PHOSPHOLIPIDS[9]

Fixation

Calcium cadmium formol:

Calcium chloride	1 g
Cadmium chloride	1 g
Formaldehyde	10 ml
Distilled water	90 ml

Paraffin sections at 6μ.

Solutions Required

A. Luxol Fast Blue Solution:

Luxol fast blue MBS (No C.I.)	0.1 g
Absolute ethyl alcohol	100.0 ml

B. 0.05 percent Lithium Carbonate.
C. 1 percent Aqueous Neutral Red (C.I. 50040).

Method

1. Sections to absolute ethyl alcohol.
2. Luxol fast blue solution for 16 hours (overnight) at 60 C.
3. Rinse in 70 percent alcohol.
4. Rinse in distilled water.
5. Differentiate in the lithium carbonate solution for 30 minutes to 2 hours.
6. Rinse in distilled water.
7. Counterstain in 1 percent Neutral red for 30 minutes.
8. Rinse in distilled water.
9. Blot dry.
10. Dehydrate rapidly through 95 percent and absolute alcohol, clear, and mount.

Results

Phospholipids	Blue
Nuclei	Red
Early lipofuchsin, elastic tissue, keratin, keratohyaline, and eosinophil granules	Blue to purple

SCHULTZ'S METHOD FOR CHOLESTEROL[10]

Fixation

Ten percent neutral formalin. Frozen sections at 10μ.

Solutions Required

A. 2.5 percent Ferric Ammonium Sulfate.
B. Glacial Acetic-Sulfuric Acid Mixture:

Glacial acetic acid	5 ml
Sulfuric acid, conc.	5 ml

Add the sulfuric acid to the glacal acetic acid very slowly and with constant stirring. Prepare immediately before use.

Method

1. Collect frozen sections into distilled water.
2. Ferric ammonium sulfate solution for 3 days at room temperature or 37 C.
3. Rinse in three changes of distilled water.
4. Float sections onto clean slides.
5. Place a drop of the *freshly* prepared glacial acetic-sulfuric acid mixture onto the section.
6. Cover with a clean coverslip.
7. Examine within a few minutes. The color reaction fades rapidly.

Results

Cholesterol	Blue to blue/green reaction
Background	Colorless

REFERENCES

1. Herxheimer G: Ueber Fettfarbstoffe, Dsch Med Wchnschr 27:607-609, 1901

2. Postgraduate Medical Study: Histochemistry, University of Kansas School of Medicine, 1959
3. Lillie RD, Ashburn LL: Supersaturated solutions of fat stains in dilute isopropanol for demonstration of acute fatty degeneration not shown by Herxheimer technic, Arch Pathol 36:432–435, 1943
4. Chiffelle TL, Putt FA: Propylene and ethylene glycol as solvents for Sudan IV and Sudan black B, Stain Technol 26:51–56, 1951
5. Cain AJ: The use of nile blue in the examination of lipoids, Q J Microsc Sci 88:383, 1947
6. Fischler F: Ueber die Unterscheidung von Neutralfetten, Fettsäuren und Seifen im Gewebe, Zentbl Allg Pathol Pathol Anat 15:913–917, 1904
7. Benda C: Eine makro-und mikrochemische Reaktion der Settgewebs-Nekrose, Arch Path Anat 161:194–198, 1900
8. Baker JR: The histochemical recognition of lipine, J Microsc Sci 87:441–470, 1946
9. Pearse AGE: Copper phthalocyanins as phospholipid stains, J Pathol Bacteriol 70:554–557, 1955
10. Schultz A: Eine Methode des mickrochemischen Cholesterinnachweises am Gewebschmitt, Zbl Allg Pathol 35:314, 1924

BIBLIOGRAPHY

Bancroft JD: Histochemical Techniques, 2nd ed. Butterworths, London, 1975

Barka T, Anderson PJ: Histochemistry: Theory, Practice, and Bibliography, Hoeber Medical Division, Harper & Row, New York, 1963

Lillie RD: Histopathologic Technic and Practical Histochemistry, 3rd ed. Blakiston Division, McGraw-Hill, New York, 1965

Pearse AGE: Histochemistry, Theoretical and Applied, 3rd ed. Little, Brown, Boston, 1968

TWENTY

Enzymes

An enzyme is an organic compound, protein in nature, that acts as a catalyst or accelerator for the chemical reactions occurring in biological systems.

Enzymes cannot be seen, but the site of enzymic activity can be demonstrated by the action of the enzyme on a specific substrate and the formation of an insoluble substance from this reaction. This substance can then be rendered opaque or colored and thus be visible under the microscope.

The initial product of the reaction between the enzyme and the substrate is called the *primary reaction product* (*PRP*). If this PRP is colored or opaque, as happens in the Diazo technique for alkaline phosphatase, it is termed *simultaneous capture*, but when the PRP is colorless and is then coupled with a colored or opaque substance it is termed a *postcoupling reaction*. This colored or opaque product is the *final reaction product* (*FRP*).

A *self-colored substrate* reaction is one employing a water-soluble dye. The dye is made insoluble when the enzyme removes a hydrophilic group leaving a colored precipitate at the site of enzyme activity. *Intramolecular rearrangement* is another type of reaction, based on the rearrangement of the molecular structure of a colorless substrate to give a colored insoluble precipitate at the site of enzyme activity.

A majority of the techniques used in current histochemistry are either of the simultaneous capture or postcoupling type of reaction. The self-colored substrate and intramolecular rearrangement type of reaction are confined to only a few methods.

Because of their labile nature, enzymes are more difficult to preserve than most other tissue constituents. With a very few exceptions, absolutely fresh tissue is essential. Different enzymes react in various ways to outside influences. Some diffuse into the cytoplasm and are damaged by freezing and thawing, while others may be damaged or destroyed during fixation. Alkaline phosphatase is better able to withstand the effects of fixation than acid phosphatase.

A definite loss of enzyme activity occurs in tissue left at room temperature. If the tissue cannot be processed or placed into the appropriate fixative immediately it is received, it must be refrigerated at 4 C. The cryostat negates some of these problems as sections of fresh tissue can be rapidly obtained and then postfixed or refrigerated. However, a supply of acetone, 95 percent alcohol, and buffered formalin or formalin calcium chloride should be kept in the refrigerator ready for use.

Control sections must always be run with the test section. A negative control is readily obtained by placing a parallel test section into boiling distilled water for 15 minutes. One test section and the negative control should be passed through the substrate and a third section should be incubated in distilled water for the same length of time. This section should give a negative result. Any positive reactions in the two sections expected to give negative results must be regarded as false, and the test repeated. Nonspecific background staining is eliminated as a source of error if both negative control sections give the expected negative result. A known positive control should also be run in parallel as a check that the reagents are working.

Many of the substrate solutions required are available commercially.*

There are approximately eighty methods for demonstrating the various enzymes. The methods presented here are restricted to those which might reasonably be requested from a routine histology laboratory.

ACID PHOSPHATASE: THE NAPHTHOL AS-BI PHOSPHATE METHOD[1]

Fixation

Ten percent buffered (pH 7.2) formalin at 4 C for 18–24 hours, or postfix cryostat-cut sections of fresh tissue. Mount frozen sections of

* The reader is referred to the catalogue of the Sigma Chemical Company, St. Louis, Missouri. The same company also produces kits for staining acid and alkaline phosphatase.

fixed tissue onto *clean* slides and allow to air-dry at room temperature for 1–2 hours.

Solutions Required

A. Substrate Solution:

Naphthol AS-BI phosphate	50 mg
N:N-Dimethylformamide	5 ml

B. Veronal Acetate Buffer, Stock Solution:

Sodium acetate ($NaC_2H_3O_2 \cdot 3H_2O$)	9.714 g
Sodium barbiturate	14.714 g
Distilled water	to 500 ml

Store in the refrigerator.

C. Sodium Nitrite, 4 percent:

Sodium nitrite	0.4 g
Distilled water	10.0 ml

Mix immediately before use.

D. Hexazotized Pararosanilin:

Pararosanilin hydrochloride	1 g
Distilled water	20 ml
Hydrochloric acid, conc.	5 ml

Dissolve the pararosanilin in the water and add the hydrochloric acid. Heat gently, cool, and filter. Store in the refrigerator.

E. Incubating Solution:

Solution A	0.5 ml
Solution B	2.5 ml
Solution C 0.4 ml, Solution D 0.4 ml } mix	0.8 ml
Distilled water	6.5 ml

The final pH should be between 4.7 and 5.0. Adjust if necessary with 0.1 N sodium hydroxide.

Method

1. Incubate sections in solution E for 15 to 60 minutes at 37 C.
2. Wash in distilled water.
3. Either
   Mount in glycerin Jelly

   OR

   Dehydrate rapidly, clear, and mount.

Results

Sites of acid phosphatase activity	Red

Note

If desired the nuclei can be stained after step 2 with either 1 percent aqueous methylene blue or 2 percent methyl green.

This is a simultaneous coupling method. The acid phosphatase hydrolyzes the naphthol AS-BI phosphate, and the released naphthol combines with the hexazotized pararosanilin to produce an azo dye.

ACID PHOSPHATASE: GOMORI'S LEAD PRECIPITATION METHOD[2]

Fixation

Precooled 10 percent buffered (pH 7.2) formalin at 4 C for 18–24 hours or postfix cryostat-frozen sections of fresh tissue.

Solutions Required

A. Veronal-Acetate Buffer, pH 5.0:

Solution A

Sodium acetate (trihydrate), $NaC_2H_3O_2 \cdot 3H_2O$ (mol wt 136.08)	1.94 g
Sodium diethyl barbiturate, $C_8H_{11}N_2O_3Na$ (mol wt 206.18)	2.94 g
Distilled water	100.00 ml

Section B

Hydrochloric acid, conc.	0.84 ml
Distilled water	100.00 ml

To obtain pH 5.0, mix:

Solution A	5 ml
Solution B	9 ml
Distilled water	9 ml

This solution may be prepared in larger quantities and stored at 4 C or made fresh for use.

B. Incubating Medium:

Veronal-acetate buffer (pH 5.0)	10 ml
Lead nitrate	20 mg

Dissolve completely and add:

Sodium β-glycerophosphate	32 mg

The pH of this solution should be in the range of 4.8–5.0. Prepare fresh for each use.

C. 1 percent Ammonium Sulfide. Prepare fresh.

Method

1. Rinse sections in distilled water.
2. Incubating solution at 37 C for ½ to 2 hours.
3. Wash in distilled water.
4. 1 percent ammonium sulfide for 2 minutes.
5. Wash well in distilled water.
6. Counterstain nuclei if desired.
7. Wash in tap water.
8. Mount in glycerin jelly

OR

Dehydrate, clear, and mount.

Results

Sites of acid phosphatase activity	Brown to black
Nuclei	As stained

The enzyme acts on a substrate containing organic phosphate in the presence of lead ions to form lead phosphate. Upon treatment with ammonium sulfide, this forms lead sulfide which is brown to black under the microscope.

ALKALINE PHOSPHATASE: THE NAPHTHOL AS-BI PHOSPHATE METHOD[3]

Fixation

Precooled 10 percent buffered formalin at 4 C for 18–24 hours or cold acetone fixed paraffin sections. Postfixed cryostat-frozen sections of fresh tissue.

Solutions Required

A. Sodium Carbonate (molar solution):

Sodium carbonate ($Na_2CO_3 \cdot 10H_2O$)	28.61 g
Distilled water	to 100.00 ml

B. 0.2 M Tris Buffer (pH 8.32):

Solution A

Tris (hydroxymethyl)-aminomethane	2.42 g
Distilled water	to 100.00 ml

Solution B

0.1 N Hydrochloric acid:

Hydrochloric acid, conc.	0.85 ml
Distilled water	to 100.00 ml

Working Solution:

Solution A	25 ml
Solution B	20 ml
Distilled water	55 ml

C. Naphthol AS-BI Stock Solution:

Naphthol AS-BI phosphate	25 mg
N:N-Dimethyl formamide	10 ml
Distilled water	10 ml
Molar sodium carbonate	2–6 drops

Mix in the order given. The sodium carbonate is added very carefully until the pH is 8.0. Then add:

Distilled water	300 ml
Tris buffer, pH 8.32	180 ml

This solution is faintly opalescent, but is stable for several months.

D. Incubating Solution:

Naphthol AS-BI stock solution	10 ml
Fast red TR (C.I. 37085)	10 mg

Shake well, filter, and use immediately.

Method

1. Sections to distilled water.
2. Incubating solution for 5–15 minutes at room temperature.
3. Wash in water.
4. Counterstain nuclei if desired.
5. Wash well in water.
6. Mount in glycerin jelly.

Results

Sites of alkaline phosphatase activity	Red

This is a simultaneous coupling reaction. The alkaline phosphatase splits the substrate releasing the naphthol AS-BI phosphate, which combines with the diazonium salt (Fast red TR) to produce an azo dye.

ALKALINE PHOSPHATASE: GOMORI'S CALCIUM-COBALT METHOD (MODIFIED)[4]

Fixation

Precooled 10 percent buffered formalin at 4 C for 18–24 hours, cold acetone at 4 C for 18–24 hours, or cold 80 percent alcohol for 24 hours.

Paraffin sections may be prepared. Postfix cryostat sections of fresh tissue.

Solutions Required

A. Incubating Medium:

2 percent sodium β-glycerophosphate	2.5 ml
2 percent sodium barbiturate, diethyl	2.5 ml
2 percent calcium nitrate	5.0 ml
1 percent magnesium chloride	0.25 ml
Distilled water	1.25 ml

The final pH of this solution should be in the range 9.0–9.4. Prepare fresh for use. The stock solutions may be kept at 4 C, but the final solution is not stable.

B. 2 percent Cobalt Nitrate.

C. 1 percent Ammonium Sulfide, fresh.

Method

1. Sections to distilled water.
2. Incubating solution at 37 C for 45 minutes to 6 hours.
3. Wash well in two changes of distilled water.
4. 2 percent cobalt nitrate for 3 minutes.
5. Wash well in two changes of distilled water.
6. 1 percent ammonium sulfide for 2 minutes.
7. Wash well in distilled water.
8. Counterstain the nuclei if desired.
9. Wash well in running tap water.
10. Mount in glycerin jelly

    OR

    Dehydrate, clear, and mount.

Results

Sites of alkaline phosphatase activity	Brown to black
Nuclei	As stained

The enzyme releases phosphate ions from the substrate that combine with the calcium to form calcium phosphate. This is in turn converted to cobalt phosphate by the action of cobalt nitrate and then into cobalt sulfide which is brown to black under the microscope. The magnesium salts are added to the substrate as an activator for alkaline phosphatase.

DOPA-OXIDASE (TYROSINASE) REACTION[5]

Fixation

Ten percent neutral formalin. Frozen or paraffin sections at 6μ.

Solutions Required

A. Phosphate Buffer Solution, pH 7.4:

Solution A

Sodium Phosphate, monobasic, $NaH_2PO_4 \cdot H_2O$ (mol wt 137.99)	27.6 g
Distilled water	to 1000.0 ml

Solution B

Sodium phosphate, dibasic, Na_2HPO_4 (mol wt 141.96)	28.4 g
Distilled water	to 1000.0 ml

Working Solution

Solution A	19.0 ml
Solution B	81.0 ml
Distilled water	100.0 ml

B. Incubating Solution:

Phosphate buffer (pH 7.4)	100.0 ml
D.L.3:4-Dihydroxyphenylalanine (DOPA)	0.1 g

C. 1 percent Aqueous Neutral Red (C.I. 50040)

Method

1. Wash sections briefly in distilled water.
2. Place into incubating solution for 45 minutes at 37 C.
3. Place into fresh incubating solution for 2–4 hours at 37 C.
4. Wash in running tap water for 5 minutes.
5. 1 percent aqueous neutral red for 1 minute.
6. Rinse in tap water.
7. Dehydrate rapidly, clear, and mount.

Results

DOPA Oxidase	Brownish black
Nuclei	Red

Dihydroxyphenylalanine is oxidized by DOPA-Oxidase (tyrosinase) to form a brown to black pigment.

ADENOSINE TRIPHOSPHATASE (ATPASE): THE CALCIUM METHOD[6]

Fixation

Fix in formol-calcium chloride for 24 hours at 4 C, or cut cryostat-frozen sections and postfix, or cut fresh frozen sections and air-dry for 30 minutes at room temperature.

Solutions Required

A. Incubating Solution:

Sodium barbiturate, 2.062 percent	20 ml
Calcium chloride, 2 percent	10 ml
Distilled water	30 ml
Adenosine triphosphate disodium salt (ATP sodium salt)	152 mg

Adjust the pH to 9.4 with 0.1 N NaOH and add distilled water to make a total volume of 100 ml. Filter if necessary.

B. 1 percent Calcium Chloride.
C. 2 percent Cobalt Chloride.
D. 1 percent Ammonium Sulfide.
E. 1 percent Aqueous Neutral Red (C.I. 50040).

Method

1. Freshly prepared incubating solution for 15 minutes to 3 hours at 37 C.
2. Wash in three changes of calcium chloride for a total of 10 minutes.
3. 2 percent cobalt chloride for 3–5 minutes.
4. Wash in distilled water, four changes, 30 seconds in each.
5. 1 percent ammonium sulfide for 1–3 minutes.
6. Rinse well in tap water.
7. 1 percent aqueous Neutral red for 1 minute.
8. Rinse in tap water.
9. Dehydrate rapidly, clear, and mount.

Results

Sites of ATPASE activity	Black
Nuclei	Red

Adenosine triphosphate is split by the triphosphatase with the release of phosphate ions which combine with calcium ions in the substrate to form calcium phosphate. This insoluble precipitate is then converted to cobalt phosphate and then to the black cobalt sulfide.

CHLOROACETATE-ESTERASE: THE NAPHTHOL AS-D CHLOROACETATE (NASD) METHOD[7]

Fixation

Smears air-dried and fixed in absolute methyl alcohol or tissue fixed in 10 percent neutral formalin.

Solutions Required

A. Hexazotized Pararosanilin:

Hydrochloric acid, conc.	1.6 ml
Distilled water	8.4 ml
Pararosanilin, acridin free*	0.4 g

B. 4 percent Sodium Nitrite. Prepare freshly for use.

C. 0.1 N Hydrochloric Acid:

Hydrochloric acid, conc.	8.35 ml
Distilled water	to 1000.00 ml

D. 0.1 M Sodium Barbital (sodium diethylbarbiturate):

Sodium barbital	10.3 g
Distilled water	to 500.0 ml

E. 0.1 N Hydrochloric Acid/0.1 M Sodium Barbital:

0.1 N Hydrochloric acid	14.6 ml
0.1 M Sodium barbital	15.4 ml

F. NASD Chloroacetate-Dimethylformamide Mixture:

Naphthol AS-D chloroacetate†	0.01 g
N:N-Dimethyl formamide	1.00 ml

G. Working Esterase Solution:

Solution A	1 drop
Solution B	1 drop

Mix *drop on drop* in a 50-ml beaker and let stand for 1 minute. Add:

Solution E	30 ml

Mix well. This solution should be colorless. Adjust the pH to 6.3 (range of 5.8–6.8 is acceptable). Add:

Solution F	1 ml

Mix well. The solution should be pink and flocculent. Filter before use.

* Available from Roboz Surgical Inst. Co. Washington, D.C. 20006.

† Available from Sigma Chemical Co., St. Louis, Missouri, 63178.

Method

1. Sections to distilled water.
2. Working esterase solution for 30 minutes at room temperature. Check under the microscope. If the reaction is not complete refilter the solution and leave for a further 30 minutes.
3. Wash in running tap water for 5 minutes.
4. Counterstain nuclei with Harris' hematoxylin for 2 minutes.
5. Wash in running tap water for 5 minutes.
6. Rinse in distilled water and blot dry.
7. Clear in xylene and mount.

Results

Nuclei	Blue
Neutrophil myeloid and mast-cell granules	Red

NONSPECIFIC ESTERASE: THE ALPHA-NAPHTHYL ACETATE METHOD[8]

Fixation

Fix smears in absolute methyl alcohol. Ten percent neutral formalin for tissue in paraffin sections.

Solutions Required

A. Phosphate Buffer, pH 7.6:

Solution A

Sodium phosphate, monobasic $NaH_2PO_4 \cdot H_2O$ (mol wt 137.99)	27.6 g
Distilled water	to 1000.0 ml

Solution B

Sodium phosphate, dibasic Na_2HPO_4 (mol wt 141.96)	28.4 g
Distilled water	to 1000.0 ml

Working Solution

Solution A	13.0 ml
Solution B	87.0 ml
Distilled water	100.0 ml

B. Hexazotized Pararosanilin (page 338).

C. Alpha-Naphthyl Acetate Solution:

Alpha-naphthyl acetate*	10 mg
Ethylene glycol monomethyl ether	0.5 ml

* Available from Sigma Chemical Co., St. Louis, Missouri.

D. 4 percent Sodium Nitrite. Prepare freshly for use.
E. Working Substrate Solution:

Solution A			8.9 ml
Solution B	0.3 ml	mix	0.6 ml
Solution D	0.3 ml		
Solution C			0.5 ml

Adjust the pH to 6.1 with 1 N sodium hydroxide (range 5.8–6.5 is acceptable). Filter before use.

Method

1. Sections to distilled water.
2. Working substrate solution for 45 minutes at room temperature.
3. Wash in distilled water.
4. Counterstain the nuclei with Harris' hematoxylin for 2 minutes.
5. Wash in running tap water for 5 minutes.
6. Rinse in distilled water and blot dry.
7. Clear in xylene and mount.

Results

Nuclei	Blue
Nonspecific esterase activity	Dark red granules in the cytoplasm of monocytes, histiocytes, and megakaryocytes.

REFERENCES

1. Barka T: A simple azo-dye method for histochemical demonstration of acid phosphatase, Nature 187:248–249, 1960
2. Gomori G: An improved histochemical technic for acid phosphatase, Stain Technol 25:81–85, 1950
3. Burstone MS: Histochemical comparison of naphthol AS-phosphatases for the demonstration of phosphatases, J Natl Cancer Inst 20:601–613, 1958
4. Gomori G: Alkaline phosphatase of cell nuclei, J Lab Clin Med 37:526–531, 1951
5. Becker SW, Praver LL, Thatcher H: An improved (paraffin section) method for the DOPA reaction, Arch Dermatol Syph 31:190–195, 1935
6. Padykula HA, Herman E: The specificity of the histochemical method for adenosine triphosphatase, J Histochem Cytochem 3:170–195, 1955

7. Leder LD: Über die selektive fermentcytochemische Darstellung von Neutrophilen Myeloishen Zellen und Gewebs mastzellen in Paraffinschnitt, Klin Wochenshr 42:553, 1964
8. Yam LT, Li CY, Crosby WH: Cytochemical identification of monocytes and granulocytes, Am J Clin Pathol 55:283–290, 1971

BIBLIOGRAPHY

Bancroft JD: Histochemical Techniques, 2nd ed. Butterworths, London, 1975

Barka T, Anderson PJ: Histochemistry: Theory, Practice, and Bibliography, Hoeber Medical Division, Harper & Row, New York, 1963

Culling CFA: Handbook of Histopathological and Histochemical Techniques, 3rd ed. Butterworth, London, 1974

Pearse AGE: Histochemistry, Theoretical and Applied, 3rd ed. Little, Brown, Boston, 1968

TWENTY-ONE

Methods for the Identification and Staining of Pigments in Tissue Sections

One of the most frequent requests that histopathology laboratories receive is for special stains to demonstrate and identify the various pigments seen in sections stained with the hematoxylin and eosin method.

Pigments occur frequently in tissues, and may be due to either natural causes or pathologic conditions. Because of the large variety of pigments we will omit those which are artifacts of fixation, a group which is covered in an earlier chapter, and limit this chapter to those pigments most frequently encountered in our day to day work

Pigments are classified into two groups: endogenous pigments and exogenous pigments.

Endogenous Pigments

Endogenous pigments form the larger of the two groups, and consist of those pigments formed within the tissue by natural means. This group can be further divided into two subclassifications: hematogenous pigments and autogenous pigments.

HEMATOGENOUS PIGMENTS

Hematogenous pigments are those that are formed by a breakdown of hemoglobin. There are five pigments in this group that are of concern to the histotechnologist. They are:

1. Hemofuscin.
2. Hemoglobin.
3. Hemosiderin (Free iron).
4. Hematoidin (Bile pigment).
5. Hemazoin (Malarial pigment).

Hemofuscin is an iron-free light brown to yellow pigment that occurs in the liver with hemosiderin in hemachromatosis. It is insoluble in hydrogen peroxide, and being iron-free does not react with ferrocyanide. It stains intensely with basic dyes.

MALLORY'S STAIN FOR HEMOFUSCIN[1]

Fixation

Ten percent neutral formalin.

Solutions Required

A. Harris' Hematoxylin (page 208).

B. Mallory's Fuscin Stain:

Basic fuchsin (C.I. 42510)	1 g
Absolute ethyl alcohol	100 ml
Distilled water	100 ml

Method

1. Sections to water.
2. Harris' hematoxylin for 2 minutes.
3. Blue in running tap water for 5–10 minutes.
4. Mallory's fuscin stain for 10–20 minutes.
5. Wash well in tap water.
6. Differentiate in 95 percent alcohol.
7. Dehydrate in absolute alcohol, clear, and mount.

Results

Nuclei	Blue
Hemofuscin	Red
Ceroid	Red
Hemosiderin	Unstained

Hemoglobin is the only pigment in this group that is normally present in tissue, for example, in the red blood-cell (erythrocyte). This is the oxygen carrying conjugated protein of the erythrocyte and consists of a colorless protein component and a pigmented portion containing iron. In pathologic conditions it is seen as yellow-brown droplets, most frequently in renal casts.

It is soluble in water and dilute alcohol and may be demonstrated by either the Patent blue method of Dunn, or by Dunn and Thompson's method.

DUNN AND THOMPSON'S METHOD FOR HEMOGLOBIN[2]

Fixation

Ten percent neutral formalin.

Solutions Required

A. Harris' Hematoxylin *minus* Acetic Acid (page 208).
B. 4 percent Ferric Ammonium Sulfate (iron alum).
C. Picro-Fuchsin Stain:

1 percent acid fuchsin (C.I. 42685)	13 ml
Picric acid, sat. aq.	87 ml

Method

1. Sections to distilled water.
2. Harris' hematoxylin (minus acetic acid) for 15 minutes.
3. Wash in running tap water for 5 minutes.
4. Mordant in 4 percent ferric ammonium sulfate for 1 minute.
5. Rinse in tap water.
6. Picro-fuchsin stain for 15 minutes.
7. Differentiate in 95 percent ethyl alcohol for 2–3 minutes.
8. Dehydrate in absolute alcohol, clear, and mount.

Results

Nuclei	Brown to purple
Hemoglobin and RBCs	Green
Collagen	Red

DUNN'S MODIFICATION OF LISON'S METHOD FOR HEMOGLOBIN[3]

Fixation

Ten percent neutral formalin.

Solutions Required

A. Leuco-Patent Blue Stock Solution:

1 percent aq. patent blue V (C.I. 42051)	100 ml
Powdered zinc	10 g
Glacial acetic acid	2 ml

Boil this mixture until it is a pale straw color. This takes approximately 10 minutes. Cool, filter, and store in a glass-stoppered bottle. The solution is stable.

B. Leuco-patent Blue Working Solution:

Leuco-patent blue stock solution	10 ml
Glacial acetic acid	2 ml
3 percent (10 vol) hydrogen peroxide	1 ml

C. 1 percent Aqueous Neutral Red (C.I. 50040).

Method

1. Sections to distilled water.
2. Leuco-patent blue working solution for 5 minutes. This must be freshly prepared.
3. Rinse in tap water.
4. 1 percent aqueous Neutral red for 1 minute.
5. Rinse in tap water.
6. Dehydrate, clear, and mount.

Results

Nuclei	Red
Hemoglobin	Blue
Oxidase granules	Blue

Note

Hemoglobin peroxidase is a relatively stable enzyme and is resistant to short fixation in formalin.

Hemosiderin may be present in tissues in certain pathologic conditions, particularly hemachromatosis, and is seen as a yellowish brown pigment in clumps or granules. It is soluble in acids, even after fixation, but is insoluble in alkalis, alcohol, and water. Although masked iron is best demonstrated by microincineration, the Prussian blue reaction is specific for free iron.

The principle of Perls' Prussian blue reaction is that potassium ferrocyanide will form Prussian blue with reactive *ferric* salts in an acid solution. Dilute hydrochloric acid is sufficient to liberate loosely bound ferric iron such as hemosiderin from protein.

The reaction is:

$$4Fe^{+++} + 3K_4Fe(CN)_6 \text{———} HCl \text{———} Fe_4[Fe(CN)_6]_3 + 12K^+$$

Iron + Potassium Ferrocyanide —— Hydrochloric Acid —— Prussian Blue + Potassium

Turnbull's blue reaction will demonstrate *ferrous* salts. The reaction is:

$$3FeCl_2 + 2K_3Fe(CN)_6 \text{——} HCL \text{——} Fe_3[Fe(CN)_6]_2 + 6KCl$$

Potassium Ferricyanide —— Ferrous Ferricyanide

PERLS' METHOD FOR HEMOSIDERIN (FERRIC SALTS)[4]

Fixation

Ten percent neutral formalin.

Solutions Required

A. 2 percent Hydrochloric Acid.
B. 2 percent Potassium Ferrocyanide.
C. Acid Ferrocyanide Mixture. Mix fresh for use:

Solution A	1 part
Solution B	1 part

D. 1 percent Aqueous Neutral Red (C.I. 50040).

Method

1. Sections to distilled water.
2. Solution C for up to 30 minutes.
3. Rinse in distilled water.
4. 1 percent aqueous Neutral red for 1–2 minutes.
5. Rinse in distilled water.
6. Dehydrate, clear, and mount.

Results

Nuclei	Red
Hemosiderin (ferric salts)	Blue

THE TURNBULL BLUE REACTION FOR FERROUS SALTS[5]

Fixation

Ten percent neutral formalin.

Solutions Required

A. Ammonium Sulfide Solution:

Ammonium sulfide, light	10 ml
95 percent ethyl alcohol	30 ml

B. 1 percent Hydrochloric Acid.
C. 20 percent Potassium Ferricyanide.
D. Acid–Ferricyanide Solution:

1 percent hydrochloric acid	1 part
20 percent potassium ferricyanide	1 part

Mix immediately before use.

E. 1 percent Aqueous Neutral Red (C.I. 50040).

Method

1. Sections to distilled water.
2. Ammonium sulfide solution for 1–3 hours.
3. Wash in distilled water.
4. Acid–ferricyanide solution for 15 minutes.
5. Rinse in distilled water.
6. 1 percent aqueous neutral red for 1–2 minutes.
7. Rinse in distilled water.
8. Dehydrate, clear, and mount.

Results

Nuclei	Red
Hemosiderin (ferrous salts)	Blue

Hematoidin occurs in a variety of forms from greenish-brown masses or granules to yellowish-brown or reddish-brown crystals, and is thought to be identical to bilirubin. It is located in the liver and sites of old hemorrhages. Although soluble in chloroform, it is insoluble in water and only slightly soluble in absolute ethyl alcohol. It may be demonstrated by Hall's method for bilirubin.

HALL'S METHOD FOR BILIRUBIN[6]

Fixation

Ten percent neutral formalin.

Solutions Required

A. Fouchet's Reagent:

25 percent trichloracetic acid	100 ml
10 percent ferric chloride	25 ml

B. Van Gieson's Stain (page 218).

Method

1. Sections to distilled water.
2. Fouchet's reagent, freshly prepared, for 5 minutes.
3. Wash in running water for 2 minutes.
4. Rinse in distilled water.
5. Van Gieson's stain for 3 minutes.
6. Rinse in distilled water.
7. Dehydrate rapidly, clear, and mount.

Results

Bilirubin	Green
Collagen	Red
Muscle	Yellow
Erythrocytes	Yellow

Note

Nuclei may be stained with Harris' hematoxylin if desired.

Hemazoin is found in cells occupied by malarial parasites and may be seen in the liver, spleen, bone marrow, and brain capillaries. It occurs as dark brown to black granules that are soluble in saturated alcoholic picric acid. Although this pigment may resemble formalin in appearance, it is easily differentiated from formalin pigment by its location and distribution.

AUTOGENOUS PIGMENTS

Autogenous pigments are nonhematogenous in origin, and a great many of them may be demonstrated in normal tissue. They may also occur in certain pathologic conditions. Perhaps one of the best examples of this is melanin, which is found in normal skin, hair, and in the eyes, but it is also present in melanomas.

The pigments in this group which concern us are:

1. Argentaffin—found in normal and pathologic tissues (page 276).
2. Chromaffin—found in normal and pathologic tissues (page 281).
3. Copper—found in pathologic conditions.
4. Lipofuscin—found in pathologic conditions.
5. Melanin—found in normal and pathologic tissues.

Copper is present in the liver and is increased in cirrhosis. It is especially abundant in cases of Wilson's disease. The rubeanic acid method is used to demonstrate it.

THE RUBEANIC ACID METHOD FOR COPPER[7]

Fixation

Ten percent neutral formalin.

Solutions Required

A. Rubeanic Acid (Dithiooxamide) Stock Solution:

Rubeanic acid	0.1 g
Absolute ethyl alcohol	100.0 ml

B. Sodium Acetate Solution:

Sodium acetate	10.0 g
Distilled water	100.0 ml

C. Staining Solution:

Solution A	2.5 ml
Solution B	50.0 ml

Method

1. Sections to distilled water.
2. Staining solution overnight at 37 C.
3. 70 percent ethyl alcohol for 15 minutes.
4. Absolute ethyl alcohol for 6 hours.
5. Clear in xylene and mount.

Results

Copper	Green to black granules

Lipofuscin is a fine yellow-brown granular pigment occurring in the liver, cardiac muscle, adrenals, and ganglion cells. This pigment is often referred to as "wear and tear pigment" or "brown atrophy." It is insoluble in water and alcohol, and formalin fixation is recommended.

Several methods may be employed for the demonstration of lipofuscin, but the method of choice is Schmorl's method (page 278), the principle of which is that ferric-*ferricyanide* is reduced to ferric-*ferrocyanide* or Prussian blue.

Lipofuscin will stain red after prolonged exposure to carbol fuchsin (Ziehl Neelson method), about one hour being necessary, followed by counterstaining with picric acid. The Sudan black method will also give good results.

Melanin occurs in normal skin, hair, and eyes, and is also found in pathologic conditions such as the melanoma. It is seen as yellow-brown to black granules or masses, depending upon the density of the deposits of melanin pigment.

The pigment is insoluble in organic solvents, weak acids, and weak alkalis. It is soluble in strong alkalis such as alcoholic sodium hydroxide, and may be bleached with either potassium permanganate for 1–12 hours followed by oxalic acid or with 10 percent (30 vol) hydrogen peroxide for 24–48 hours.

Melanin may be demonstrated by several staining methods, but for demonstration to be diagnostic it should be bleached from a parallel section and stained in another.

The recommended staining methods are Schmorl's method (page 278), Fontana's ammoniacal silver nitrate method, and the DOPA reaction (page 343). The initials DOPA stand for dihyroxyphenylalanine, which was originally thought to be the precursor of melanin, and the DOPA oxidase reaction is thought to be responsible for the conversion of tyrosine into melanin.

FONTANA'S METHOD FOR MELANIN[8]

Fixation

Ten percent neutral formalin.

Solutions Required

A. Fontana's Ammoniacal Silver Nitrate Solution:

To 5 percent silver nitrate add concentrated ammonia, drop by drop, until the resultant precipitate is just dissolved. Add a few drops of 5 percent silver nitrate until the solution remains slightly opalescent. Filter before use.

B. 0.2 percent Gold Chloride.

C. 5 percent Sodium Thiosulfate.
D. 1 percent Aqueous Neutral Red (C.I. 50040).

Method

1. Sections to distilled water. Four changes of 30 minutes each.
2. Ammoniacal silver nitrate solution for 12–18 hours in the dark.
3. Wash in several changes of distilled water.
4. 0.2 percent gold chloride for 10 minutes.
5. Wash in distilled water.
6. 5 percent sodium thiosulfate for 5 minutes.
7. Wash in running tap water for 5 minutes.
8. 1 percent aqueous Neutral red for 1–2 minutes.
9. Rinse in water.
10. Dehydrate rapidly, clear, and mount.

Results

Nuclei	Red
Melanin	Black

Exogenous Pigments

Exogenous pigments usually have their origin outside the body and gain admittance to the tissue by either ingestion, injection, or inhalation. These extraneous materials are often colored, opaque, or crystalline, and are completely different in origin and structure to the endogenous pigments.

Those most commonly present in tissue are:

1. Asbestos bodies
2. Carbon
3. Silica
4. Tattoo pigment

Asbestos bodies may be found in the lungs and associated glands of asbestos workers. The body has a characteristic appearance with a shape somewhat resembling a dumb-bell or bar-bell. The characteristic shape and its light golden brown color make it easily identifiable in sections stained with the hematoxylin and eosin method. It may also be demonstrated by Perls' method, because of the iron deposits that become deposited on it, particularly at the ends. Although it is doubly refractile it is not anisotrophic and therefore cannot be demonstrated by polarized light, except in the rare instances when it collects a coating of silica.

Carbon is seen as jet black granules or masses, and is usually located in the lungs and associated lymph nodes. It is so common, and the deposits are frequently so heavy, that it can be seen macroscopically in most lung tissue. The pigmentation is totally insoluble and cannot be bleached.

Silica occurs as grayish crystals and is anisotrophic. Like carbon it is usually seen in the lungs and associated lymph nodes, particularly those of stone masons and miners. It may be demonstrated histologically by microincineration or by polarized light.

Tattoo pigment may be a variety of colored pigments found just under the skin and sometimes in associated glands. One of the common pigments used in tattooing is carbon. It is easily identifiable on gross examination of the specimen.

REFERENCES

1. Mallory FB, Parker F, Nye RN: Experimental pigment cirrhosis due to copper and its relation to hemachromatosis, J Med Res 42:461–490, 1921
2. Dunn RC, Thompson ECA: A new hemoglobin stain for histologic use: A slightly modified Van Gieson stain, Arch Pathol 39:49–50, 1945
3. Dunn RC: A simplified stain for hemoglobin in tissue or smears using Patent blue, Stain Technol 21:65–67, 1946
4. Perls M: Nachweis von Eisenoxyd in gewissen Pigmenten, Virchows Arch 39:42–48, 1867
5. Schmeltzer W: Herstellung von Trockenpräparaten aus Schleimhäuten usw. zur Betrachtung ihrer Oberflächengestaltung im auffallenden Licht mettells Binokularmikrockop, Z Wiss Mikrosc 50:335–339, 1934
6. Hall MJ: A staining reaction for bilirubin in sections of tissue, Am J Clin Pathol 34:313–316, 1960
7. Howell JS: Histochemical demonstration of copper in copper-fed rats and in hepatolenticular degeneration, J Pathol Bacteriol 77:473–484, 1959
8. Fontana A: Über die Silberdarstellung des Treponema pallidum und anderer Mikroorganismen in Ausstrichen, Dermatol Z 46:291–293, 1925

TWENTY-TWO

Methods for the Demonstration of Microorganisms, Fungi, Virus Inclusion Bodies, and Parasites

Microorganisms

Microorganisms are microscopic living organisms. Those of medical interest are the bacteria that cause disease.

In histologic technique we cannot identify specific bacteria, that is the responsibility of the microbiology laboratory, but we can demonstrate their presence in tissue. We can also demonstrate whether the bacteria are cocci (spherical bodies), bacilli (rod shaped bodies), or spirochetes (spiral shaped bodies), and whether, on being stained, the organism is *Gram positive* (blue/black), *Gram negative* (red), or *acid fast* (resistant to decolorization with an acid). Spirochetes are normally demonstrated by silver impregnation methods, but some may be stained by the Giemsa method.

A simple stain to demonstrate the presence of bacteria in tissue is methylene blue. The section is flooded with stain for approximately a minute and then rinsed in 70 percent alcohol, dehydrated, cleared, and mounted. Bacteria stain blue. While this method does not differentiate between the Gram positive and Gram negative organisms it does show if bacteria are present, and is especially useful on rapid frozen sections.

JENSEN'S MODIFICATION OF GRAM'S METHOD[1]

Fixation

Any fixative.

Solutions Required

A. 1 percent Aqueous Methyl Violet (C.I. 42535).

B. Gram's Iodine:

Iodine, resublimed	1 g
Potassium iodide	2 g
Distilled water	100 ml

Dissolve the potassium iodide in a little of the distilled water, add the iodine and dissolve. Add the remainder of the distilled water.

C. Iodine/Alcohol:

Tincture of iodine	1 ml
Absolute ethyl alcohol	99 ml

D. Tincture of Iodine:

Iodine, resublimed	2 g
Potassium iodide	2 g
Distilled water	2 ml
90 percent ethyl alcohol	74 ml

Dissolve the potassium iodide in the alcohol with gentle heat on an electric hotplate. Add the iodine and dissolve.

E. 1 percent Aqueous Neutral Red (C.I. 50040).

Method

1. Sections to water.
2. 1 percent aqueous methyl violet for 3 minutes.
3. Gram's iodine for 3 minutes.
4. Rinse well in tap water.
5. Differentiate in iodine/alcohol until no more color comes away freely.
6. Wash in running tap water for 5 minutes.
7. 1 percent aqueous Neutral red for 2 minutes.
8. Rinse in tap water.
9. Rinse rapidly in absolute ethyl alcohol to remove the excess Neutral red. Blot dry.
10. Rinse in xylene, blot dry. Repeat until the section is cleared.
11. Mount.

Results

Gram-positive organisms	Blue/black
Gram-negative organisms	Red
Nuclei	Red

Note

Acetone may be used to differentiate the Gram-positive organisms instead of iodine/alcohol, but the stain bleeds out so rapidly that often complete decolorization occurs. Iodine/alcohol is slower but much safer.

BROWN AND BRENN'S METHOD FOR BACTERIA[2]

Fixation

Ten percent neutral formalin is best.

Solutions Required

A. Crystal Violet/Sodium Bicarbonate Mixture:

1 percent aq. Crystal violet (C.I. 42555)	10.0 ml
5 percent sodium bicarbonate	2.5 ml

B. Gram's Iodine (page 361).
C. Ether–Acetone: equal parts.
D. 0.025 percent Aqueous Basic Fuchsin (C.I. 42510).
E. 0.1 percent Picric Acid in Acetone.

Method

1. Sections to water.
2. Crystal violet/sodium bicarbonate mixture for 1 minute. Mix and filter immediately before use.
3. Wash in tap water.
4. Gram's iodine for 1 minute.
5. Rinse in tap water.
6. Blot dry.
7. Differentiate in equal parts of ether and acetone until no more color comes away freely. This must be watched closely.
8. Rinse in tap water.
9. 0.025 percent basic fuchsin for 1 minute.
10. Rinse in tap water. Blot nearly dry.
11. Dip once into acetone.
12. Differentiate in 0.1 percent picric acid in acetone until sections are yellowish pink. Dip into fresh acetone.

13. Dip into a mixture of acetone and xylene in equal parts.
14. Clear in three changes of xylene and mount.

Results

Gram-positive organisms	Blue/black
Gram-negative organisms	Red
Nuclei	Red
Background	Yellow

BROWN-HOPPS MODIFICATION OF THE HUMBERSTONE GRAM METHOD[3]

Fixation

Ten percent neutral formalin.

Solutions Required

A. 1 percent Crystal Violet (C.I. 42555).
B. Gram's Iodine (page 361).
C. Methyl Cellosolve (ethylene glycol monomethyl ether).
D. 0.5 percent Basic Fuchsin (C.I. 42510).
E. Gallego's Differentiating Solution:

Distilled water	50 ml
Formaldehyde (37–40%)	1 ml
Glacial acetic acid	0.5 ml

F. 1.5 percent Tartrazine (C.I. 19140).

Method

1. Sections to distilled water.
2. Place the sections on a staining rack. Flood the slides with 1 percent Crystal violet for 2 minutes.
3. Rinse in distilled water.
4. Gram's iodine for 5 minutes.
5. Rinse in distilled water.
6. Differentiate in methyl cellosolve until no more color streams away freely, approximately 5–10 seconds.
7. Quickly rinse in distilled water.
8. 0.5 percent basic fuchsin for $2\frac{1}{2}$ minutes.
9. Rinse in distilled water.
10. Gallego's differentiating solution for 5 minutes. This differentiates and "fixes" the basic fuchsin.

11. Rinse thoroughly in distilled water.
12. Blot gently to remove the excess water. Do *not* dry.
13. 1.5 percent tartrazine for 3–5 seconds. *Immediately* blot away excess stain, but do *not* dry.
14. Three changes of methyl cellosolve, 6 dips in each.
15. Clear in three changes of xylene and mount.

Results

Gram-positive organisms	Blue/black
Gram-negative organisms	Red
Background	Yellow

Note

Steps 6, 7, 13, and 14 are critical.

BROWN AND HOPPS NEW GRAM STAIN[4]

Fixation

Ten percent neutral formalin, Bouin's fluid, glutaraldehyde, and Helly's fluid.

Solutions Required

A. 1 percent Crystal Violet (C.I. 42555).
B. Gram's Iodine (page 361).
C. Basic Fuchsin, Stock Solution:

Basic fuchsin (C.I. 42510)	0.25 gm
Distilled water	100.0 ml

Filter through Whatman No. 40 filter paper.

Solution A (For use with formalin, glutaraldehyde, and Bouin's fluid fixed tissues):

Basic fuchsin stock solution	1.0 ml
Distilled water	25.0 ml

Solution B (For use with Helly's fluid fixed tissues):

Basic fuchsin stock solution	5.0 ml
Distilled water	25.0 ml

D. Gallego's Differentiating Solution (page 363).
E. 0.05 percent Picric Acid in Acetone.
F. Acetone–Xylene: equal parts.

Method

1. Sections to distilled water.
2. 1 percent Crystal violet for 2 minutes.
3. Rinse thoroughly in tap water.
4. Gram's iodine for 5 minutes.
5. Wash in tap water for 2 minutes.
6. Blot lightly to remove excess water. Do *not* dry.
7. Differentiate in acetone until color stops streaming from the section. This is very rapid and only requires a few seconds. Dip into a coplin jar.
8. Quickly rinse in distilled water to stop the differentiation.
9. Basic fuchsin solution for 5 minutes.
10. Rinse in tap water.
11. Gallego's differentiating solution for 5 minutes.
12. Wash thoroughly in tap water.
13. Blot lightly to remove excess water. Do *not* dry.
14. Acetone, three quick dips.
15. 0.05 percent picric acid in acetone, three quick dips.
16. Acetone, three quick dips.
17. Acetone–xylene, five quick dips.
18. Agitate in xylene for 10 seconds.
19. Clear in fresh xylene and mount.

Results

Gram-positive organisms	Blue/black
Gram-negative organisms	Red
Nuclei	Light red
Background	Usually yellow

Note

The stains and Gram's iodine should be applied to sections on a staining rack and not in coplin jars. The acetone, picric–acetone, and acetone–xylene should be in coplin jars for quick dipping.

MACCALLUM-GOODPASTURE METHOD FOR GRAM POSITIVE AND NEGATIVE ORGANISMS[5]

Fixation

Any well-fixed tissue.

Solutions Required

A. Goodpasture's Solution:

Basic fuchsin (C.I. 42510)	0.6 g
Aniline	1.0 ml
Phenol crystals, melted	1.0 ml
30 percent ethyl alcohol	100.0 ml

B. Formaldehyde (37–40%).

C. Saturated Aqueous Picric Acid.

D. Stirling's Crystal Violet Solution:

Crystal violet (C.I. 42555)	5.0 g
Absolute ethyl alcohol	10.0 ml
Aniline	2.0 ml
Distilled water	88.0 ml

E. Gram's Iodine (page 361).

F. Aniline–Xylene: equal parts.

Method

1. Sections to distilled water.
2. Goodpasture's solution for 10 minutes.
3. Rinse in distilled water.
4. Formaldehyde for a few minutes, until the bright red color turns pink. This differentiates and fixes the Goodpasture solution.
5. Wash in running tap water for 3 minutes.
6. Saturated aqueous picric acid for 3–5 minutes.
7. Rinse in distilled water.
8. 95 percent ethyl alcohol for 30 seconds (differentiation).
9. Rinse in distilled water.
10. Stirling's Crystal violet solution for 3 minutes.
11. Rinse in distilled water.
12. Gram's iodine for 1 minute.
13. Rinse in distilled water.
14. Blot lightly to remove the excess water. Do *not* dry.
15. Differentiate in aniline–xylene with constant agitation until the section appears a light purplish-red.
16. Clear in two changes of fresh xylene.
17. Mount.

Results

Gram-positive organisms	Blue/black
Gram-negative organisms	Red
Other elements	Shades of red to purple

Methods for Acid-Fast Bacteria

ZIEHL-NEELSEN METHOD FOR ACID-FAST BACTERIA (MODIFIED)[6]

Fixation

Any well-fixed tissue.

Solutions Required

A. Carbol Fuchsin Solution:

3 percent alcoholic basic fuchsin	10 ml
5 percent aqueous phenol	90 ml

Filter before use.

B. 1 percent Hydrochloric Acid in 70 percent Ethyl Alcohol

OR

1 percent Sulfuric Acid.

C. 1 percent Aqueous Methylene Blue (C.I. 52015).

Method

1. Sections to water.
2. Carbol fuchsin solution for 1 hour at room temperature or for 5 minutes at 60 C (preheated).
3. Wash in tap water.
4. Differentiate in 1 percent acid-alcohol or 1 percent sulfuric acid until the sections are pale pink, approximately 5 minutes.
5. Wash in running tap water for 5 minutes.
6. 1 percent aqueous methylene blue for 30 seconds.
7. Rinse in distilled water.
8. Dehydrate rapidly, clear, and mount.

Results

Acid-fast bacilli	Bright red
Nuclei	Blue
Background	Pale blue
RBCs	Pink to red

Note

For lepra bacilli proceed as follows:

1. Steps 1–3 as above.
2. Differentiate slides one at a time in 1 percent sulfuric acid until sections are a faint pink. This will take about 1–2 minutes.
3. Wash in running tap water for 5 minutes.

4. 1 percent aqueous methylene blue for 15–30 seconds.
5. Rinse well in tap water to remove excess methylene blue.
6. Either drain and air dry, or blot dry with filter paper.
7. Dip into xylene until cleared. Steps 6 and 7 may need repeating several times until the section is fully cleared.
8. Mount.

Results

Lepra bacilli	Red
Acid-fast bacilli	Red
RBCs	Pink to red
Nuclei	Blue
Background	Pale blue

FITE'S METHOD FOR ACID-FAST ORGANISMS[7]

Fixation

Ten percent neutral formalin or Zenker's fluid.

Solutions Required

A. Fite's New Fuchsin Stain:

New fuchsin (C.I. 42520)	0.5 g
Phenol crystals, melted	5.0 ml
Absolute alcohol, ethyl or methyl	10.0 ml
Distilled water	85.0 ml

Filter before use.

B. 2 percent Hydrochloric Acid in 95 percent Ethyl Alcohol.
C. Formaldehyde (37–40%, reagent grade). *Neutralized*.
D. 1 percent Potassium Permanganate.
E. 2 percent Oxalic Acid.
F. Harris' Hematoxylin (page 208).
G. Modified Van Gieson's Stain:

Acid fuchsin (C.I. 42685)	0.01 g
Picric acid	0.1 g
Distilled water	100.0 ml

Method

1. Sections to water.
2. Fite's New fuchsin stain for 24–48 hours at room temperature (overnight will usually suffice).

OR

12–24 hours at 60 C (overnight will suffice).

3. Wash in tap water for 5 minutes.
4. Neutral formaldehyde for 5 minutes. Sections will turn blue.
5. Wash in tap water for 5 minutes.
6. 1 percent potassium permanganate for 2–5 minutes.
7. Rinse thoroughly in tap water.
8. 2 percent oxalic acid for 1 minute.
9. Wash in running tap water for 5 minutes.
10. Harris' hematoxylin for 2 minutes.
11. Wash in running tap water for 5 minutes.
12. Modified Van Gieson's stain for 3 minutes.
13. Rinse in 95 percent alcohol.
14. Dehydrate, clear, and mount.

Results

Acid-fast bacilli	Blue to blue/black
Collagen	Red
Smooth muscle	Yellow
Nuclei	Brown

AURAMINE/RHODAMINE FLUORESCENT METHOD FOR ACID-FAST BACTERIA[8]

Fixation

Ten percent neutral formalin.

Solutions Required

A. Auramine–Rhodamine Solution:

Auramine O (C.I. 41000)	15.0 g
Rhodamine B (C.I. 45170)	7.5 g
Glycerol	750.0 ml
Phenol crystals, melted	100.0 ml
Distilled water	500.0 ml

B. 0.5 percent Hydrochloric Acid in 70 percent Ethyl Alcohol.*

C. 0.5 percent Potassium Permanganate.

* For lepra bacilli: 0.5 percent aqueous hydrochloric acid.

Method

1. Sections to distilled water.
2. Filtered Auramine–rhodamine solution for 10 minutes at 60 C.
3. Wash in running tap water for 2 minutes.
4. Differentiate in 0.5 percent acid–alcohol for 2 minutes (0.5 percent aqueous hydrochloric acid for lepra bacilli).
5. Wash in running tap water for 2 minutes.
6. Differentiate in 0.5 percent potassium permanganate for 2 minutes. This step quenches background fluorescence.
7. Wash in running tap water for 2 minutes.
8. Dehydrate in 95 percent ethyl alcohol, followed by two changes of absolute ethyl alcohol.
9. Clear in xylene and mount.
10. Examine under the fluorescence microscope using the 40× objective with a UG1 or UG2 exciter filter, and a colorless uv barrier filter.

Results

Acid-fast bacilli	Orange/yellow fluorescence

Methods for Spirochetes

LEVADITI'S METHOD FOR SPIROCHETES[9]

Fixation

Ten percent neutral formalin for 24 hours. Tissue should be as fresh as possible and must *not* exceed 1 mm in thickness.

Solutions Required

A. 1.5 (or 3) percent Silver Nitrate.*
B. Reducing Solution:

Pyrogallic acid	4 g
Formaldehyde (37–40%)	5 ml
Distilled water	95 ml

Method

1. Wash block of fixed tissue in running tap water for 6 hours.
2. Place into 95 percent ethyl alcohol for 24 hours.

* *Note*. 1.5 percent silver nitrate is recommended for autopsy tissue and 3 percent silver nitrate is recommended for surgical tissue.

3. Wash in many changes of distilled water over 24 hours.
4. Place into the appropriate silver nitrate solution for 3 days at 37 C in the dark. Change the silver solution daily.
5. Wash in distilled water for 30 minutes.
6. Place into the reducing solution for 48 hours.
7. Wash in distilled water for 30 minutes.
8. Process the tissue block and embed in paraffin wax.
9. Cut sections at 4μ.
10. Mount and dry.
11. Decerate, rinse in clean xylene, and mount.

Results

Spirochetes	Black
Background	Golden brown

WARTHIN-STARRY METHOD FOR SPIROCHETES (MODIFIED)[10,11]

Fixation

Ten percent neutral formalin. Fixatives containing chromates *must* be avoided.

Solutions Required

A. Distilled Water (triple distilled, or water for injection):
   Acidify 1000 ml with 1 percent citric acid to a pH of 4.0.

B. 1 percent Silver Nitrate in acidulated water.

C. 2 percent Silver Nitrate in acidulated water.

D. 5 percent Gelatin Solution:

Gelatin, high-grade Difco granular or sheet	10.0 g
Acidulated water	200.0 ml

E. Hydroquinone Solution:

Hydroquinone (photographic grade)	0.3 g
Acidulated water	200.0 ml

F. Developer Solution:
   Prewarm solutions C, D, and E to 54 C and combine in the order given:

Solution C	1.50 ml
Solution D	3.75 ml
Solution E	2.00 ml

   Prepare immediately before use.

Method

1. Sections to triple-distilled water.
2. 1 percent acidulated silver nitrate for 30 minutes at 43 C. Prepare the developing solution during this step.
3. Place the sections on a staining rack that has been laid over a 60 C water bath. Flood the sections with developing solution and allow to develop until the sections appear yellow to light brown, 6–8 minutes. Check a known positive control under the microscope. The developing time may need to be extended for the demonstration of Donovan bodies.
4. Quickly place into hot (56 C) tap water and wash thoroughly.
5. Rinse in distilled water.
6. Dehydrate, clear, and mount.

Results

Spirochetes	Black
Donovan bodies	Black
Background	Golden brown

STEINER AND STEINER METHOD FOR SPIROCHETES[12]

Fixation

Ten percent neutral formalin.

Solutions Required

A. 1 percent Uranyl Nitrate.
B. 1 percent Silver Nitrate.
C. Silver Nitrate–Sodium Potassium Tartrate Solution:

Silver nitrate	2 g
Distilled water, boiling	1000 ml

Dissolve the silver nitrate in the boiling water. To this boiling solution add:

Sodium potassium tartrate powder	1.65 g

Filter into an amber glass bottle. The solution will have a milky appearance.

D. 2.5 percent Gum Mastic in Absolute Ethyl Alcohol:

The gum mastic takes approximately 24 hours to dissolve in the alcohol, and the solution should be aged for a week prior to use. Filter until clear.

E. 1.8 percent Hydroquinone.
F. Reducing Solution:

Solution D	20 ml
Into this solution pour:	
Solution C	20 ml
Do not reverse this order. Immediately prior to use add:	
Solution E	60 ml

Method

1. Sections to distilled water.
2. 1 percent uranyl nitrate for 3 minutes.
3. Wash in two changes of distilled water.
4. 1 percent silver nitrate at 56 C for 2 hours.
5. Wash in distilled water.
6. Rinse in two changes of 95 percent ethyl alcohol.
7. Rinse in two changes of absolute ethyl alcohol.
8. 2.5 percent gum mastic solution for 5 minutes.
9. Reducing solution for 5–15 minutes. Check the slides after 5 minutes and then at short intervals. The sections should turn a light brown.
10. Wash in two changes of distilled water.
11. Dehydrate, clear, and mount.

Results

Spirochetes	Black
Donovan bodies	Black
Bacteria and fungi	Black
Background	Yellow to brown

Fungi

Fungi are a class of vegetable organism of a low order of development. The fungi causing disease may be classified according to their morphology (appearance) in living tissue. They fall into three groups:

1. Those with filaments (hyphae),
2. Those with rounded bodies, and
3. Those with both hyphae and rounded bodies.

Most, but not all, fungi can be cultured, and are identified by their cultural characteristics and morphology. We in the histology laboratory are required to demonstrate the presence or absence of fungi in tissue sections; we are not expected to identify the specific fungus. The majority of fungi are P.A.S. positive and may also be demonstrated by one of the Gram methods: hyphae, staining Gram positive; spores, Gram negative. The standard methods for demonstrating fungi are the Gridley method and the methenamine silver method.

GRIDLEY'S METHOD FOR FUNGI[13]

Fixation

Any well-fixed tissue.

Solutions Required

A. 4 percent Chromic Acid.
B. Coleman's Feulgen Reagent.

Basic fuchsin (C.I. 42510)	1 g
Sodium metabisulfite	2 g
N Hydrochloric acid	10 ml
Distilled water	200 ml

Bring the water to the boil, remove from the heat and add the basic fuchsin. When completely dissolved cool and add the sodium metabisulfite and N hydrochloric acid. Allow to stand for 24 hours. Add:

Activated charcoal	0.5 g

Shake thoroughly and filter through coarse filter paper. The filtrate should be colorless. Store in the refrigerator.

C. Sulfurous Acid Rinse:

N Hydrochloric acid	5 ml
10 percent Sodium metabisulfite	6 ml
Distilled water	100 ml

D. Aldehyde Fuchsin (page 232).
E. Metanil Yellow Solution:

Metanil yellow (C.I. 13065)	0.25 g
Distilled water	100.00 ml
Glacial acetic acid	0.25 ml

Method

1. Sections to distilled water.
2. 4 percent chromic acid for 1 hour.
3. Wash in running tap water for 5 minutes.

4. Rinse in distilled water.
5. Coleman's feulgen solution for 15 minutes.
6. Rinse in three changes of sulfurous acid, 2 minutes in each.
7. Wash in running tap water for 15 minutes.
8. Rinse in 70 percent ethyl alcohol.
9. Gomori's aldehyde fuchsin solution for 30 minutes.
10. Wash in two changes of 95 percent ethyl alcohol.
11. Rinse in distilled water.
12. Metanil yellow solution for 1 minute.
13. Rinse well in distilled water.
14. Dehydrate, clear, and mount.

Results

Hyphae	Deep blue
Condidia (spores)	Rose to purple
Elastic fibers	Deep blue
Mucin	Deep blue
Background	Yellow

GROCOTT'S METHENAMINE-SILVER NITRATE METHOD FOR FUNGI[14]

Fixation

Ten percent neutral formalin.

Solutions Required

A. 5 percent Chromic Acid.
B. 1 percent Sodium Bisulfite.
C. Methenamine-Silver Nitrate Solution:

Stock Solution

5 percent silver nitrate	5 ml
3 percent methenamine	100 ml

On mixing, a white precipitate forms. This dissolves immediately on shaking. Store in the refrigerator.

Working Solution

Stock solution	25 ml
Distilled water	25 ml
5 percent sodium borate (Borax)	2 ml

Make fresh for each use.

D. 0.1 percent Gold Chloride.
E. 2 percent Sodium Thiosulfate.
F. Light Green Solution:

Stock Solution

Light green S.F. yellowish (C.I. 42095)	0.2 g
Distilled water	100.0 ml
Glacial acetic acid	0.2 ml

Working Solution

Stock solution	10 ml
Distilled water	50 ml

Method

1. Sections to distilled water.
2. 5 percent chromic acid for 1 hour.
3. Rinse thoroughly in tap water.
4. 1 percent sodium bisulfite for 1 minute to remove any residual chromic acid.
5. Wash in running tap water for 5 minutes.
6. Wash in four changes of distilled water.
7. Working methenamine solution at 60 C for 1 hour, or until sections turn yellow-brown. If this change does not occur make up fresh chromic acid.
8. Rinse in six changes of distilled water.
9. 0.1 percent gold chloride for 2–5 minutes.
10. Rinse in distilled water.
11. 2 percent sodium thiosulfate (hypo) for 5 minutes. This removes any unreduced silver.
12. Wash in running tap water for 5 minutes.
13. Counterstain in the working solution of Light green for 30 seconds.
14. Rinse in tap water.
15. Dehydrate, clear, and mount.

Results

Fungi	Black
Background	Pale green
Mucin	Gray

Note

When the sections turn brown (step 7), examine the control under the microscope to check the staining.

Inclusion Bodies

Inclusion bodies may be found in the cytoplasm, the nucleus, or occasionally in both simultaneously. Their formation is induced by viruses, and, in some instances, by lead poisoning.

Most inclusion bodies may be stained by Lendrum's method, but this will not demonstrate Negri bodies. These may be demonstrated by the Giemsa or Macchiavello method.

LENDRUM'S PHLOXINE-TARTRAZINE METHOD FOR INCLUSION BODIES[15]

Fixation

Ten percent neutral formalin or Zenker's fluid.

Solutions Required

A. Harris' Hematoxylin (page 208).

B. Phloxine Solution:

Phloxine B (C.I. 45410)	1 g
Calcium chloride	1 g
70 percent ethyl alcohol	200 ml

C. Saturated Solution of Tartrazine (C.I. 19140) in Cellosolve (ethylene glycol monoethyl ether).

Method

1. Sections to water.
2. Harris' hematoxylin for 2 minutes.
3. Wash in running tap water for 5 minutes.
4. Phloxine solution for 30 minutes.
5. Rinse in distilled water.
6. Differentiate in saturated tartrazine in cellosolve until the inclusion bodies are red and the background is yellow. Continue applying tartrazine until the RBCs are colored yellow. Control the staining under the microscope.
7. Dehydrate, clear, and mount.

Results

Nuclei	Blue/black
Inclusion bodies	Red
RBCs	Yellow
Background	Yellow

PHOSPHOTUNGSTIC ACID-EOSIN METHOD FOR NEGRI BODIES[16]

Fixation

Ten percent neutral formalin.

Solutions Required

A. Harris' Hematoxylin (page 208).
B. 0.5 percent Hydrochloric Acid.
C. Dilute Lithium Carbonate:

Saturated aq. lithium carbonate	1 ml
Distilled water	200 ml

D. Phosphotungstic Acid-Eosin:

Eosin Y (C.I. 45380)	1.0 g
Phosphotungstic acid	0.7 g
Distilled water	10.0 ml
Sat. aq. Lithium carbonate	2 drops
Absolute ethyl alcohol	190.0 ml

Method

1. Sections to distilled water.
2. Harris' hematoxylin for 2 minutes.
3. Wash in running tap water for 5 minutes.
4. 0.5 percent hydrochloric acid, 8 quick dips.
5. Wash in running tap water for 5 minutes.
6. Dilute lithium carbonate for 1 minute.
7. Wash in running tap water for 10 minutes.
8. Dehydrate through 50, 70, 80, 90, 95 percent to absolute ethyl alcohol, giving 10 dips in each grade of alcohol.
9. Phosphotungstic acid-eosin for 8 minutes.
10. Wash in running tap water for 5 minutes.
11. Dehydrate as in step 8.
12. Absolute ethyl alcohol, three changes with 4 minutes in each.
13. Blot dry.
14. Clear and mount.

Results

Negri bodies	Red
Nucleoli	Dark blue
RBCs	Rose

MACCHIAVELLO'S METHOD FOR RICKETTSIAE AND INCLUSION BODIES (MODIFIED)[17]

Fixation

Ten percent neutral formalin or Zenker's fluid.

Solutions Required

A. 0.25 percent Basic Fuchsin (C.I. 42510), pH 7.2.
B. 0.5 percent Citric Acid.
C. 1 percent Methylene Blue (C.I. 52015).

Method

1. Sections to distilled water.
2. 0.25 percent basic fuchsin for 30 minutes.
3. Differentiate rapidly in 0.5 percent citric acid for approximately 3 seconds.
4. Wash quickly in tap water.
5. 1 percent methylene blue for 15–30 seconds.
6. Rinse thoroughly in tap water.
7. Dehydrate, clear, and mount.

Results

Rickettsia	Red
Inclusion bodies	Red
Nuclei	Blue
Background	Pale blue

Parasites

The parasites most frequently encountered in tissue sections are malarial parasites, ova of helminths and nematodes, and amoeba. Ova and amoeba may be demonstrated by the P.A.S. method and the Heidenhain iron hematoxylin method. Malarial parasites and other blood parasites may be demonstrated by the Giemsa stain.

REFERENCES

1. Jensen V: Üeber eine Modifikation der Gram färbung, besonders mit Rücksicht auf die Gonokokkendiagnose, Berlin Klin Wschr 49:1663–1665, 1912

2. Brown JH, Brenn LA: A method for the differential staining of gram positive and gram negative bacteria in tissue sections, Bull Johns Hopkins Hosp 48:69–73, 1931
3. Brown RC, Hopps HC: Geographic Pathology Division, Armed Forces Institute of Pathology, Washington, D.C.
4. Brown RC, Hopps HC: Staining of bacteria in tissue sections: a reliable gram stain method, Am J Clin Pathol 60:234–240, 1973
5. MacCallum WG: A stain for influenza bacilli in tissues. A combination of Goodpasture's and Weigert's stains, J Am Med Assoc 72:193, 1919
6. Neelsen F: Ein casuistischer Beitrag zur Lehre von Tuberkulose, Zentralbl Med Wissensch, Ensch 21:497–501, 1883
7. Fite GL: The fuchsin-formaldehyde method of staining acid-fast bacilli in paraffin sections, J Lab Clin Med 25:743–744, 1940
8. Kuper SWA, May JR: Detection of acid-fast organisms in tissue sections by fluorescence microscopy, J Pathol Bacteriol 79:59–68, 1960
9. Levaditi C, Manouellen Y: Nouvelle méthode rapide pour la coloration de spirochetes sur coupes, C R Soc Biol 60:134–136, 1906
10. Warthin AS, Starry AC: A more rapid and improved method of demonstrating spirochetes in tissues, Am J Syph Gon Ven Dis 4:97, 1920
11. Parker AJ: The Warthin-Starry re-examined, AFIP Symosium on Histopathologic Technique, Silver Springs, Md, October, 1970
12. Steiner G, Steiner G: New simple silver stain for demonstration of bacteria, spirochetes, and fungi in sections from paraffin embedded tissue blocks, J Lab Clin Med 29:868–871, 1944
13. Gridley MF: A stain for fungi in tissue sections, Am J Clin Pathol 23:303–307, 1953
14. Grocott RG: A stain for fungi in tissue sections and smears using Gomori's methenamine-silver nitrate technic, Am J Clin Pathol 25:975–979, 1955
15. Lendrum AC: The phloxine-tartrazine method as a general histological stain and for the demonstration of inclusion bodies, J Pathol Bacteriol 59:399–404, 1947
16. Massignani AM, Malferrari R: Phosphotungstic acid-eosin combined with hematoxylin as a stain for Negri bodies in paraffin sections, Stain Technol 36:5–8, 1961
17. Macchiavello A: Estudios sobre tifus exantematico. III. Un nuevo metodo para tenir Rickettsia, Rev Chil Hig Med Prev 1:101–106, 1937

TWENTY-THREE

Methods for the Nervous System

The nervous system is composed of a complicated network of cells and fibers and may be divided into three interconnected systems; the brain and spinal cord forming the *central nervous system* (CNS); the *peripheral nervous system* consisting of 12 pairs of cranial nerves and 31 pairs of spinal nerves connecting the brain and the spinal cord with organs in the periphery; and the *autonomic nervous system*, which supplies the nerves to glands, blood vessels, involuntary muscles (cardiac and smooth muscle), and the viscera. These latter nerves are mainly involved in the unconscious reflex actions in the body, whereas the peripheral nervous system is involved with transmitting and receiving impulses produced by stimulation, either internal or external, carrying them to and from the central nervous system and the organs concerned.

The brain and spinal cord are composed of gray matter and white matter. The gray matter consists of the nerve cells (*neurones*) and neuroglial cells, and the white matter consists of myelinated nerve fibers. The peripheral nerves consist of bundles of nerve fibers (*axons*), most of which are surrounded by a *myelin sheath* (myelinated). Axons may be very long, and end by branching into a series of fine fibers that pass impulses to the next neurone by means of the fine branching fibers (*dendrites*) radiating from the cell body (Figure 1).

Neuroglial cells consist of *astrocytes*, both fibrous and protoplasmic, and *oligodendrocytes*. The function of the astrocytes is probably to supply nutrition to the nerve cells by acting as an intermediary between the blood supply and the cells, and in forming a rigid support network for the brain tissue. They also lay down a dense network of glial fibers when the tissue is diseased or injured. The fibrous astrocytes are found principally in the white matter, while the protoplasmic astrocytes are found principally in the gray matter. Oligodendrocytes (oligodendroglia) are found in both the gray and the white matter, making up almost 75 percent of the glial cells. They are smaller than astrocytes and are located alongside the fiber tracts. Their function is to produce, replace, repair, and supply nutrition to the myelin.

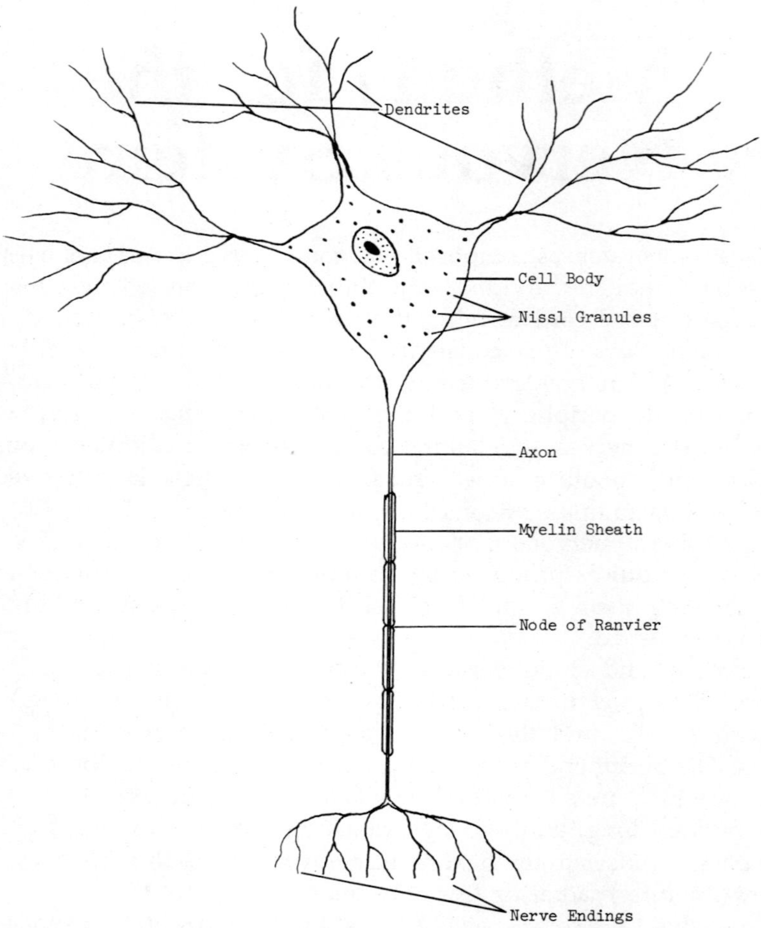

Figure 23-1. Simple diagram of a neurone.

Microglia, which are present in addition to the neuroglial cells, do not affect the normal functioning of the nervous tissue. They are of a different origin than the neuroglial cells and are regarded as part of the reticuloendothelial system.

Methods for Demonstrating Myelin

BUSCH'S METHOD FOR DEGENERATE MYELIN[1]

Fixation

Five percent formalin.

Solution Required

Busch's Fluid:

Solution A

Osmium tetroxide (osmic acid)	1.0 g
Distilled water	100.0 ml

Solution B

Sodium iodate	1.5 g
Distilled water	100.0 ml

For use mix:

Solution A	1 part
Solution B	2 parts

Method

1. Wash thin pieces (3 mm in thickness) of fixed tissue in running tap water for 6 hours.
2. Transfer to Busch's fluid for 5–7 days in the dark.
3. Wash in running tap water for 3–6 hours.
4. Process the tissue through dehydration, clearing, and impregnation. Embed in paraffin wax.
5. Cut sections and mount onto slides.
6. Decerate, rinse in clean xylene, and cover.

Results

Degenerate myelin	Black
Other tissue structures	Unstained

LOYEZ'S HEMATOXYLIN METHOD FOR NORMAL MYELIN[2]

Fixation

Ten percent neutral formalin.

Solutions Required

A. 4 percent Ferric Ammonium Sulfate.
B. Loyez's Hematoxylin:

Hematoxylin (C.I. 75290)	1 g
Absolute ethyl alcohol	10 ml

Dissolve on an electric hotplate.

Lithium carbonate	4 g
Distilled water	90 ml

Dissolve and add to the hematoxylin solution. This solution must be made up fresh for each use.

C. 1 percent Hydrochloric Acid in 70 percent Alcohol.

Method

1. Sections to distilled water.
2. Mordant in 4 percent ferric ammonium sulfate for 24 hours.
3. Wash in several changes of distilled water.
4. Loyez's hematoxylin for 2–4 hours at 60 C.
5. Wash in running tap water.
6. Differentiate in 1 percent acid-alcohol, controlling under the microscope.
7. "Blue" in running tap water for 10 minutes.
8. Dehydrate, clear, and mount.

Results

Normal myelin	Black to blue
RBCs	Black
Nuclear chromatin	Black (does not always stain)
Other structures	Unstained

Note

This method is recommended for celloidin sections.

THE LUXOL FAST BLUE METHOD FOR NORMAL MYELIN[3]

Fixation

Ten percent neutral formalin.

Solutions Required

A. Luxol Fast Blue:

Luxol fast blue MBS (C.I. None)	0.1 g
95 percent ethyl alcohol	100.0 ml
10 percent acetic acid	0.5 ml

This solution is stable for years.
Filter before use.

B. 0.05 percent aqueous Lithium Carbonate.
C. 70 percent Ethyl Alcohol.
D. Counterstain of choice.

Method

1. Sections to 95 percent ethyl alcohol.
2. Luxol fast blue overnight at 60 C.
3. Rinse in 95 percent ethyl alcohol.
4. Rinse thoroughly in distilled water.
5. 0.05 percent lithium carbonate for a few seconds.
6. Differentiate in 70 percent ethyl alcohol until the gray matter appears colorless. Steps 6 and 5 may need repeating several times. Control under the microscope.
7. Wash thoroughly in distilled water.
8. Counterstain as desired.
9. Dehydrate, clear, and mount.

Results

Normal myelin	Blue
Other structures	As stained

Note

This method is particularly suitable for paraffin sections.

Methods for Nerve Cells and Fibers

BODIAN'S METHOD FOR NERVE FIBERS AND NERVE ENDINGS[4]

Fixation

Ten percent neutral formalin.

Solutions Required

A. Protargol Solution:

Protargol	1 g
Glass-distilled water	100 ml

Sprinkle the protargol onto the surface of the water and allow it to dissolve without shaking or mixing.

B. Reducing Solution:

Hydroquinone	1 g
Sodium sulfite	5 g
Glass-distilled water	100 ml

Dissolve the hydroquinone in the water and add the sodium sulfite.

C. 1 percent Gold Chloride. Add 3 drops of glacial acetic acid to each 100 ml.

D. 2 percent Oxalic Acid.

E. 5 percent Sodium Thiosulfate.

Method

1. Paraffin sections to distilled water.
2. Add approximately 2.5 g of *clean* copper shot to 50 ml of 1 percent protargol. Leave the slides in this solution for 48 hours at 37 C.
3. Wash in three changes of distilled water.
4. Place into the reducing solution for 10 minutes.
5. Rinse in three changes of distilled water.
6. Tone in 1 percent gold chloride solution for 10 minutes.
7. Wash in three changes of distilled water.
8. Develop in 2 percent oxalic acid until the background is gray and the nerve fibers stand out black, approximately 3–5 minutes. Control under the microscope.
9. Wash in three changes of distilled water.
10. 5 percent sodium thiosulfate for 5 minutes.
11. Wash in distilled water.
12. Dehydrate, clear, and mount.

Results

Nerve fibers and nerve endings	Black
Nuclei	Black
Other tissue structures	Unstained

BIELSCHOWSKY METHOD FOR NERVE CELLS AND THEIR PROCESSES[5]

Fixation

Ten percent neutral formalin. Cut frozen sections at 10μ–15μ.

Solutions Required

A. 4 percent Silver Nitrate.

B. Bielschowsky's Ammoniacal Silver Nitrate Solution:

To 5 ml of 20 percent silver nitrate add 6 drops of 40 percent sodium hydroxide. Add concentrated ammonia (5 ml usually required), drop by drop, until the precipitate is *just* dissolved. Make up to a final volume of 25 ml with distilled water. Filter before use. This solution must be prepared fresh each time.

C. 4 percent *Neutral* Formalin.

D. 0.2 percent Gold Chloride.

E. 5 percent Sodium Thiosulfate.

Method

1. Frozen sections are collected into distilled water.
2. 4 percent silver nitrate for 24–48 hours in the dark.
3. Rinse in distilled water.
4. Bielschowsky's ammoniacal silver nitrate solution for 3–10 minutes, until the sections turn brown.
5. Wash rapidly in distilled water.
6. 4 percent *neutral* formalin for 10 minutes.
7. Wash in several changes of distilled water for 15–20 minutes.
8. Tone in 0.2 percent gold chloride until the sections appear gray.
9. Rinse in distilled water.
10. 5 percent sodium thiosulfate for 1 minute.
11. Mount sections onto clean slides.
12. Dehydrate, clear, and mount.

Results

Axis cylinders	Black
Neurofibrils	Black
Dendrites	Black
Other structures	Light brown to gray

GLEES AND MARSLAND'S MODIFICATION OF BIELSCHOWSKY'S METHOD: FOR PARAFFIN SECTIONS[6]

Fixation

Ten percent neutral formalin.

Solutions Required

A. 20 percent Silver Nitrate.
B. 10 percent Neutral Formalin.
C. Ammoniacal Silver Nitrate Solution:

20 percent silver nitrate	30 ml
Absolute ethyl alcohol	20 ml

Add concentrated ammonia, drop by drop, until the resultant precipitate is just dissolved. Add 5 more drops of ammonia.

D. 0.2 percent Gold Chloride.
E. 5 percent Sodium Thiosulfate.

Method

1. Sections to distilled water.*
2. 20 percent silver nitrate for 30 minutes at 37 C.
3. Rinse in distilled water.
4. 10 percent neutral formalin for 10 seconds. Two rinses.
5. Rinse off with ammoniacal silver nitrate solution. Flood the slide with ammoniacal silver nitrate solution for 30 seconds.
6. Pour off the ammoniacal silver nitrate solution and flood slide with two changes of 10 percent neutral formalin, 1 minute each.
7. Examine microscopically. If impregnation is insufficient, repeat steps 5 and 6.
8. Rinse in distilled water.
9. Tone in 0.2 percent gold chloride for up to 10 minutes.
10. Rinse in distilled water.
11. 5 percent sodium thiosulfate for 5 minutes.
12. Wash well in tap water.
13. Dehydrate, clear, and mount.

Results

Axons	Black
Dendrites	Black
Other structures	Light gray (*light brown if the section was not toned*)

* If sections tend to float off of slides they may be celloidinized prior to staining.

PHOSPHOTUNGSTIC ACID HEMATOXYLIN METHOD FOR GLIAL FIBERS[7]

Fixation

Ten percent neutral formalin.

Solutions Required

A. Acidified Potassium Permanganate:

0.3 percent potassium permanganate	100.0 ml
Sulfuric acid, conc.	0.1 ml

Prepare fresh for use.

B. 5 percent Oxalic Acid.

C. 4 percent Ferric Ammonium Sulfate.

D. Phosphotungstic Acid Hematoxylin (PTAH) (page 253).

Method

1. Paraffin sections to distilled water.*
2. Oxidize in acidified potassium permanganate for 15 minutes.
3. Wash thoroughly in running tap water for 5 minutes.
4. Bleach until colorless in 5 percent oxalic acid.
5. Rinse in three changes of tap water.
6. Rinse in distilled water.
7. Mordant in 4 percent ferric ammonium sulfate for 2 hours.
8. Wash in three changes of distilled water.
9. PTAH for 2 hours.
10. Rinse in 95 percent ethyl alcohol.
11. Dehydrate in absolute ethyl alcohol, clear, and mount.

Results

Neuroglia	Blue/black
Myofibrils	Blue/black
Axons	Paler blue/black
Collagen	Red
Astrocytes	Paler red
RBCs	Blue/black

* It may be necessary to celloidinize the sections if they tend to lift off of the slide.

NAOUMENKO AND FEIGIN'S METHOD FOR ASTROCYTES IN PARAFFIN SECTIONS[8]

Fixation

Formalin-ammonium-bromide or 10 percent neutral formalin. Paraffin sections at 15μ-20μ.

Solutions Required

A. Formalin-Ammonium-Bromide Solution:

Ammonium bromide	0.6 g
Formaldehyde (37-40%)	14.0 ml
Distilled water	100.0 ml

B. Gold Chloride Solution:

1 percent gold chloride	8.0 ml
Distilled water	40.0 ml
5 percent mercuric chloride	6.4 ml

Mix thoroughly. Prepare immediately before use.

C. 5 percent Sodium Thiosulfate.

Method

1. Sections to distilled water.
2. Formalin-ammonium-bromide solution for 1-3 days.
3. Rinse quickly in distilled water.
4. Gold chloride solution for 6 hours in the dark at room temperature.
5. Wash in distilled water for 2-5 minutes.
6. 5 percent sodium thiosulfate for 5 minutes.
7. Wash in distilled water for 2-5 minutes.
8. Dehydrate, clear, and mount.

Results

Astrocytes	Dark purple
Background	Pink

CAJAL'S GOLD SUBLIMATE METHOD FOR ASTROCYTES[9]

Fixation

Formalin-ammonium-bromide or 10 percent neutral formalin. Cut frozen sections at 15μ-20μ. Formalin-fixed sections should be mordanted in FAB overnight.

Solutions Required

A. Gold Sublimate Solution:

Mercuric chloride	0.4 g
Distilled water	60.0 ml

Dissolve with gentle heat and add:

1 percent gold chloride (brown)	10.0 ml

Mix immediately before use.

B. 5 percent Sodium Thiosulfate.

Method

1. Frozen sections to distilled water. Formalin-fixed sections should be mordanted in F.A.B. overnight.
2. Wash in two changes of distilled water.
3. Gold sublimate solution for 4–10 hours in the dark, or until the sections are a deep purple.
4. Rinse rapidly in distilled water.
5. 5 percent sodium thiosulfate for 5 minutes.
6. Wash in distilled water.
7. Mount onto clean slides.
8. Blot nearly dry with fluffless filter paper.
9. Dehydrate, clear, and mount.

Results

Astrocytes	Deep ruby to purple
Background	Light purple

HOLZER'S METHOD FOR GLIAL FIBERS[10]

Fixation

Ten percent neutral formalin. Paraffin sections at 6μ.

Solutions Required

A. Phosphomolybdic-Alcohol Solution:

0.5 percent phosphomolybdic acid	1 part
95 percent ethyl alcohol	2 parts

B. Alcohol-Chloroform Solution:

Absolute ethyl alcohol	2 parts
Chloroform	8 parts

C. Crystal Violet Solution:

Crystal violet (C.I. 42555)	5 g
Absolute ethyl alcohol	20 ml
Chloroform	80 ml

D. 10 percent Potassium Bromide.

E. Differentiating Solution:

Aniline oil	8 parts
Chloroform	12 parts

Method

1. Sections to distilled water.
2. Blot nearly dry.
3. Mordant for 3 minutes in the phosphomolybdic acid-alcohol solution.
4. Drain off the mordanting solution and rinse with absolute ethyl alcohol.
5. Clear in the alcohol-chloroform solution: 30 seconds.
6. Crystal violet solution for 30 seconds.
7. Flush the slide with 10 percent potassium bromide until no more greenish scum can be seen.
8. Blot with fluffless filter paper.
9. Differentiate in freshly made aniline-chloroform until the section is a lilac color. Control under the microscope.
10. Wash with several changes of xylene and mount.

Results

Glial fibers	Deep violet
Background	Pale violet

Note

If the section is blotted thoroughly in step 8 there should be no crystal violet precipitate. However, if it is present it may be removed by washing the slide in aniline oil.

TOLUIDINE BLUE METHOD FOR NISSL GRANULES[11]

Fixation

Ten percent neutral formalin.

Solution Required

1 percent Aqueous Toluidine Blue (C.I. 52040).

Method

1. Sections to distilled water.
2. 1 percent toluidine blue for $1\frac{1}{2}$ hours.
3. Rinse quickly in tap water.
4. Blot almost dry with fluffless filter paper.
5. Differentiate and dehydrate rapidly in absolute ethyl alcohol.
6. Clear in xylene and mount.

Results

Nissl granules	Blue
Background cytoplasm	Unstained
Nuclei	Blue

EINARSON'S GALLOCYANINE METHOD FOR NISSL GRANULES[12]

Fixation

Ten percent neutral formalin, Carnoy's fluid, or Zenker's fluid.

Solution Required

Gallocyanine Solution:

Gallocyanine (C.I. 51030)	0.3 g
Chromium potassium sulfate (chrome alum)	10.0 g
Distilled water	200.0 ml

Dissolve the alum in the water with gentle heat. Add the dye and bring to the boil and keep boiling for 15 to 20 minutes. Stand for 16–24 hours and filter. The solution will keep for about a month.

Method

1. Sections to distilled water.
2. Gallocyanine solution for 16–48 hours at room temperature or for 2–4 hours at 60 C.
3. Rinse in distilled water.
4. Dehydrate, clear, and mount.

Results

Nissl granules	Deep blue
Nuclei	Deep blue
Background	Unstained

REFERENCES

1. Busch CK: Ueber eine Färbungsmethode secundärer Degenerationen der Nervensystems mit Osmiumsäure, Neurol Zentralbl 17:476, 1898
2. Loyez M: Coloration des fibres nerveuses par la méthode à l'hématoxyline au fer après inclusion à la celloïdine, C R Seanc Soc Biol 69:511, 1910
3. Margolis G, Pickett JP: New applications of the luxol fast blue myelin stain, Lab Invest 5:459–474, 1956
4. Bodian D: The staining of paraffin sections of nervous tissue with activated protargol. The role of fixatives, Anat Rec 69:153–162, 1937
5. Bielschowsky M: Eine Modifikation meines Silberimprägnationsverfahrens zur Darstellung der Neurofibrillen, J Psychol Neurol (Lepizig) 12:135–137, 1909
6. Marsland TA, Glees P, Erikson LB: Modification of the Glees silver impregnation for paraffin sections, J Neuropathol Exp Neurol 13:587, 1954
7. Clark G, Powers JM: A consistent phosphotungstic acid hematoxylin stain for glial fibers, Stain Technol 51:227–229, 1976
8. Naoumenko J, Feigin I: A modification for paraffin sections of the Cajal gold-sublimate stain for astrocytes, J Neuropathol Exp Neurol 20:602–604, 1961
9. Cajal SRy: El proceder del oro-sublimado para la coloración de la Neuroglia, Trab Lab Invest Biol Univ Madrid 14:155, 1916
10. Holzer W: Über eine neve Methode der Gliofaser-Farbung, Z Neurol Psychiatr 69:354, 1921
11. Irugalbandara ZE: Simplified differentiation of Nissl granules stained by toluidine blue in paraffin sections, Stain Technol 35:47–48, 1960
12. Einarson L: A method for progressive selective staining of Nissl and nuclear substance in nerve cells, Am J Pathol 8:295–307, 1932

BIBLIOGRAPHY

Gasser G: Basic Neuropathological Technique, Blackwell, Oxford, 1961

Ráliš HM, Beesley RA, Ráliš ZA: Techniques in Neurohistology, Butterworth, London, 1973

Appendices

APPENDIX 1

Laboratory Glassware

All glassware should be handled with care, and any that is chipped or cracked should be disposed of immediately. A lacerated hand is false economy for salvaging a chipped beaker and pipettes with chipped tips are no longer accurate. Measuring cylinders and coplin jars with broken bases will tip easily, spilling their contents over the bench or technician, as well as being a source of lacerations.

BEAKERS

These are usually manufactured from heat-resistant glass and range in capacity from 5 to 5000 ml. Most have a spout for pouring. Some beakers have graduations up the side, but these are only for guidance and should *never* be used for measuring volumes.

FLASKS

Flasks are also manufactured from heat-resistant glass and range in capacity from 10 to 6000 ml.

Erlenmeyer flasks are conical in shape and are useful for making solutions, especially if evaporation is to be kept at a minimum. Some have an arm protruding from the side. This is for attaching to a vacuum pump to assist in filtration.

Flat-bottomed round flasks are convenient for heating liquids in the preparation of solutions. They should always be stood on an asbestos mat when being heated.

Round-bottomed flasks (boiling flasks) can withstand higher temperatures than flat-bottomed flasks and may be heated with a naked flame. They may also be placed in heating mantles.

Volumetric flasks are dome-shaped, flat-bottomed flasks with a long, narrow neck that will have a graduation ring engraved on it. Also engraved on the flask is its capacity, eg, *TC 100 ml 20 C*. This means that when read at the graduation mark (with the bottom of the meniscus) the flask will *contain* 100 ml of solution at 20 C. Volumetric flasks are frequently fitted with a ground-glass stopper.

MEASURING CYLINDERS

Measuring cylinders are tall, graduated cylinders with a molded base for standing. They range in capacity from 5 to 2000 ml. All readings are taken from the bottom of the meniscus against the graduation. In addition to the graduations they may carry the inscription *TC × ml 20 C*, or *TD × ml 20 C*. This means that they will *contain* or *deliver* × ml at 20 C. The cylinder marked TD must be drained against the side of the receiving container for 15 seconds after its contents have been poured out. All readings of measurement must be made at *eye level*.

Some cylinders may be fitted with a ground-glass stopper.

PIPETTES

There are two types of pipette: the graduated type, which is calibrated up its length, and the bulb type, which has a single calibration mark of capacity. Some graduated pipettes may *not* be calibrated to their tip.

As with the measuring cylinders, pipettes may be marked *TC* or *TD*. The delivery pipette (*TD*) must be drained against the side of the receiving vessel for 15 seconds in order that its contents are delivered accurately. The residual drop in the tip is discarded. The pipette calibrated to contain (*TC*) a given volume of liquid must be washed out in order to deliver its contents accurately. The rinsings are added to the contents of the receiving vessel.

FUNNELS

There are two types of funnel: the filter funnel and the separating funnel.

Filter funnels are used to support filter paper during filtration and for pouring liquids into narrow-necked containers.

Separating funnels, which are pear shaped, are used for separating liquids that are not miscible, ie, ether and water. The flask is half filled with the mixture and allowed to stand so that the two liquids separate. The lower liquid is then drained off by opening the tap at the bottom of the funnel.

CLEANING OF GLASSWARE

The cleaning of glassware is made a lot easier if it is rinsed out immediately after use and placed into a container of soapy water. For general use glassware is washed in hot soapy water or detergent and brushed thoroughly to remove all traces of stain or reagent. It is then thoroughly rinsed in clean tap water and finally rinsed with three changes of distilled or deionized water. After rinsing it is inverted to drain and dry.

Some glassware, such as that used for silver techniques, should be chemically or acid cleaned. After washing and rinsing, the glassware is steeped in either of the following solutions for several hours:

Solution A

Potassium dichromate	10 g
Distilled water	75 ml
Sulfuric acid, conc.	25 ml

Solution B

Distilled water	400 ml
Hydrochloric acid, conc.	1200 ml
Nitric acid, conc.	400 ml

Prepare in a fume cupboard and allow the fumes to abate before closing the bottle.

Caution must be exercised and rubber gloves should be worn when using either of the above solutions.

After steeping in either solution the glassware is rinsed thoroughly with several changes of tap water followed by at least three changes of distilled water. It is then allowed to drain and dry.

APPENDIX 2

Table of Measurements

WEIGHT:

1 mg	=	0.001 g	250 mg	=	0.25 g				
10 mg	=	0.01 g	500 mg	=	0.5 g				
25 mg	=	0.025 g	750 mg	=	0.75 g				
50 mg	=	0.05 g	1000 mg	=	1.0 g				
75 mg	=	0.075 g	1000 g	=	1.0 kg				
100 mg	=	0.1 g							

VOLUME:

1 ml	=	0.001 liter
10 ml	=	0.01 liter
100 ml	=	0.1 liter
500 ml	=	0.5 liter
1000 ml	=	1.0 liter

LINEAR:

1 Å (Angstrom)	=	1/10,000	micron (μ)	=	0.0001μ
10 Å	=	1/1000	micron	=	0.001 μ
100 Å	=	1/100	micron	=	0.01 μ
1000 Å	=	1/10	micron	=	0.1 μ
10,000 Å	=	1	micron	=	1.0 μ
1 μ	=	1/1000	mm	=	0.001 mm
10 μ	=	1/100	mm	=	0.01 mm
100 μ	=	1/10	mm	=	0.1 mm
1000 μ	=	1	mm	=	1.0 mm
1 mm	=	1/10	cm	=	0.1 cm
10 mm	=	1	cm	=	1.0 cm
100 cm	=	1 meter			
1000 meter	=	1 kilometer			

APPENDIX 3

Preparation of Solutions

A percentage solution is parts per 100 ml. For example: a 10 percent solution is 10 parts (g or ml) in a *total* volume of 100 parts (10 parts + 90 parts for liquids, or 10 g + 100 ml for solids).

TO MAKE SOLUTIONS FROM SOLIDS

Example

To make a one percent solution of a solid take:

Solid	1 g
Solvent	100 ml

Note. In chemistry the solvent is added *to a total volume of 100 ml*. For routine purposes, dyes do not require chemical accuracy, and for histologic stains and solutions the full volume of solvent is used.

TO MAKE SOLUTIONS FROM LIQUIDS

Example

To make a one percent solution of a liquid take:

Liquid	1 ml
Solvent	99 ml

DILUTIONS

A dilution may be stated as a percentage solution or, for instance, as 1:10 (1:10 means 1 part in 10 parts or 1 part + 9 parts = 10 parts).

It is often necessary to make a more dilute solution from a more concentrated or stronger solution.

To dilute a solution of a high strength to a lower strength, dilute with the solvent required as follows:

Example

A 35 percent solution is required from an 80 percent solution:

Solution	35 ml
Solvent	*to* 80 ml

Example

A 20 percent solution is required from a 95 percent solution:

Solution	20 ml
Solvent	*to* 95 ml

If one exact amount is required, for example, 200 ml of 20 percent solution from an 80 percent solution, use the following equation: let X = the volume required of the original concentration, V = the final volume required, R = the required concentration, O = the original concentration. Then

$$X = \frac{V \times R}{O}.$$

For our example we have

$$X = \frac{200 \times 20}{80} = \frac{400}{8} = 50.$$

Therefore, 50 ml of 80 percent solution is required to make 200 ml of a 20 percent solution.

MOLAR SOLUTIONS

A molar solution of a chemical is a 1 g molecular weight of that chemical dissolved in a solvent to make a total volume of 1 liter of solution.

Example

To make a molar solution of sodium chloride, find the molecular weight of sodium chloride (formula NaCl):

Na	mol wt: 22.997
Cl	mol wt: 35.457
	58.454

Dissolve 58.454 g of sodium chloride in distilled water to make a final *total* volume of 1 liter (1000 ml).

Example

To make a molar solution of sodium hydroxide, find the molecular weight of sodium hydroxide (formula NaOH):

Na	mol wt: 22.997
O	mol wt: 16.000
H	mol wt: 1.008
	40.005

Dissolve 40.005 g of sodium hydroxide in distilled water to make a final *total* volume of 1 liter (1000 ml).

Note

The molecular weight, or formula weight, of a chemical is normally listed on the bottle or may be found in a chemical catalog.

Normal Solutions

A normal solution (N) of a chemical is a solution containing 1 g molecular weight of the chemical divided by the hydrogen equivalent (valency) of the chemical in a liter of solvent.

This rule applies to solid chemicals only. Liquid chemicals must also be divided by the specific gravity (density) and the concentration of the chemical in solution.

Example

To make a normal solution of a solid chemical, in this case sodium hydroxide, first find the molecular weight of the formula. As stated under molar solutions, this figure is given as the formula weight (FW) on the label of the bottle. Then find the valency. Divide the molecular weight by the valency to arrive at the number of grams required in 1 liter of solvent.

Sodium hydroxide (NaOH) has a molecular weight of 40.005 and a valency of 1:

$$\frac{\text{Mol wt}}{\text{Valency}} = \frac{40.00}{1} = 40.00 \text{ g.}$$

Dissolve 40 g of sodium hydroxide in distilled water to a final *total* volume of 1 liter (1000 ml).

Example

A normal solution of potassium permanganate ($KMnO_4$) has a molecular weight of 158.03 and a valency of 5.

$$\frac{\text{Mol wt}}{\text{Valency}} = \frac{158.03}{5} = 31.6 \text{ g.}$$

Dissolve 31.6 g of potassium permanganate in distilled water to a final *total* volume of 1 liter (1000 ml).

Example

To make a normal solution of a liquid chemical, in this case hydrochloric acid, first find the molecular weight, then the specific gravity (sp gr), the valency, and the concentration.

Hydrochloric acid (HCl) has a molecular weight of 36.4, a valency of 1, a specific gravity of 1.18, and a concentration of 37 percent:

$$\frac{\text{Mol wt}}{\text{Valency} \times (\text{Sp Gr}) \times \text{Concentration}} = \frac{36.4}{1 \times 1.18 \times 0.37}$$

$$= 83.37 \text{ ml.}$$

Add 83.37 ml of hydrochloric acid to distilled water for a final *total* volume of 1 liter (1000 ml).

Example

Sulfuric acid (H_2SO_4) has a molecular weight of 98.08, a valency of 2, a specific gravity of 1.84, and a concentration of 97 percent.

$$\frac{\text{Mol wt}}{\text{Valency} \times (\text{Sp Gr}) \times \text{Concentration}} = \frac{98.08}{2 \times 1.84 \times 0.97}$$

$$= 27.48 \text{ ml.}$$

Add 27.48 ml of sulfuric acid to distilled water for a final *total* volume of 1 liter (1000 ml).

The following list of chemicals gives the information required to make a normal solution, and the amount required per liter.

ACETIC ACID, GLACIAL (CH_3COOH)

Mol Wt, 60.05; Valency, 1; Sp Gr, 1.05; Conc, 99.7%	*57.19 ml*

FORMIC ACID (HCOOH)

Mol Wt, 46.03; Valency, 1; Sp Gr, 1.22; Conc, 97.0%	*38.91 ml*
Mol Wt, 46.03; Valency, 1; Sp Gr, 1.22; Conc, 90.0%	*41.85 ml*
Mol Wt, 46.03; Valency, 1; Sp Gr, 1.22; Conc, 88.0%	*43.02 ml*

HYDROCHLORIC ACID (HCl)	
Mol Wt, 36.46; Valency, 1; Sp Gr, 1.19; Conc, 38.0%	*80.63 ml*
Mol Wt, 36.46; Valency, 1; Sp Gr, 1.18; Conc, 36.5%	*84.65 ml*
NITRIC ACID (HNO_3)	
Mol Wt, 63.01; Valency, 1; Sp Gr, 1.42; Conc, 70%	*63.39 ml*
Mol Wt, 63.01; Valency, 1; Sp Gr, 1.50; Conc, 90%	*46.67 ml*
OXALIC ACID	
$H_2C_2O_4 \cdot 2H_2O$	
Mol Wt, 126.07; Valency, 2	*63.03 g*
$H_2C_2O_4$	
Mol Wt, 90.04; Valency, 2	*45.02 g*
POTASSIUM DICHROMATE ($K_2Cr_2O_7$)	
Mol Wt, 294.21; Valency, 6.	*49.04 g*
POTASSIUM HYDROXIDE (KOH)	
Mol Wt, 56.11; Valency, 1	*56.11 g*
POTASSIUM PERMANGANATE ($KMnO_4$)	
Mol Wt, 158.03; Valency, 5	*31.60 g*
SODIUM ACETATE:	
$NaC_2H_3O_2 \cdot 3H_2O$	
Mol Wt, 136.08; Valency, 1	*136.08 g*
$NaC_2H_3O_2$	
Mol Wt, 82.03; Valency, 1	*82.03 g*
SODIUM CARBONATE:	
$Na_2CO_3 \cdot H_2O$	
Mol Wt, 124.00; Valency, 2	*62.00 g*
Na_2CO_3	
Mol Wt, 105.99; Valency, 2	*52.99 g*
SODIUM HYDROXIDE (NaOH)	
Mol Wt, 40.00; Valency, 1	*40.00 g*
SODIUM THIOSULFATE:	
$Na_2S_2O_3 \cdot 5H_2O$	
Mol Wt, 248.19; Valency, 1	*248.19 g*
$Na_2S_2O_3$	
Mol Wt, 158.11; Valency, 1	*158.11 g*
SULFURIC ACID (H_2SO_4)	
Mol Wt, 98.07; Valency, 2; Sp Gr, 1.55; Conc, 65%	*48.67 ml*
Mol Wt, 98.07; Valency, 2; Sp Gr, 1.84; Conc, 96.5%	*27.62 ml*

Note

Much of the information required for preparing both molar and normal solutions is to be found on the labels of the bottles of chemicals. However, some manufacturers/suppliers do not put the specific gravity or the concentration of liquid chemicals on their labels, and none list the valency. Although the suggestion has been submitted to some of the companies, *none* put the formula for the required amount of reagent necessary to make a liter of a normal solution on their labels. It would be extremely helpful to all laboratory staff if they did.

APPENDIX 4

Acids, Bases, pH, and Buffers

Contributed by

John P. Koski, B.Sc, HT(ASCP)

Product Specialist in Cellular Chemistry

HARLECO, Gibbstown, New Jersey.

The physiologic life functions occurring in the body depend upon water. Even when tissue specimens have been processed in paraffin, most histologic procedures require that we deparaffinize (decerate) the section and hydrate before staining certain elements. The successful reproducibility of staining procedures depends upon many chemical factors, the most critical of which is pH.

The term pH describes a mathematical scale introduced by the Danish analytical chemist Sørenson in the late nineteenth century. This discussion specifically excludes the nature of computations used to derive pH. While the mathematics are important to the pure chemist, they are not of use to the histologist.

Acids, Bases, and Salts

Water is a simple compound with an empirical formula of H_2O. It may also be written as H—OH. Water is a partially ionizable compound able to break up or *dissociate* into ions. This occurs to a minor extent until the ions begin recombining to form water. This condition of simultaneous dissociation and recombination is called equilibrium:

$$H{-}OH \rightleftharpoons H^+ + OH^-$$

The ions formed are charged particles. The hydrogen ion is represented as H^+ and the hydroxide ion as OH^-. At equilibrium, the number of hydrogen and hydroxide ions is equal, and the water is said to be *neutral*. What would happen if we were able to add either hydrogen or hydroxide ions from another source?

Acids are compounds that ionize in water to give hydrogen ions. The other ion that balances it in charge must be something besides hydroxide. Hydrochloric acid is such an example:

$$\underset{\text{(hydrogen chloride)}}{HCl} \xrightarrow{H_2O} \underset{\text{(hydrogen ion)}}{H^+} + \underset{\text{(chloride ion)}}{Cl^-}$$

If hydrochloric acid is mixed in water, we will see an excess of hydrogen ions which have no hydroxide to recombine or neutralize them. Thus when acids are dissolved in water, the water is no longer neutral but acidic.

Bases are compounds that ionize in water to give hydroxide ions. The positive ion that balances the hydroxide must be something other than hydrogen. Sodium hydroxide is such a base:

$$NaOH \xrightarrow{H_2O} Na^+ + OH^-$$

The hydroxide furnished by a base will find no hydrogen ion with

TABLE I
Common Acids and Bases

Compound Name	Formula	Cation	Anion	Class
Hydrochloric acid	HCl	H^+	OH^-	acid
Nitric acid	HNO_3	H^+	NO_3^-	acid
Acetic acid	$HC_2H_3O_2$	H^+	$C_2H_3O_2^-$	acid
		commonly recognized as		
	HAc	H^+	Ac^-	acid
Formic acid	HCOOH	H^+	$HCOO^-$	acid
Monobasic potassium phosphate[a]	KH_2PO_4	K^+	$H_2PO_4^-$	
	$H_2PO_4^-$	H^+	HPO_4^-	acid
Dibasic sodium phosphate[a]	Na_2HPO_4	$2Na^+$	HPO_4^-	base
Sodium hydroxide	NaOH	Na^+	OH^-	base
Ammonium hydroxide	NH_4OH	NH_4^+	OH^-	base

[a] Phosphate salts act as complex acids and bases. See text discussion on buffers.

which to recombine. Solutions that have excess hydroxide ions are said to be basic. Table I gives a listing of the common acids and bases.

When acids and bases are mixed, the hydrogen and hydroxide ions react with each other to form water. This reaction is called neutralization. The ions that remain balance each other in charge and can be isolated from the water as a salt. The following reaction shows the ionization and neutralization between hydrochloric acid and sodium hydroxide.

$$HCl \longrightarrow H^+ + Cl^-$$
$$NaOH \longrightarrow Na^+ + OH^-$$
$$\overline{\qquad\qquad\qquad}$$
$$H_2O + NaCl$$

The sum of all ions is represented by water and the salt. The reaction between an acid and a base, called neutralization, results in the formation of water and a salt.

The pH Scale

Sørenson's range of pH in whole numbers went from 0 to 14. By definition, the midpoint of 7 was neutral. Adding acid to the solution causes the pH to fall; the more acid added, the lower the pH will be. Adding base causes the pH to rise; the more base added, the higher the pH becomes:

MORE ACID (Acid) NEUTRAL (Alkaline) MORE BASIC
1—2—3—4—5—6———7———8—9—10—11—12—13—14

Because of the mathematics involved, it is difficult to explain why concentrated acids and bases will not fit in this range. The pH scale is important because it is the range in which most biologic phenomenon occurs. Common acids include orange juice, soda drinks, coffee, and beer. Basic substances include tap water, soaps, milk, and bicarbonates. The vast majority of bodily functions occurs in the pH range of 6 to 7.

Earlier we said that some substances that dissolve in water were ionized. Most acids and bases completely ionize when dissolved in water. The components of tissue sections do not fully ionize unless the pH is carefully adjusted.

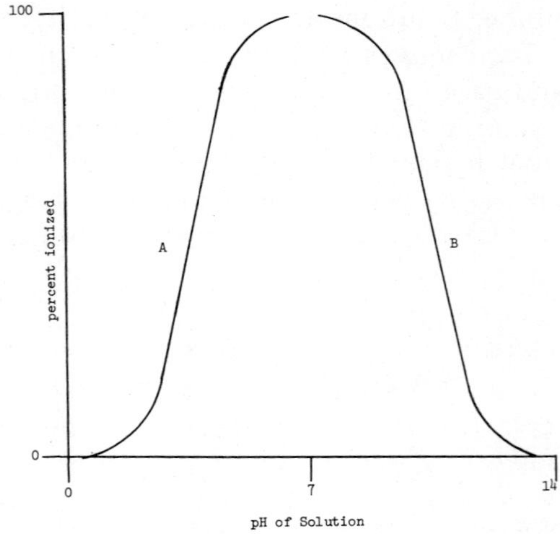

The line drawing above demonstrates curves for two hypothetical substances. For substance A, increasing the pH of the solution increases the amount of substance that is ionized or charged. Substance B acts in the opposite manner and increasing the pH will decrease the amount of substance ionized. The singular point to be made is that the pH of a solution regulates the extent to which substances become ionized or charged.

Staining solutions and rinse solutions often contain acids. The pH or acid level suggested has been selected to ensure that a maximum

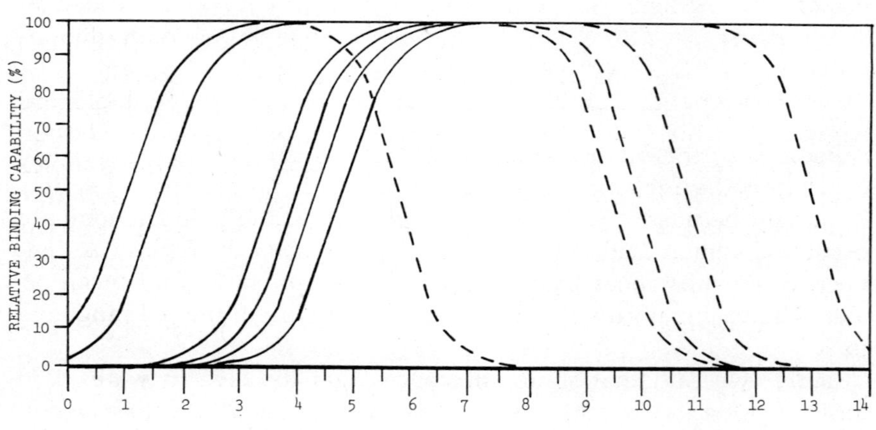

Figure 4-1. Functional group dissociation curves in salt-dye.

amount of dye molecule and a maximum amount of tissue component are ionized. When the dye and tissue element are oppositely charged, successful dye-binding occurs.

Bases are used in stain rinses and in silver solutions. In the first case, basic solutions serve one or both of two functions. In the hematoxylin and eosin stain, nuclei bind hematoxylin best at acidic pH. The dye molecule however is red-violet. An alkaline rinse restores the blue-black color. Bases may thus serve as color developers. Second, by increasing the pH, bases cause electrostatic (charge) binding of the dye with the element to be stained. Figure 1 shows the ionization curve for phosphodiester (nuclear) phosphate. Although ionization occurs at low pH, formal salt linkages occur when the section is rinsed in a medium of high pH.

Continuous use of acid and base solutions consumes these materials. Hydrochloric and acetic acids and ammonium hydroxide are volatile and escape from solution. In both cases, a decrease in the concentration of acid or base changes the pH of the solution. Some reagents are *buffered* to prevent changes in pH.

Buffer Systems

Buffers are aqueous solutions that absorb acids or bases added to them, thus preventing any change in pH. The initial pH is determined by the relative concentrations of buffer salts added.

The salts used to form a buffer are a mixture of a weak acid with the salt of a strong base. The anion, or negative ion, in each salt is common to both. A common buffer system is formed by mixing the weak *acetic acid* with the salt *sodium acetate*. Such a mixture is called an *acetate buffer* because the acetate anion is common to both components.

Buffers are most commonly used for procedures using biological systems. Enzyme and immunofluorescence techniques are based upon interactions of proteins. Silver protargol is a protein-silver complex used in neurologic tissue demonstrations. Protein molecular structure is sensitive to pH changes. The mechanism of protein interactions is highly dependent upon its three dimensional structure and indirectly upon pH.

The consuming of excess acid and base becomes intricate. Weak acids do not fully ionize in solution even though they have dissolved in water. Acetic acid presents such a case:

$$HAc \rightleftharpoons H^+ + Ac^-$$

The reversible arrow indicates that after a certain point ions recombine to form the neutral water-soluble acid molecule. If a base were added, hydrogen ions would be consumed by the neutralization reaction. More acetic acid would ionize to replace the hydrogen.

If acid were added, the hydrogen ion would combine with the acetate and form the neutral molecule. Little acetate is initially present from the acetic acid. In the acetate buffer system, sodium acetate becomes the source of Ac^-.

When acetic acid and sodium acetate are mixed in aqueous solution, all of the sodium acetate ionizes. Only part of the acetic acid ionizes. The solution becomes an intricate and intimate mixture:

$$HAc \rightarrow H^+ + Ac^-$$

$$NaAc \rightarrow Na^+ + Ac^-$$

$$\overline{HAc + H^+ + Na^+ + Ac^- + Ac^-}$$

When base is added, H^+ is consumed and HAc further ionizes to replace it. When acid is added, Ac^- combines with H^+ to form HAc. Of course there is a limit to the amount of acid or base that may be added. Buffers are usually used once and discarded to avoid the possibility of exceeding their capacity.

The phosphate buffer system is somewhat more complex. Rather than define all equilibrium reactions present in that buffer, let us define the terminology used. All components are derivatives of phosphoric acid which ionizes in three stages:

$$(1) \quad H_3PO_4 \rightarrow H^+ + H_2PO_4^-$$

$$(2) \quad H_2PO_4^- \rightarrow H^+ + HPO_4^=$$

$$(3) \quad HPO_4^= \rightarrow H^+ + PO_4^{\equiv}$$

Phosphoric acid is a liquid. Whenever it is dissolved in water all of the above ions exist to some extent. If this acid is neutralized by sodium hydroxide, a mixture of the following salts is recovered:

NaH_2PO_4	monobasic sodium phosphate
Na_2HPO_4	dibasic sodium phosphate
Na_3PO_4	trisodium phosphate

The terms monobasic and dibasic describe whether one or two of the available hydrogens were neutralized by base.

Monobasic sodium phosphate is slightly acid in aqueous solution. Dibasic sodium phosphate is alkaline. The two salts enter into equilibrium and consume excess acid or base with no net change in pH.

Phosphate buffers are used in 10 percent formalin and in diastase enzyme solutions. Citrate buffers can be used for certain endogenous enzymes and protargol solutions. Less commonly used buffers include cacodylate, Tris, Veronal and phthalate.

Measurement of pH

Histologists are not required to calculate pH for the same reasons that graduate chemists do. The molar concentrations of acid or base which comprise the pH scale are so low that they require large decimal numbers.

Notice that large decimal numbers may be expressed as some power of 10. This abbreviation, called *scientific notation*, is more familiar to use with whole numbers. For example, the number 1000 may be expressed as 10^3 (ten to the third power or ten cubed).

The logarithm (log) of any number is the power to which 10 must be raised to obtain that number. Thus the log of 1000 is 3 because $10^3 = 1000$. The familiar system of exponents becomes reversed with decimals:

$$0.0000100 = 1.0 \times 10^{-5}$$

$$0.0000054 = 5.4 \times 10^{-6}$$

$$0.0000010 = 1.0 \times 10^{-6}$$

In the case of the above numbers, shifting the decimal place to the right would convert the decimal to a whole number. The number of places is expressed in the exponent; Sørenson's mathematical expression for pH is given as:

$$\text{pH} = -\log_{10}[\text{H}^+]$$

where *log* stands for logarithm and $[H^+]$ represents the molar concentration of the hydrogen ion. The laws of the mathematics of logarithms are too detailed to be discussed here. Moreover, we would not have any practical use for them. The pH of a solution can be electronically calculated by an instrument called a pH meter.

The pH meter is similar to a battery. In both, an electrical current of known voltage and amperage flows when the circuit is completed. Both have electrodes; both have known chemical mechanisms. The pure chemist uses a standard hydrogen electrode in a pH meter. Hydrogen is explosive and quite unsuitable under routine laboratory conditions. Moreover, the hydrogen electrode must be operated with painstaking detail and precision. For this reason most biomedical laboratories use the glass-electrode system.

We are not certain about the chemistry of glass electrodes, though we know that they are responsive to the hydrogen ion. They are somewhat inaccurate, but the error is overcome by adjusting the readings electrically to match known standard values.

A wide range of reference buffers are available commercially. They are prepared by standardizing against a hydrogen electrode and by standardizing the buffer salts against material from the National Bureau of Standards.

The operation of each instrument varies with the manufacturer. In general, each instrument has a balance point at which the pH on the scale is an accurate reading of the pH in solution. The balance point is adjusted by a balance control knob while the electrodes are immersed in a solution of the established reference buffer.

A *slope* adjustment is also necessary. The slope adjustment is an electronic balance that corrects electrode error in the pH range between the balance point and a higher or lower reference pH. If the solution to be measured has a pH lower than the balance point, a reference buffer of even lower pH should be used. If the solution to be measured has a pH higher than the balance point, an even higher pH reference buffer will be used to adjust the slope.

Most pH meters are accurate to two decimal places. They are exceedingly accurate for histologic work. At the current level of technology there is no further excuse to depend upon indicator solutions, which are inaccurate for a number of reasons.

Indicators are pH sensitive organic dyes that change from one color to another. Being dyes, they are unsuitable for testing the pH of biologic stain solutions. When used on colorless differentiating solutions or buffers they may give false results. The pH must be estimated by judging the color of the indicator. The human eye is not sensitive enough to distinguish color changes occurring over a range of 0.5 pH units where most dyes are in the uncertain species area. In other words, a blue dye that changes to yellow may be green at its inflection point. The end point for color change may therefore be in error by 0.5 pH units. Our demand upon buffers is for much greater accuracy.

Acids, bases, salts, buffers, and pH have been discussed here to give the reader a sense of accuracy demanded in histologic technique. For as much as has been said, more has not. The fundamental ideas are, however, important for further study.

APPENDIX 5

Buffer Tables

WALPOLE'S ACETIC ACID–SODIUM ACETATE BUFFER (pH RANGE 3.6–5.6)

Solutions Required

Solution A

0.2 M Sodium Acetate ($NaC_2H_3O_2$, mol wt 82.03)

Sodium acetate	16.4 g
Distilled water	to 1000.0 ml

OR

0.2 M Sodium Acetate ($NaC_2H_3O_2 \cdot 3H_2O$, mol wt 136.08)

Sodium acetate	27.2 g
Distilled water	to 1000.0 ml

Solution B

0.2 M Acetic Acid (CH_3COOH, mol wt 60.05)

Glacial acetic acid	12.0 ml
Distilled water	to 1000.0 ml

pH	Soln A	Soln B	Dist Water
3.6	3.7 ml	46.3 ml	50.0 ml
3.8	6.0 ml	44.0 ml	50.0 ml
4.0	9.0 ml	41.0 ml	50.0 ml
4.2	13.2 ml	36.8 ml	50.0 ml
4.4	19.5 ml	30.5 ml	50.0 ml
4.6	24.5 ml	25.5 ml	50.0 ml
4.8	30.0 ml	20.0 ml	50.0 ml
5.0	35.2 ml	14.8 ml	50.0 ml
5.2	39.5 ml	10.5 ml	50.0 ml
5.4	41.2 ml	8.8 ml	50.0 ml
5.6	45.2 ml	4.8 ml	50.0 ml

0.1 M PHOSPHATE BUFFER (pH RANGE 5.7–8.0)

Solutions Required

Solution A

0.2 M Monobasic Sodium Phosphate ($NaH_2PO_4 \cdot H_2O$, mol wt 137.99)

Sodium phosphate, monobasic	27.59 g
Distilled water	to 1000.00 ml

Solution B

0.2 M Dibasic Sodium Phosphate (Na_2HPO_4, mol wt 141.96)

Sodium phosphate, dibasic	28.39 g
Distilled water	to 1000.00 ml

OR

0.2 M Dibasic Sodium Phosphate ($Na_2HPO_4 \cdot 7H_2O$, mol wt 268.07)

Sodium phosphate, dibasic	53.6 g
Distilled water	to 1000.0 ml

pH	Soln A	Soln B	Dist Water
5.7	93.5 ml	6.5 ml	100 ml
5.8	92.0 ml	8.0 ml	100 ml
5.9	90.0 ml	10.0 ml	100 ml
6.0	87.7 ml	12.3 ml	100 ml
6.1	85.0 ml	15.0 ml	100 ml
6.2	81.5 ml	18.5 ml	100 ml
6.3	77.5 ml	22.5 ml	100 ml
6.4	73.5 ml	26.5 ml	100 ml
6.5	68.5 ml	31.5 ml	100 ml
6.6	62.5 ml	37.5 ml	100 ml
6.7	56.5 ml	43.5 ml	100 ml
6.8	51.0 ml	49.0 ml	100 ml
6.9	45.0 ml	55.0 ml	100 ml

7.0	39.0 ml	61.0 ml	100 ml
7.1	33.0 ml	67.0 ml	100 ml
7.2	28.0 ml	72.0 ml	100 ml
7.3	23.0 ml	77.0 ml	100 ml
7.4	19.0 ml	81.0 ml	100 ml
7.5	16.0 ml	84.0 ml	100 ml
7.6	13.0 ml	87.0 ml	100 ml
7.7	10.5 ml	89.5 ml	100 ml
7.8	8.5 ml	91.5 ml	100 ml
7.9	7.0 ml	93.0 ml	100 ml
8.0	5.3 ml	94.7 ml	100 ml

0.2 M TRIS–HYDROCHLORIC ACID BUFFER (pH RANGE 7.2–9.1)

Solutions Required

Solution A

0.2 M Tris(hydroxymethane)Aminomethane [$H_2NC(CH_2OH)_3$, mol wt 121.14]:

Tris	24.22 g
Distilled water	to 1000.00 ml

Solution B

0.1 N Hydrochloric Acid (HCl, mol wt 36.46, Sp Gr 1.18)

Hydrochloric acid, conc	8.4 ml
Distilled water	to 1000.0 ml

pH	Soln A	Soln B	Dist Water
7.19	25 ml	45.0 ml	30.0 ml
7.36	25 ml	42.5 ml	32.5 ml
7.54	25 ml	40.0 ml	35.0 ml
7.66	25 ml	37.5 ml	37.5 ml
7.77	25 ml	35.0 ml	40.0 ml
7.87	25 ml	32.5 ml	42.5 ml
7.96	25 ml	30.0 ml	45.0 ml
8.05	25 ml	27.5 ml	47.5 ml
8.14	25 ml	25.0 ml	50.0 ml
8.23	25 ml	22.5 ml	52.5 ml
8.32	25 ml	20.0 ml	55.0 ml
8.41	25 ml	17.5 ml	57.5 ml
8.51	25 ml	15.0 ml	60.0 ml
8.62	25 ml	12.5 ml	62.5 ml
8.74	25 ml	10.0 ml	65.0 ml
8.92	25 ml	7.5 ml	67.5 ml
9.10	25 ml	5.0 ml	70.0 ml

0.05 M TRIS-MALEIC ACID BUFFER (pH RANGE 5.2-8.6)

Solutions Required

Solution A

0.2 M Tris(hydroxymethane)Aminomethane [$H_2NC(CH_2OH)_3$, mol wt 121.14]-Maleic acid ($HO_2CCH:CHCO_2H$, mol wt 116.08):

Tris	24.22 g
Maleic acid	23.22 g
Distilled water	to 1000.00 ml

Solution B

0.2 M Sodium Hydroxide (NaOH, mol wt 40.0):

Sodium hydroxide	8.0 g
Distilled water	to 1000.0 ml

pH	Soln A	Soln B	Dist Water
5.2	50 ml	7.0 ml	143.0 ml
5.4	50 ml	10.8 ml	139.2 ml
5.6	50 ml	15.5 ml	134.5 ml
5.8	50 ml	20.5 ml	129.5 ml
6.0	50 ml	26.0 ml	124.0 ml
6.2	50 ml	31.5 ml	118.5 ml
6.4	50 ml	37.0 ml	113.0 ml
6.6	50 ml	42.5 ml	107.5 ml
6.8	50 ml	45.0 ml	105.0 ml
7.0	50 ml	48.0 ml	102.0 ml
7.2	50 ml	51.0 ml	99.0 ml
7.4	50 ml	54.0 ml	96.0 ml
7.6	50 ml	58.0 ml	92.0 ml
7.8	50 ml	63.5 ml	86.5 ml
8.0	50 ml	69.0 ml	81.0 ml
8.2	50 ml	75.0 ml	75.0 ml
8.4	50 ml	81.0 ml	69.0 ml
8.6	50 ml	86.5 ml	63.5 ml

VERONAL-ACETATE BUFFER (pH RANGE 3.6-9.2)

Solutions Required

Solution A

Veronal (sodium diethylbarbiturate)-Sodium Acetate Solution:

Sodium acetate ($NaC_2H_3O_2 \cdot 3H_2O$)	1.94 g
Veronal	2.94 g
Distilled water	to 100.00 ml

Solution B

0.1 N Hydrochloric Acid:

Hydrochloric acid, conc	8.4 ml
Distilled water	to 1000.0 ml

pH	Soln A	Soln B	Dist Water
3.6	5.0 ml	14.0 ml	4.0 ml
3.8	5.0 ml	13.0 ml	5.0 ml
4.0	5.0 ml	12.5 ml	5.5 ml
4.2	5.0 ml	12.0 ml	6.0 ml
4.4	5.0 ml	11.0 ml	7.0 ml
4.5	5.0 ml	11.0 ml	9.0 ml
4.6	5.0 ml	10.0 ml	8.0 ml
4.8	5.0 ml	9.5 ml	8.5 ml
5.0	5.0 ml	9.0 ml	9.0 ml
5.2	5.0 ml	8.5 ml	9.5 ml
5.4	5.0 ml	8.0 ml	10.0 ml
6.2	5.0 ml	7.0 ml	11.0 ml
6.8	5.0 ml	6.5 ml	11.5 ml
7.0	5.0 ml	6.0 ml	12.0 ml
7.2	5.0 ml	5.5 ml	12.5 ml
7.4	5.0 ml	5.0 ml	13.0 ml
7.6	5.0 ml	4.0 ml	14.0 ml
8.0	5.0 ml	3.0 ml	15.0 ml
8.2	5.0 ml	2.0 ml	16.0 ml
8.6	5.0 ml	0.75 ml	17.25 ml
8.9	5.0 ml	0.5 ml	19.5 ml
9.2	5.0 ml	0.25 ml	17.75 ml

APPENDIX 6

Biologic Stains: Their Color Index and Synonyms

Biologic Stain	Color Index	Synonyms
ACID FUCHSIN[a]	42685	Acid Magenta, Acid Rubin, Fuchsin S, Rubin S
Alcian Blue	74240	ALCIAN BLUE 8GX, Ingrain Blue I
ALIZARIN RED S	58005	Alizarine Carmine, Alizarin Red (Wat Sol), Alizarin Sodium Monosulfonate, Alizarin-sulfonate Sodium
ANILINE BLUE (Wat Sol)	42755	Blackley Blue, Bleu de Lyon, China Blue, Cotton Blue, Marine Blue, Soluble Blue, Water Blue
AURAMINE O	41000	Canary Yellow, Pyoktanin Yellow, Pyoktaninum Aureum
AZOCARMINE B, BX	50090	Basalan Carmine BE, Rosinduline 2B
BIEBRICH SCARLET WS	26905	Crocein Scarlet, Double Scarlet BSF, Ponceau B, Scarlet 3B
Brilliant Crocein MOO	27290	Blackley Scarlet, Crocein Scarlet MOO, Scarlet MOO, WOODSTAIN SCARLET
CARMINIC ACID	75470	Acid Carminic, Cochineal, Natural Red 4

[a] *Note*. The names printed in capitals are those by which the dye is commonly known. (Source: Brown GG: The Synonym Cross Reference For Biological Stains. Gibbstown, NJ, Harleco, 1976).

Biologic Stain	Color Index	Synonyms
CELESTIN BLUE B	51050	Coreine 2R
CHROMOTROPE 2R	16570	Acid Phloxine GR, Acid Red 29, Azofuchsin 4G, Carmoisine XL-6R, Fast Fuchsin, XL Carmoisine 6R
CONGO RED	22120	Congo, Congo Red 4B, Cosmos Red, Cotton Red, Direct Red
Crystal Ponceau 6R	16250	BRILLIANT CRYSTAL SCARLET 6R, Ponceau 6R
CRYSTAL VIOLET	42555	Gentian Violet, Hexamethyl Violet, Methyl Violet 10B, Violet C, G, 7B
EOSIN B	45400	Caesar Red, Eosin BN, Eosin Scarlet, Imperial Red, Napalin G, Safrosin, Scarlet J, JJ, V
EOSIN Y, WG, G	45380	Bromo Acid, J, TS, XL, XX, Bromofluorescein, Bronze Bromo ES, Eosin B extra, Eosin J
ETHYL VIOLET	42600	Basic Violet 4, Ethyl Purple 6B
FAST GARNET GBC	37210	Bordeaux Salt II, Garnet GBC
FAST RED B	37125	Echtrotsalz B, Fast Red 5NA, Kernechtsalz B, Naphthanil Diazo Red B, Red B
FAST RED GG	37035	Fast Red 2J, Michrome Red Salt 610, Nitrazol CF, Nitrosamine Red, Parared, Para-Nitraniline Red, Red GG, 2GS
FAST RED TR	37085	Red TA, TR, TRS
Gallein	45445	ALIZARIN VIOLET, Pyrogallolphthalein
GALLOCYANIN	51030	Alizarin Blue RBN, Chrome Blue GCB, Fast Red B, Fast Violet
HEMATOXYLIN	75290	Logwood crystalline
LIGHT GREEN SF (Yellowish)	42095	Acid Green, Acid Green F, Fast Acid Green, Fast Green N, Light Green 2G, Lissamine Green SF
LUXOL FAST BLUE MBS	None	Azosol Fast Blue HLR, MLB, Solvent Blue 38
MALACHITE GREEN	42000	Aldehyde Green, Benzaldehyde Green, China Green, Diamond Green, Emerald Green, Light Green N, New Victoria Green, Solid Green O, Victoria Green B
MARTIUS YELLOW	10315	Fast Yellow, Manchester Yellow, Naphthol Yellow, Naphthylamine Yellow

Biologic Stain	Color Index	Synonyms
METANIL YELLOW	13065	Acid Yellow R, Orange MNO, Soluble Yellow OL, Tropaeolin G, Victoria Yellow, Yellow M
METHYL BLUE	42780	Bavarian Blue, Cotton Blue, Helvetia Blue, Ink Blue, Poirrier Blue
METHYL GREEN	42585	Double Green SF, Light Green
Methyl Violet	42535	Aniline Violet, Dahlia B, Gentian Violet, METHYL VIOLET 2B, 3B, 6B, Methyl Violet R, Paris Violet, Pyoktanin Blue, Pyoktanin Coeruleum
METHYLENE BLUE	52015	Swiss Blue
NEW FUCHSIN	42520	Basic Violet 2, Iso Rubin, Magenta III, New Magenta
NILE BLUE A, BX	51180	Nile Blue Sulfate
OIL RED O	26125	Sudan Red 5B
ORANGE II	15510	Acid Orange, Mandarin G, Orange II Beta Naphthol, Tropaeolin 000-2
ORANGE G	16230	Acid Orange G, Crystal Orange, Wool Orange 2G
ORCEIN	None	Lichen
PATENT BLUE V	42051	Acid Blue, Alphazurin 2G, Blue V, Patent Blue, Pontacyl Brilliant Blue, Xylene Blue VS
PHLOXINE B	45410	Cyanocin, Cyanosine, Eosin 10B, Magdala Red (Tech), Phloxine BB, BP, N, RB, TA, TB
PICRIC ACID	10305	Trinitrophenol
Pyronin Y	45005	PYRONIN G Extra
RHODAMINE B	45170	Brilliant Pink B, Rhodamine O
Rosanilin	42510	Aniline Red, BASIC FUCHSIN, Basic Rubin, Brilliant Fuchsin, Diamant Fuchsin, Diamond Fuchsin, Fuchsin, Fuchsin Basic, Fuchsin RFN, Leifson, Magenta I, Rosanilin Hydrochloride, Roseine, Rubin
RUBEANIC ACID	None	Dithioozamide
SAFFRON	75100	Natural Yellow 6
SAFRANIN O	50240	Aniline Rose, Cotton Red, Gossypimine
SIRIUS RED F3B	35780	Chlorantine Fast Red 7BLN, Durazol Red B, Pontamine Fast Red 7BNL

Biologic Stain	Color Index	Synonyms
Spirit Blue	42775	ANILINE BLUE (alc sol), Bleu de Lyon (alc sol), Bleu de Nuit, Bleu Lumiere, Gentian Blue, Light Blue, Lyon Blue, Opal Blue, Paris Blue, Poirrier Blue.
Sudan IV	26105	Fat Ponceau LB, Fettponceau, Lipid Crimson, Oil Red 4B, Scarlet B, Scarlet R, Scarlet Red, Scharlach, SCHARLACH R, Sudan Red BB
TARTRAZINE	19140	Acid Yellow 23, Yellow T
THIOFLAVIN T, TCN	49005	Thioflavin TG
THIONIN	52000	Lauth's Violet
Toluidine Blue	52040	Methylene Blue T, TOLUIDINE BLUE O

APPENDIX 7

Control Blocks for Staining Methods

Method, or Substance To Be Stained	Control Material
Acid-fast organisms	Tissue known to be infected with acid-fast organisms
Amyloid	Tissue known to contain amyloid
Argentaffin granules	Formalin-fixed appendix
Argyrophillic granules	Formalin-fixed intestine
Axons, dendrites, and nerve fibers	Cerebrum
Gram-positive and Gram-negative organisms	Infected appendix or other known lesion
Basement membrane	Normal kidney
Bile	Liver with obstructed bile duct
Chromaffin granules	Chromate fixed adrenal
Cholesterol	Artery or gall bladder with cholesterolosis
Collagen	Liver
Copper	Liver with Wilson's disease
Cross-striations in muscle	Cardiac or skeletal muscle
DNA	Lymph node—plasma cells
RNA	Lymph node—plasma cells, or normal spinal cord (Nissl)
Elastic fibers	Skin or artery
Fibrin	Blood clot—less than 72 hours old
Fungi	Tissue known to be infected
Glycogen	Liver

Method, or Substance To Be Stained	Control Material
Hyaluronic acid	Normal skin
Iron	Liver with hemochromatosis or spleen
JG granules	Normal kidney
Mast cells	Skin, lymph node, and bone marrow
Melanin	Negroid skin
Mucin	Appendix and small intestine
Myelin	Normal spinal cord
Nissl granules	Normal spinal cord
Phospholipids	Normal spinal cord and cerebrum
Plasma cells	Lymph node
Reticulum	Liver and lymph node
Smooth muscle	Stomach wall
Trichrome stains	Stomach or appendix
Uric acid	Gusty joint articulations

APPENDIX 8

Glossary

Acidophilic	Readily stained with acid dyes.
Alcoholic	A solution in which the solvent is alcohol.
Amphoteric	Capable of acting as both an acid or a base.
Angstrom	1/10,000 of a micron or 1/10,000,000 of a millimeter. Usually designated by the symbol Å.
Anion	An ion carrying a negative charge. Acidic.
Anisotropic	Doubly refractile and having polarizing power.
Aqueous	A solution in which the solvent is water. Watery.
Autolysis	Destruction of the tissue by enzymes that are produced by the tissues.
Basophilic	Readily stained with basic dyes.
Biconcave	Having two concave surfaces, that is two surfaces hollowed or rounded inwards.
"Blueing"	Washing sections in tap water or an alkaline solution causing hematoxylin to stain blue. This process normally follows differentiation in acid/alcohol.

Cation	An ion carrying a positive charge. Basic.
"Chatters"	Horizontal thick and thin ridges appearing in sections.
Chuck	The block holder on a microtome.
Clearing	The removal of the dehydrating agent and its replacement with a substance that is miscible with the embedding or mounting medium to be used.
Cytoplasm	The protoplasm of the cell external to the nucleus.
Decalcification	The removal of calcium salts from the tissue following fixation.
Decerate	To remove paraffin wax from sections.
Decolorization	The removal of color from a stained section, to differentiate.
Dehydration	The removal of water from tissue or sections.
Deliquescent	Capable of becoming liquid by absorbing moisture from the air.
Dessication	Drying, the removal of water.
Dichroism	Presenting one color in reflected light and another color in transmitted light.
Differentiation	The washing out of excess stain until the required color, shade, or combination of colors is obtained.
Dura mater	The outermost and toughest of the three membranes surrounding the brain and spinal cord.
Embedding	Placing a specimen into an embedding medium and causing it to solidify. It is often referred to as casting or blocking.
Fixation	The preservation of fresh tissue.
Aim of	To preserve cell and tissue constituents in as lifelike a manner as possible after death.
Effect of	To render cell and tissue constituents resistant to damage and distortion during subsequent processing.
Fixative	A reagent or combination of reagents used to fix tissue.

Cytoplasmic — A fixative designed to preserve the cytoplasmic detail of cells, often at the expense of destroying the nuclear substances and the overall picture of the tissue.

Microanatomic — A fixative designed to preserve the microscopic anatomy of tissue.

Nuclear — A fixative designed to preserve the nuclear detail of cells, often destroying cytoplasmic substances in the process.

Heel — As applied to a microtome knife, the end to which the handle is attached.

Honing — The action of sharpening a knife by grinding the cutting edge, either on a stone or with an abrasive compound.

Hypo — Synonym for sodium thiosulfate.

Impregnation
1. The saturation of tissue with an embedding medium.
2. The deposition of salts of heavy metals on or around tissue fibers during a staining reaction.

Metachromatic — A reaction in which a substance is stained a different color to that of the stain employed. This phenomenon is only found in basic aniline dyes.

Micron — 1/1000 of a millimeter (1/25,000 of an inch), and is the unit of measurement for the thickness of sections, the diameter of cells, and the size of bacteria. It is denoted by the symbol μ.

Microtome — The machine on which sections are cut.

Mordant — A substance that causes a staining reaction to take place by forming an insoluble lake between the dye and the tissue.

Nucleus — The darkly staining body within the cell containing the hereditary characteristics of the cell and composed of nucleoprotein.

Orientation — The precise positioning of tissue in a block, aligning the block on the microtome, or placing a section on a slide.

Pawl A pivoted tongue adapted to fall into notches on a ratchet wheel, thus permitting rotation in one direction only.

Pigment Color or particles imparted to cells and tissue.

Artifact Particles or crystals deposited during processing, usually during fixation, eg, mercuric chloride pigment or deposit.

Endogenous Pigments formed within the tissue by natural means, eg, melanin.

Exogenous Pigments within the tissue but having their origin outside the body, eg, tattoos.

Planoconcave Having one flat side and one concave side (hollowed).

Protoplasm The main constituent of all cells. It is a homogenous translucent substance containing water with salts and sugars in true solution, proteins in colloidal solution, and inorganic salts.

Putrefaction Decomposition, especially enzymic decomposition of proteins.

Quenching The rapid freezing of tissue during freeze-drying as a means of preservation.

Ratchet wheel A toothed wheel turned by means of an engaging pawl.

Refractive index The ratio of the velocity of light in air to the velocity of light in a substance.

Scores Tears across a section due to dirt, foreign bodies in the tissue, or a "nick" in the knife.

Sections Extremely thin slices of tissue, usually 4μ–15μ in thickness.

Smear A thin layer of cells spread onto a microscope slide or coverslip.

Stain A dye or mixture of dyes used to impart color to a substance.

Staining The process of coloring cells, cellular constituents, and tissue fibers to facilitate optical differentiation by microscopic examination.

Progressive	Staining each constituent to a precise color or density without overstaining and differentiating.
Regressive	The process of overstaining and subsequently differentiating to the required shade or color.
Stropping	The process of polishing the cutting edge of a knife on leather or canvas after honing.
Toe	In reference to microtome knives: the end furthest away from the handle.
Vacuum embedding	Embedding under negative pressure.

APPENDIX 9

Laboratory Suppliers

MAJOR LABORATORY SUPPLY HOUSES—MAIN OFFICES

Fisher Scientific Co.
711 Forbes Avenue
Pittsburgh, PA 15219

Curtin Matheson Scientific Inc.
4220 Jefferson Avenue
P.O. Box 1546
Houston, TX 77001
Telex 77-5624. Cable "REAGENT"

V.W.R. Scientific
P.O. Box 3200
San Francisco, CA 94119
Cable "VANROG"

Scientific Products
1430 Waukegan Road
McGaw Park, IL 60085

Arthur H. Thomas Co.
Vine Street at Third
P.O. Box 779
Philadelphia, PA 19105
Cable "BALANCE"

EQUIPMENT FOR HISTOPATHOLOGY

Automatic Tissue Processors

Technicon Instruments Corp.
Tarrytown, NY 10591
Cable "TECHINLAB"

Automatic Tissue Processors, Stainers, and Knife Sharpeners

Shandon Southern Instruments, Inc.
515 Broad Street
Sewickley, PA 15143

Cryostats and Microtomes

International Equipment Co.
300 Second Avenue
Needham Heights, MA 02194

Embedding Systems, Cryostats, and Knife Sharpeners

Lab-Tek Products
Division Miles Laboratories, Inc.
30 W. 475 N. Aurora Road
Naperville, IL 60540

Knife Sharpeners and Microtomes

Hacker Instruments, Inc.
Box 657
Fairfield, NJ 07006

Manufactures of Equipment and Supplies for Pathology

Lipshaw Manufacturing Corp.
7446 Central Avenue
Detroit, MI 48210

Microtomes

Ivan Sorvall Inc.
Newton, CT 06470

Microtomes, Cryostats, Automatic Tissue Processors, Knife Sharpeners, and Microscopes

American Optical Co.
Scientific Instrument Division
Buffalo, NY 14215

Microtomes and Microscopes

Ernst Leitz
GmbH, Wetzlar, Germany

Microtomes and Ultramicrotomes

Cambridge Medical Instruments Ltd.
Rustat Road
Cambridge, CB4 3JA, United Kingdom

Microtome Knives: Sharpening and Reconditioning

C.L. Sturkey
P.O. Box 59
Perkiomenville, PA 18074

Ultramicrotomes

LKB Instruments, Inc.
12221 Parklawn Drive
Rockville, MD 20852

Water Baths and Ovens

Blue M Electric Co.
Blue Island, IL 60406

CHEMICAL SUPPLY HOUSES

J.T. Baker Chemical Co.
222 Red School Lane
Phillipsburg, NJ 08865
Cable "BACHEMCO"

Eastman Organic Chemicals
Eastman Kodak Co.
Rochester, NY 14650

Fisher Scientific Co.
711 Forbes Avenue
Pittsburgh, PA 15219

Mallinckrodt
Second and Mallinckrodt Streets
P.O. Box 5439
St. Louis, MO 63160

Matheson, Coleman, and Bell
Manufacturing Chemists
2909 Highland Avenue
Norwood, OH 45212

Sigma Chemical Co.
P.O. Box 14508
St. Louis, MO 63178
Cable "SIGMACHEM"

DYES AND STAINING REAGENTS

Chroma—Grubler Biological Stains

Roboz Surgical Instrument Co., Inc.
810 18th Street N.W.
Washington, DC 20006

Harleco Dyes and Stains

Harleco
480 Democrat Road
Gibbstown, NJ 08027

Eastman Dyes, Stains, and Indicators

Eastman Organic Chemicals
Eastman Kodak Co.
Rochester, NY 14650

National Aniline Dyes

National Aniline Division
Allied Chemical and Dye Corp.
40 Rector Street
New York, NY 10001

Edward Gurr, Ltd., and George T. Gurr, Ltd. —Dyes and Stains

Bio/Medical Specialties
P.O. Box 1687
Santa Monica, CA 90406

GLASSWARE

Laboratory Glassware

Wheaton Scientific
1000 North Tenth Street
Millville, NJ 08332

Kimble Products
Owens-Illinois, Inc.
P.O. Box 1035
Toledo, OH 43666

Laboratory Glassware, Microscope Slides, and Coverslips

Corning Glass Works
Laboratory Products Dept.
Corning, NY 14830

Microscope Slides and Coverslips

Richard-Allan Medical Industries, Inc.
P.O. Box 351
8850 M-89
Richmand, Mich 49083

Index